THE
DANGEROUS SKY

A history of aviation medicine

THE
DANGEROUS SKY

A history of aviation medicine

DOUGLAS H. ROBINSON M.D.

UNIVERSITY OF WASHINGTON PRESS
SEATTLE

Library of Congress Cataloging in Publication Data

Robinson, Douglas Hill, 1918–
    The dangerous sky; a history of aviation medicine.

    Bibliography: p.
    1. Aviation medicine—History.   I. Title.
RC1052.R62   616.9'80213   68-11049
ISBN 0-295-95304-7

AUTHOR'S DEDICATION

To Merle
Whose love, encouragement and understanding
have inspired me through the years.

CONTENTS

ILLUSTRATIONS

1. Cut-away view of Paul Bert's pressure chamber, 1878. Bert is conducting an experiment on himself, breathing from a bag containing oxygen-enriched air.
2. German oxygen equipment for high altitude balloon flights of about 1908.
3. Stratosphere balloon *Explorer II* in the Stratobowl near Rapid City, South Dakota, on the morning of 11 November 1935.
4. Inside the *Explorer II* gondola.
5. Captain A. W. Stevens in the hatchway of the spherical Dowmetal gondola of *Explorer II*.
6. Major David B. Simons (MC) in pressure suit just prior to Man High II flight on 20 August 1957.
7. The first fatality in powered flight: Lieut. Thomas E. Selfridge (left) about to take off at Fort Myer in the Army Signal Corps Wright 'A' on 17 September 1908. Orville Wright at the controls.
8. A few moments later and the aircraft has crashed.
9. A Bleriot monoplane, Type XI, similar to the one in which M. Bleriot first crossed the English Channel on 25 July 1909.
10. British S.E. 5a fighter in Palestine.
11. Rumpler C-VII.
12. Oxygen equipment in a British D.H. 4 squadron.
13. Observer in the forward cockpit of a Gotha G-IV German bomber.
14. Observer and pilot in a Handley-Page 0/400, September 1918.
15. Flight crew of an F.E.2b night bombing squadron dressing in electrically heated suits, boots and gloves, January 1918.
16. The German Heinicke parachute under test at McCook Field, U.S.A. in 1919.
17. The Packard-LePere LUSAC II flown by Major Rudolph Schroeder to a new altitude record of 33,115 feet on 27 February 1920, and by Lieut. John Macready to 34,510 feet on 28 September 1921.
18. Lieut. John A. Macready dressed for a high altitude flight.
19. Lieut. Macready alongside the XCO5-A high altitude aircraft in which he reached a record height of 38,704 feet on 29 January 1926.
20. The first high altitude chamber at the medical research laboratory at Mineola, New York, 1918.
21. The first human centrifuge at the Aero Medical Laboratory, Wright Field, in 1935.

"A hundred necks have to be broken before all the sources of accident can be ascertained and guarded against."
Sir George Cayley to W. S. Henson. October 14, 1846.

AUTHOR'S PREFACE

Man is a terrestrial animal. For perhaps half a million years he has walked erect on the face of the earth, transporting himself on his two feet at a slow but steady four miles per hour on suitable surfaces, and able to carry a load on his back of approximately one hundred pounds. His conquest of the seas, the skies, and space result not from special adaptations such as flippers and feathers, but from the development of a sophisticated technology deriving from the evolution of a superior intelligence and of the hand as a prehensile tool. His ships, aircraft and even rockets transport great loads at velocities unattainable through human strength, drawing on the power of the sun, released through the combustion of fossil fuels and the fission of the atom. More and more he controls them through automatic devices, rather than by means of his inadequate mind and senses.

The air, like the sea, can be lethal to the human animal stripped of his artificial protections. Adapted to breathing air at sea level density and pressure, he loses consciousness and dies at great altitudes where the pressure of the atmosphere is too low to force life-giving oxygen through his lungs and into his blood stream. With his bones, muscles, and blood vessels designed to maintain function against the normal pull of gravity (1 G), he is unable to move under the force of gravity four times multiplied, and at 6 G he loses consciousness. Colliding head-on with another man at running speed, he may knock himself unconscious: with velocity and impact forces enormously multiplied in flying, abrupt deceleration in a plane crash can have a violently disruptive and disintegrating effect on human flesh and bone.

In the realm of the 'special' senses, man is found deficient. Migratory birds are possessed of a homing mechanism not yet understood, bats can locate insect prey in the dark through high-frequency echolocation. Man must substitute radio navigation aids and radar for these natural attributes of the 'lower' species who are more fortunate in this respect. In orienting himself without sight of the ground, man is superior through having produced gyroscope-driven instruments; lacking a corresponding natural sense, birds walk or roost when fog obscures the landscape.

Yet man through all the ages has dreamed of soaring through the heavens, free like the birds, and the realization within our own time of the fantasy of flight has been partly in response to profound emotional drives rooted deep in the collective unconscious of us all. Trade, transportation and war have caused vast sums to be invested in research into aerodynamics and in the production of aircraft of ever-increasing size and speed: yet the emotional appeal, the liberation from the bonds of earth, the ecstasy of realizing long-forgotten infantile dreams of omnipotence and power, enthrall the airline pilot and the week-end flyer alike. God may not have built man to fly; yet today, borne aloft by the power of thousands of horses, he soars through the heavens as one returned to an ancient domain, the land of fantasy now made real. In the process, he has learned not only to fashion the vehicles and to unlock the power of modern fuels, but also to overcome a variety of biological handicaps which emphasize the terrestrial origin of his body.

The history of how man has overcome these handicaps necessarily falls into two parts: the development of aviation in general, and of aircraft design in particular, since it is progress in aircraft capability which has created the physiological and psychological stresses affecting the human pilot and his passengers; and the medical research, and practical application of the knowledge obtained, which protects the human occupants of the aircraft against the adverse effects of the flying environment. Aviation, and its accompanying medical history, customarily is divided into eras, with emphasis on the pioneering period and the two world wars; thus each of the seven chapters following will include an historical sketch of aviation development and operation during the period, together with a matching description of medical solutions and events in relation to the problems that occurred. This necessarily multi-disciplined approach may explain why nobody has previously essayed a history of medicine in aviation. On the aviation side, I have been interested in aviation history for many years, have published a number of books and articles, hold private power and glider licences and fly my own aircraft. On the medical side, while I have never practised aviation medicine, I have been interested in the subject since my medical school days, when I bought a new copy of the first edition of Armstrong's *Principles and Practice of Aviation Medicine*.

I am not qualified to write a textbook of aviation medicine, and have included medical information only where it is indispensable to explaining problems encountered historically. While I hope that physicians will read with profit and enjoyment of the feats of their predecessors, I aim to attract readers with a broad interest in aviation and aviation history, particularly those who fly themselves.

Considerations of space require that certain limits be set: the book is intended to be a history of medicine in aviation, and I shall have to leave to others the history of space medicine. I have further chosen to limit myself to the in-flight medical problems of air crew and passengers, arbitrarily omitting consideration of a number of conditions generally included in textbooks of aviation medicine such as transmission of disease by aircraft in international commerce, and medical evacuation of the sick and wounded; while only passing attention has been given to the aviation physical examination. In general, I have taken the view that any agency which causes death, injury or impairment of function in aircrew or passengers is of medical interest.

Many persons have assisted me in the writing of this book, both from the historical and from the medical aspect. I am deeply indebted to Captain Ashton Graybiel (MC) USN, Director of Research at the US Navy School of Aviation Medicine, Pensacola, Florida, who arranged for me to visit the school, to make full use of the library, gave me much of his time and loaned me books and periodicals unobtainable elsewhere. I am grateful also for assistance from the librarians, Misses White and Denton, and Warrant Officer Dowd. Colonel C. V. Glines USAF, Directorate of Information Services, arranged for me to take the three-day pressure chamber indoctrination course at the Physiological Training Unit, Carswell AFB, Texas. Personnel who made this visit highly rewarding and instructive were Captain Philip Leatherwood MSC, Captain William J. Sears MSC, AIC Tyree, AIC Williams and AIC Michael Weston. While in Fort Worth, I spent a fascinating afternoon with Captain John W. Joyce (MC) USAF, Flight Surgeon of the 43rd Bomb Wing equipped with the supersonic B-58 Hustler. I also consulted with Mr William F. Funk, Design Safety Specialist, General Dynamics/Fort Worth, and spent some hours with Dr John S. Minnett discussing medical problems of airline pilots.

Commander Malcolm D. Ross USNR, the late Major General Orvil A. Anderson USAF, and Vice Admiral T. G. W. Settle USN wrote to me at length concerning their high altitude balloon flights. Many others helped with narrations of their own aero-medical experiences, including Oberst a.D. Martin Dietrich and many other former members of the German Naval Airship Division of World War I, and the late Raymond A. Watts, formerly of No. 84 Squadron, RAF. Captains Leonard Morgan, Robert Ross, Robert Regis, and Flight Engineer Jack Maxwell of Braniff International Airways briefed me on problems of airline flight personnel.

Major Royal Frey of the Air Force Museum, Wright-Patterson

AFB, Ohio, provided invaluable documents concerning aviation medicine in the air service of the US Army in World War I and the XC05-A high altitude research aircraft.

Miss Kathryn E. McCray, curator of the Edward H. White II Memorial Museum at Brooks Air Force Base, generously provided photographs and documents from this institution uniquely devoted to the history of aviation medicine.

My son Bruce, Naval Aviator #V-29555, helped with information on escape equipment.

My instructors, Mr C. L. Diedrich and Mrs Joan Bertles, have taught me some of the capabilities as well as the limitations of the human mechanism in aviation.

Dr Robin D. S. Higham, Dr A. D. Topping, Captain Garland Fulton USN, and Messrs Leonard Morgan, Peter Grosz, the late Thomas G. Miller and the late Willis L. Nye have read portions of the manuscript and have given suggestions and advice.

I am grateful to my editor, Mr John Hassell, for his assistance and support in publishing this book.

I wish to acknowledge the kind permission of the following publishers for allowing me to quote from works published by them:

Knorr & Hirth Verlag GMBH, München-Ahrbeck, West Germany

The Stephen Greene Press, Brattleboro, Vermont, U.S.A.

Librairie Plon, Paris, France.

Superior Publishing Co., Seattle, Washington, U.S.A.

Robert J. Benford M.D. and Charles C. Thomas Co., Springfield, Illinois, U.S.A.

AGARD-NATO (Advisory Group for Aeronautical Research & Development, North Atlantic Treaty Organization), and Butterworth Scientific Publications Ltd., London, England.

Macmillan, Basingstoke, England.

Collins and A. D. Peters & Co., London, England.

McGraw-Hill Book Co., New York, U.S.A.

E. P. Dutton & Co., Inc., New York, U.S.A.

Koehlers Verlagsgesellschaft MBH, Herford, West Germany

Doubleday & Co., Inc., New York, U.S.A.

Houghton Mifflin Co., Boston, U.S.A.

The University of Chicago Press, Chicago, U.S.A.

Oxford University Press, London, England.

J. P. Lippincott Co., New York, U.S.A.

George Allen & Unwin Ltd., London, England.

W. H. Allen & Co., Ltd., London, England.

AEROSPACE HISTORIAN, Manhattan, U.S.A.

Stackpole Books, Harrisburg, U.S.A.

Harper & Row Publishers Inc., New York, U.S.A.

HM Stationery Office, London, England.

Major General Harry G. Armstrong (MC) USAF and Williams & Wilkins Co., Baltimore, U.S.A.

Putnam & Co., Ltd., London, England.

Aerospace Medical Association, Washington, U.S.A.

National Geographic Magazine, Washington, U.S.A.

U.S. Government Printing Office, Washington, U.S.A.

DOUGLAS H. ROBINSON M.D.

INTRODUCTION

THE OLD AND THE NEW AT THE EDGE OF SPACE

On the morning of 4 May 1961 two Navy officers wearing pressure suits gazed out through their plastic face plates at the void of space. Beneath their feet spread the panorama of the eastern Gulf of Mexico. Puffy clouds far below hid the coast of Texas. As they slowly rotated, they saw, firstly, the port cities of New Orleans and Mobile, a hundred and forty miles apart but separated by a mere glance. A scratch on the face of the continent, the Mississippi River, divided New Orleans and could be traced as far north as Vicksburg. The entire state of Florida was compassed by their gaze, which extended as far up the Atlantic coast as Savannah, Georgia. Directly below, the 888-foot aircraft carrier USS *Antietam* was barely identifiable at the end of a white wake. Four hundred miles away the sea met the sky. Above the distant horizon a narrow band of whitish-blue indicated the presence of the earth's atmosphere, which in fact lay largely below them. Above the strip of blue sky the colour rapidly darkened to the blackness of airless space.

The officers were Commander Malcolm D. Ross USNR and Lieutenant Commander Victor A. Prather Jr (MC) USN, participating in the Navy's high altitude project STRATO-LAB HIGH V. Their mission was to test the pressure suits for their ability to maintain life and normal function in space. And this they were doing, for their altitude was 113,740 feet. Nor was this an instantaneous achievement, for of the eight hours and fifty-four minutes they were in the air on this day, over one and a half hours was above 100,000 feet. No rocket-propelled space capsule, no experimental aircraft was being used in this operation. Ross and Prather were being borne aloft to the edge of space by man's oldest aerial vehicle, the balloon, whose history went back a hundred and seventy-eight years, to 1783.

So sophisticated was this aerostat that the original ballooning pioneers, the brothers Montgolfier and Professor J. A. C. Charles, would hardly have comprehended the relationship. The secret of high altitude flight is lightness, and the balloon, with a full capacity of ten million cubic feet, had been manufactured by Winzen Research Inc. of Minneapolis of transparent plastic only fifteen ten-thousandths of an inch thick. Before dawn of 4 May the inflation had commenced on the deck of the *Antietam*—chosen as a launching base because, running with the speed and direction of the wind, there would be no 'felt wind' on her flight deck to whip and tear the fragile plastic. Yet only a fraction—about 30,000 cubic feet—of the full capacity of the bag had been filled with helium. This, at the altitude that Ross and Prather expected to reach, would expand and fill the balloon completely to the shape of a giant onion. Any more helium would have been valved off and wasted during the ascent.

Thus, as *Antietam* steamed down-wind, the balloon, 411 feet tall, soared high above her deck. A small bubble of helium dilating the transparent top of the bag, and empty folds of plastic narrowing down to the base, gave it a resemblance to a gigantic spermatozoon. Beneath the bag was attached a parachute seventy feet in diameter, and beneath the parachute was made fast the gondola containing the two aeronauts, the entire incredible apparatus having an overall height at takeoff of 483 feet. The gondola itself, also built by Winzen, was a simple little affair as high-altitude gondolas go, for it must be remembered that there was no intention of carrying a pressurized cabin—the men were to test their pressure suits in conditions approximating to outer space. A platform measuring five by six feet, it was surrounded on top and all four sides by homely Venetian blinds which could be turned over by remote control—black sides out to absorb solar heat, white sides out to reflect it. The blinds in front of the aeronauts could be raised to provide a 'picture window' view of space outside. Within, Ross and Prather sat before consoles of instruments, their bulky pressure suits covered in turn with outer cold-weather clothing. Electrodes cemented to their bodies picked up biological rhythms which were broadcast from individual biomedical data antennae. Liquid oxygen containers pressurized both suits and aeronauts. A radio in a pressurized container relayed messages to *Antietam*. One hundred and twenty-five pounds of steel shot served as ballast, and electrical control wires led upward to the valve in the top of the balloon. Batteries underneath the gondola floor could be released as added ballast, and blocks of styrofoam were intended to keep the gondola afloat in a water landing. A 276-foot drag rope, with a float on the end, was designed to hold the balloon above the surface. Everything had worked well in a test flight on 28 April, the gondola floating two hundred feet above the water while Ross and Prather relaxed and smoked cigarettes. It had been intended for *Antietam* to get ahead of the balloon and let it drift over the flight deck, but the wind being weak and variable on this day, the carrier had in the end backed up to the balloon and the flight deck crew had merely reeled in the rope as the balloon was slowly valved down to the deck.

Today, however, would be the real test. At the altitudes for which they were heading, instant death would ensue from at least four distinct and separate causes if the men were exposed unprotected to the atmosphere. At sea level Ross and Prather were under an air pressure equal to that of 760 millimetres of mercury. At 100,000 feet, above the greater part of the atmosphere, the pressure would be equal to only 8 mm of mercury. Although the percentage of oxygen in the air would remain an approximate twenty per cent throughout, the partial pressure of the oxygen, required to force the life-giving gas through the lungs and into the blood stream, would drop far below the level compatible with life.

Breathing one hundred per cent oxygen through face masks, they would have been fully efficient to 40,000 feet. With pressure breathing—an uncomfortable process—normal function would be maintained up to 43,000 feet. At 50,000 feet, death would result, even breathing pure oxygen, because, with a pressure of only 87 mm of mercury, the carbon dioxide and water vapour, always present in the lungs, would expand to fill them completely and no oxygen would reach the blood stream.

In addition, beyond 30,000 feet, the drop in air pressure would permit nitrogen, the inert gas constituting eighty per cent of the atmosphere, to come out of solution in the blood stream and body fluids, forming bubbles like those in a soda bottle whose cap is released. Symptoms caused by the bubbles, 'the bends,' could range from the annoying itching and crawling sensations under the skin, pain in joints wherein the bubbles would feel like gravel, to the serious 'chokes,' a sensation of suffocating with dry coughing, caused by bubbles in the lung circulation, and from bubble formation in blood vessels of the brain causing headache, paralysis, convulsions and death.

At 63,000 feet—the 'Armstrong Line,' named for its discoverer, the distinguished American pioneer of aviation medicine—the barometric pressure, 47 mm, equals the pressure of water vapour at body temperature, and the blood and body fluids boil.

At all altitudes, low temperature—the lowest recorded on the 4 May flight was −94 degrees F—would in itself have promptly caused death. In addition, with the sun's rays forming relatively large amounts of poisonous ozone at 70,000 to 80,000 feet, Ross and Prather could not have breathed this atmosphere even if it had been compressed and delivered to them.

Hence, the only practical, personal environment in which the two aeronauts could survive at great altitudes was the fully pressurized suit, wherein the pressure is maintained with one hundred per cent oxygen at a constant level of at least 141 mm, equivalent to an altitude of 40,000 feet. Constricting and uncomfortable as it is, rendering it difficult to move the limbs and impossible to turn the head freely, the suit, made of a gas-tight and inelastic fabric, enables oxygen to be delivered to the closed helmet, and hence to the lungs, at pressures that will preserve life and function in space itself.

And today Ross and Prather were going to the edge of space.

Hours of preparation by the men of the Winzen launching crew were matched by hours of preparation by the aeronauts. Before dressing, Ross and Prather submitted to having electrodes cemented to their skin to transmit a record of heart beat, temperature, brain waves and respiration to recording machines below ('it took weeks to get that stuff off,' Ross remarked). Then they drew on two sets of underwear, and with the help of attendants, worked their way into the full pressure suits, ending with the attachment of helmets and face plates to the collars of their suits. Over the suits—complete with gloves and boots—was fastened special cold-weather clothing that could be ripped off piecemeal, and then individual parachutes and harnesses. Thus loaded, they had to be assisted to their seats in the gondola, where, connected up with the oxygen supply, they breathed the gas for a half hour or more, to reduce the amount of nitrogen in the blood stream and thereby minimize the possibility of suffering from 'the bends.'

At 7.08 am four small explosive squibs, fired simultaneously by electricity, severed the tie-downs holding the gondola to the deck. Rapidly the balloon floated upwards from the gulf. In sixteen minutes it had reached 26,000 feet. Here, to prevent the possible development of 'the bends,' the barometric controls automatically inflated the pressure suits with oxygen. At 35,000 feet the ascending aerostat had reached the level of the fiercely blowing jet streams, where wind-shears at the interface of high-velocity currents could rip to pieces their fragile bag of transparent polyethylene, rendered brittle by a temperature of −40 degrees F. But today there were no perceptible currents. Apprehension developed when, at 45,000 feet, Ross heard a hissing sound as if his pressure suit were leaking. Should this be true, it would be fatal for him to ascend higher. At the same time radio contact faded, and the rate of climb slowed. At first Ross feared that the balloon was leaking, but instruments showed that it was in an inversion—a warmer, high-level layer of air in which its lift was reduced. Presently the rate of ascent returned to 750 feet per minute, radio contact came back strong and clear, and Ross found his suit was holding pressure. At 71,000 feet, Commander Prather was warned by an officer monitoring instruments aboard *Antietam* that his electrically-heated plastic face plate was overheating, with the risk that it might melt and rupture. A warning light in the gondola had failed! Nearing the ceiling of the flight, the temperature rose to −41 degrees F at 95,000 feet. 'Conditions in the gondola were pleasant,' Ross recalled, 'and I could resist no longer. I had to see outside.' A switch raised the Venetian blinds in front of the two aeronauts, and they gasped at the fantastic view through their 'picture window.'

Comfortable as they were, they could not linger. The liquid oxygen supply would not last indefinitely, and they must be down below 15,000 feet before it was exhausted. Ross pressed the valve control button to release helium from the top of the bag, carefully at first, knowing that the balloon's descent would accelerate on reaching warmer air. But at first nothing happened. The sun was warming and expanding the gas, and increasing its lift, as fast as it was valved off. After half an hour, the balloon was sinking at only seventy feet per minute, and Ross, desperately aware that they would be dead before reaching lower levels, valved for fifteen minutes more. Now, at 600 feet per minute, they could be sure that their oxygen would hold out, but the descent was too fast. At 28,000 feet the downward rate was 1140 feet per minute. To slow the balloon for a safe landing, Ross and Prather began to release ballast—first, their 125 pounds of steel shot and their batteries. This was followed, progressively, by radio equipment, oxygen converters, and the drag rope. At 15,000 feet they opened the face plates of their pressure suits and again breathed air. The rate of descent slowed to 560 feet per minute. The aeronauts lit cigarettes and calmly awaited the landing. With a splash, the gondola struck the surface of the gulf, and explosive squibs detached the 400-foot balloon. The flight was ended, and helicopters from the *Antietam,* only a mile and a half away, were on the scene at once.

Ross and Prather had been to the top of the atmosphere—they had survived, thanks to their pressure suits, on the near-airless threshold of space, where, had failure occurred, they would have died instantly in a way that no man can die on earth. Now, ironically, in the last step from the lightly-floating gondola to the broad deck of the *Antietam,* tragedy struck. The helicopters lowered cables with rescue hooks. Stepping onto the hook, Malcolm Ross, fatigued, weighted down by his suit and equipment, slipped, was dragged through the water, held on with his hands, wrapped his legs around the cable, and was hauled into the safety of the helicopter. His companion fell out of the sling, became entangled in the shroud lines of the gondola parachute, and, struggling feebly, sank, the sea flowing into the open face plate of his pressure suit. A Navy frogman dived from a helicopter, disentangled him, brought him to the surface, and he was flown to the carrier, where he was pronounced dead ninety minutes later.

Victor Prather, flight surgeon, was not the first, nor will he be the last, to give his life in the line of duty, that other men may survive in safety the perils of the Dangerous Sky.

1

The Balloon at High Altitude

Literally at one bound, man in the year 1783 realized his dream of ascending to the heavens. The vehicle was the balloon, a simple displacement craft exploiting the Archimedean principle that a body immersed in a fluid acquires an upward thrust equal to the weight of the fluid displaced, less its own mass. This required that the balloon be filled with a substance lighter than air: in the beginning there were two competing materials, hot air and hydrogen gas.

In the rudimentary state of science in the eighteenth century this discovery had been a long time coming. As early as 8 August 1709 the Jesuit, Bartholomeu Laurenco de Guzmaon, had demonstrated before the King of Portugal a device anticipating the hot-air balloon. The hydrogen balloon was foreshadowed by Cavendish's isolation of the gas—which he called 'inflammable air'—in the year 1766. Tiberius Cavallo, an Italian residing in England, caused soap bubbles to rise in the air when inflated with hydrogen in 1781.

It was the brothers Montgolfier, Joseph and Jacques-Etienne, wealthy paper makers of Annonay near Lyons, who during the next two years harnessed the lighter-than-air principle to serve man. Yet their progress was entirely empirical, deriving in no way from the work of the earlier savants, and in fact, following a false lead—the belief that smoke had magic ascending powers. They failed to appreciate that heating the air created the lift of their aerostats, and for some time a particular virtue was attached to the heavy smoke produced by damp straw. At Annonay on 5 June 1783 they publicly exhibited a balloon thirty-five feet in diameter, 23,000 cubic feet in volume, fabricated of linen rendered air-tight by a lining of paper, and inflated over a smelly, smoky fire of chopped straw and wool. This aerostat was found to have a lifting force of 500 pounds, and when released from above the fire, soared up to six or seven thousand feet and fell a mile and a half away. There followed the famous 19 September ascent in Paris before King Louis XVI of a 'Montgolfière' carrying a sheep, a cock and a duck. Now it was only a question of time before man would go aloft. In a balloon seventy-four feet high and forty-eight feet in diameter, painted a gaudy blue and decorated with intricate figures in gold, and

1

equipped with a brazier for carrying its fire aloft, the world's first aeronaut, Jean François Pilatre de Rozier (a surgeon by profession) ascended from Paris with the Marquis d'Arlandes on 21 November 1783. The flight, to an altitude of not more than 3000 feet, lasted only twenty-five minutes and carried the aeronauts five miles from their starting point. One can hardly conceive today of the bravery, the daring, required of these men in a superstitious age to take leave of Mother Earth for the first time and trust their lives to a completely new element. Regardless of their physical condition, the two young Frenchmen obviously possessed in abundance the *sine qua non* of the successful flyer—courage and a love of flying—qualities which unimaginative medical examiners have tended to discount or ignore in their pettifogging pursuit of the perfect physical specimen.

The contemporary development of the rival hydrogen balloon was a scientific achievement of the first order, contrasting with the blundering serendipity of the *frères* Montgolfier, and stands to the credit of the physicist Jacques Alexander Cesar Charles.[1] Familiar with the experiments with hydrogen of Cavendish and Cavallo, he first sent up a small balloon thirteen feet in diameter, inflated with hydrogen, on 27 August 1783. There followed the first manned ascent of a hydrogen balloon on 1 December 1783, the aeronauts being professor Charles himself and one of the brothers Robert, who had constructed the balloon. This, with remarkable foresight, anticipated in almost every detail the features of the standard gas balloon used for nearly a hundred and fifty years. Spherical in shape, twenty-seven feet in diameter, the balloon had an open filling tube, or appendix, at the bottom, to permit the escape of gas (the small demonstration balloon had burst from the expansion of the hydrogen at high altitude), and at the top of the bag, a valve permitting the aeronaut to release gas to descend. From a cord netting covering the bag depended a car, or boat-shaped gondola, ornately carved. Through the action of sulphuric acid on iron filings—a procedure used for a hundred years in ballooning—the hydrogen was produced over a three-day period. The initial ascent, with both aeronauts, lasted an hour and three-quarters, during which the balloon rose to 6000 feet and travelled twenty-seven miles. Landing at Nesle, Robert left the balloon. Charles, determined to go on alone, could not obtain more than three or four pounds of dirt for ballast, and as a result the balloon, when released, shot up with great speed. There followed an impressive experience, not without medical significance. In Charles' words:

In twenty minutes I was 1500 toises (10,000 feet) high, out of sight of terrestrial objects. The globe, which had been flaccid, swelled insensibly; I drew the valve from time to time, but still continued to ascend. For myself, though exposed to the open air, I passed from the warmth of spring to the cold of winter: a sharp, dry cold, but not too much to be borne. In the first moment I felt nothing disagreeable in the change. In a few minutes my fingers were benumbed by the cold, so that I could not hold my pen. I was now stationary as to rising and falling, and moved only in a horizontal direction. I rose up in the middle of the car to contemplate the scenery around me. When I left the earth, the sun had set on the valleys; he now rose for me alone; he presently disappeared, and I had the pleasure of seeing him set twice on the same day. . . . In the midst of my delight I felt a violent pain in my right ear and jaw, which I ascribed to the dilatation of the air in the cellular construction of these organs as much as to the cold of the external air. I was in a waistcoat and bare-headed; I immediately put on a woollen cap, yet the pain did not go off till I gradually descended.[2]

Thus did the learned professor, unaware of the need to vent his ears during changes of altitude, become the first victim of aero-otitis media. A savant rather than an explorer, Charles never made another flight. To a new breed of adventurer, recklessly disdainful of death, eager to risk their lives daily for the applause of the populace, belonged the fame and glory of the new aerial age. On 7 January 1785 Jean-Pierre Blanchard and his passenger, the American-born physician John Jeffries, who paid 700 pounds for the privilege, crossed the English Channel from Dover to the Forest of Guines in France. Stung to rivalry, de Rozier resolved to make the over-water journey in reverse, building for the purpose, against the advice of more learned men, a combined hot-air and hydrogen balloon. On 15 June 1785, shortly after the takeoff, the expected tragedy took place. Hydrogen escaping during the ascent took fire from the brazier of the hot-air balloon, and de Rozier and his companion, Pierre-Ange Romain, plunged to their deaths on the shore. They were the first victims of the air age, and their fate was typical, 'injuries, multiple, extreme.'

For some years a bitter rivalry continued between the hot-air 'Montgolfière' and the hydrogen-filled 'Charlière,' while the public dreamed extravagant dreams of steerable balloons directed by oars and sails, of intercontinental commerce in passengers and freight, and of aerial exploration of the ends of the earth. In time came disillusionment, as it became clear that the balloon, at the mercy of the wind and controllable only in the vertical plane, could not proceed from place to place under the direction of its pilot. Despite the efforts of many inventors, 'dirigibility' had to await the evolution of the internal combustion engine at the end of the next century.

The hot-air balloon, cheaper to inflate but with less lift for the same volume, and dangerous in the air by virtue of the open fire borne aloft, tended to give way more and more to the gas-filled aerostat. During the nineteenth century its only real employment was at country fairs and carnivals, where the ascent of the 'professor,' to perform gymnastics above the heads of the crowd before descending via a primitive parachute, delighted small boys and mesmerized their elders. In our own day the hot-air balloon has enjoyed a revival with Raven Industries' development of the 'Vulcoon,' with a 30,000 cubic foot bag standing fifty feet high and forty feet in diameter, its envelope fabricated of polyester plastic and rip-stop nylon (the lowest portion of fireproof fiberglass fabric), and in place of the Montgolfiers' fire of straw in an open brazier, a propane-fed burner permitting delicate adjustments of lift.[3] Carrying one man, these simply-operated craft are becoming increasingly popular for sport flying and balloon racing.

Into the late nineteenth century the gas balloon varied little in construction and rigging from the original hydrogen aerostat of Professor Charles. The balloon-cloth bag, with manœuvring valve on top, and an open appendix below; the hemp cord netting with lines led down to the car (latterly a wicker basket), and the sand ballast carried in bags, were much the same as in the 'Charlière' of 1783. To ascend, sand was dropped, and to descend, gas was released through the upper valve opened by a rope reaching to the car. The lift of the gas constantly varied depending on its temperature—sunlight warming and expanding it, and clouds or darkness contracting it and causing a descent. When the supplies of gas and of sand were at an end, the aeronauts had to land. Experienced pilots conserved both with the cunning of a miser, releasing sand in small handfuls, and Jeffries asserts, 'I verily believe, between five and six pounds of urine' saved him and Blanchard from a premature landing on the Channel flight.[4] For nearly a hundred years, varnish (John Wise, a pioneer American aeronaut, recommended boiled linseed oil cut with turpentine) was a favourite material used to render balloon silk or muslin gas-tight. 'Caoutchouc,' or crude latex, dissolved in turpentine, was used to some extent, and with the rise of the modern rubber industry and the introduction of the spreading machine at the end of the nineteenth century, rubberized balloon fabric came generally into use. Notable improvements included the guide-rope, credited to the English aeronaut William Green, which, trailing on the water or ground, tended to check the rise and fall of the balloon with fluctuations in lift;[5] and the ripping panel, invented in its generally accepted form in 1893 by Major Gross of the Prussian Airship Battalion. This, actually a large segment of the balloon, could be opened up instantly during a landing to release all the gas at once. The rope which opened the ripping panel was customarily dyed red, lest it be confused with the valve-rope and inadvertently pulled in the air.

The rise of the commercial gas industry in the mid-nineteenth century made available an abundant supply of a lifting gas much cheaper and more readily available than hydrogen, and to Green goes the credit for first using coal gas in a balloon. With a specific gravity relative to air of 0·4–0·48, compared to 0·09–0·1 for hydrogen, coal gas, or 'carburetted hydrogen,' naturally required the use of larger balloons to obtain the same lifting power. But it is safe to say that the great majority of balloon flights in the last century were made using this gas.

The military, however, used hydrogen exclusively, though this imposed on them the handicap of having to carry heavy hydrogen-generating equipment along with the balloon train. Throughout its history, and particularly in stationary and siege-like operations, the balloon enjoyed intermittent popularity as a means of observation. Revolutionary enthusiasm for the new science led the French to develop a balloon corps as early as 1794, and with a hydrogen-filled spherical balloon let up on a long rope, a disproportionate result was achieved at Fleurus against the Austrians, who panicked in the belief that their every move was noted by the observers in the sky. Napoleon, however, had no use for the lumbering balloon train in his lightning thrusts across the continent of Europe. Another revival occurred early in the American Civil War, when the Union Army included a balloon corps commanded by the aeronaut Thaddeus S. C. Lowe. His improvements included horse-drawn hydrogen generating wagons which accompanied the armies in the field, and the use of the newly-developed telegraph to communicate between the balloon observer and ground headquarters. Yet the Union Army balloon corps did not find universal acceptance, and was disbanded before the end of the war. One drawback was the unsuitability of the classic spherical balloon for ground-tethered observation service. In a moderate wind it oscillated violently on the end of its mooring line, causing air-sickness in the observer, and rendering observation impossible; in a high wind the drag of the balloon forced it nearly to the ground. The invention in 1892 of the kite balloon, by Major August von Parseval, August Riedinger the balloon builder, and Hauptmann Bartsch von Sigsfeld of the Prussian Army, provided an apparatus which, like the kite, soared stably aloft in a high wind; and the German *Drachen,* together with Allied copies, served as the 'eyes of the artillery' during the trench warfare in France from 1914 to 1918. What really condemned the observation balloon as a military weapon was its unhandiness in a war of movement. It is astonishing to read today that a Prussian 'Airship Battalion' of 1914, equipped with two kite balloons but able to operate only one at a time, carried on its roster a total of 232 officers and men and 123 horses, of which 19 were riding animals for the officers and non-coms and 72 pulled a dozen gas wagons. Each of these carried twenty high-pressure cylinders of hydrogen, weighing 132 pounds each.[6]

Mention should be made of the balloon service out of Paris during the 1870–71 siege by the Prussian Army. With all other means of communication cut, the besieged government in Paris manufactured and sent out sixty-two spherical free balloons, carrying Government officials, private and official mail, and carrier pigeons for sending back messages reduced photographically to microfilm size. One early balloon, the 'Armand Barbes,' carried on 7 October 1870, the Minister of the Interior, Leon Gambetta, who by his energy and patriotic zeal succeeded in raising in the provinces a new army that significantly prolonged the war. Eight balloons landed in enemy-controlled territory; three disappeared, presumably falling in the sea; the rest came down all over Western Europe, one 1400 miles from Paris in northern Norway near Narvik. 'The siege of Paris gave a great impetus to all aerostatical inquiries.'[7]

The greatest number of balloon flights were sporting events, and perhaps the maximum interest shown in these was in the period between 1890 and 1914. The Gordon Bennett contest in particular, coinciding with the rise of intense national rivalry in the larger industrial countries, stimulated balloon racing on the basis of national prestige. In competition for the cup put up by the American publisher in 1906, national teams of balloonists raced yearly until 1914, and from 1920 to 1938. The winner was the country whose team flew the longest distance, and the winning nation played host in the following year to the other competitors. The original cup was retired in 1924 after three straight wins by the Belgian, Ernest Demuyter. A second cup, offered by the Belgians, was won permanently by the Americans in 1928. The United States took the third cup in 1932, the Poles a fourth one in 1935, and the fifth cup was still in competition when World War II broke out, preventing the race scheduled to start on 3 September 1939 from Lwow in Poland.[8]

The parachute was first developed in connection with balloon flights at fairs and public spectacles. The Frenchman, André J. Garnerin, is credited with being the first to make general use of the parachute, with a first public descent on 22 October 1797. The modern form of parachute canopy, of wedge-shaped gores of fabric with shroud lines attached around the outer margin, was quickly evolved (Garnerin's 'chute, twenty-three feet in diameter and made up of 32 gores of canvas, approximated to modern designs). There was some variation in the way in which the parachutist was carried, Garnerin enclosing himself in a small basket four feet high and two feet three inches wide. The 'professors' performing at mid-nineteenth century country fairs developed the early body parachute harness. By the time of World War I, and long before parachutes were being used by aeroplane pilots, many kite balloon observers were saving their lives by parachute drops from their burning 'sausages.' Here the 'chute, made of silk, was carried in a bag outside the balloon basket, the shroud lines attached to a body harness, and by leaping over the side the wearer pulled the 'chute from its container.

The balloon introduced a number of medical problems. It was possible to be asphyxiated by hydrogen or coal gas while working underneath the bag during inflation. Even more subtly dangerous was the risk of being fatally poisoned by minute amounts of very toxic gases present as impurities. Stabsarzt Dr Flemming of the Prussian Airship Battalion records that, in the period immediately after its founding on 1 June 1884, the battalion suffered a number of mysterious deaths in personnel merely working in the balloon shed, or sometimes operating the hydrogen generators in the open. The onset of symptoms was insidious, with malaise and mild headache developing gradually over several hours during which the man might continue on duty. Then came dizziness, shortness of breath, and a feeling of itching or numbness in the skin. This was followed by progressive weakness, uncontrollable vomiting of green, yellow and black material, circulatory collapse, and death. There could be no question of simple asphyxia, as the men were breathing the gas only in very low concentration. Investigation revealed the presence, in small but lethal amounts, of arsine, a deadly contaminant of the hydrogen. In turn, it was determined that arsenic was present as an impurity in the sulphuric acid used to produce hydrogen by reacting on iron filings. Sometimes antimony and selenium contributed to the problem by developing poisonous gaseous compounds in the same reaction. At considerably higher expense, arsenic-free sulphuric acid was obtained for generating hydrogen, and eventually, when large amounts of hydrogen were made available by the electrolysis of water, arsine poisoning became a thing of the past.[9]

The occupants of the balloon did not feel the wind while in the air, as they moved with it and were part of the air stream. Indeed, even in cold air at considerable altitude, the sun might beat down so hotly that the occupants of the balloon removed clothing and suffered sunburn as a result. On landing, however, the strength of the wind became apparent, and many serious accidents resulted from the basket, with its occupants, being dragged at high speed across rough ground. Thus, one of the great pioneers of German ballooning, Hauptmann Bartsch von Sigsfeld, was killed near Antwerp in 1902 when, while trying to land in a sixty-mile-an-hour gale, he was thrown from the basket and sustained a fatal skull fracture. The French balloonists Wilfred de Fonvielle and Gaston Tissandier describe a typical high-wind landing in the year 1869:

The 'Swallow' approaches the ground, and the car goes down with a terrible bump. Tissandier hangs to the valve-rope, and observes that Fonvielle is covered with blood. The hoop of the balloon has struck him on the head and caused a deep wound. The car had come to the ground like a bullet, but we rose again immediately, and had to undergo several similar contusions. Our anchor fled over the ground and would not take hold of anything; it was like a cork at the end of a piece of string. We seemed to be the sport of some invisible power, that first raised us into the air and then bumped us against the earth.

We were being dragged along by the force of a furious gale! ...

Holding onto the valve-rope with all his strength, and squatting at the bottom of the car, Tissandier pulled away lustily; whilst the 'Swallow' jumped about from one tree to the other. The branches of the trees bent beneath the car, the wind whistled in our ears; the balloon appeared to have lost some gas, but a sudden gust carried it from the wood again, and down it came with a hard bump upon the open plain beyond. The wind now hollowed the balloon into a kind of cup, or basin, and carried us vigorously across ploughed land, until finally some men ran up and caught hold of the guide-rope.[10]

This landing would have been much less injurious had the ripping panel then been invented. By instantly releasing all the gas in the balloon, this would have prevented its acting as a large surface for the wind to act on, and the aeronauts would have been dragged only a short distance.

Catastrophic falls from high altitude were rare. On occasion, the balloon might burst from overpressure of expanding gas during an ascent. In theory, the open filling tube, or appendix, at the bottom of the bag, would permit free escape of expanding gas, but in practice, the appendix might be too small in diameter, or it might have been unwisely tied shut to prevent the gas from mixing with air. Yet even if the balloon burst, the aeronauts might escape with their lives. Held in shape by the netting, the ruptured bag filled with air and descended slowly like a parachute. With great daring, John Wise, the American aeronaut, deliberately exploded his balloon during an ascent from Easton, Pennsylvania, on 11 August 1838, and although he was thrown ten feet from the car by the force of the landing, he was not injured.[11]

Fire in the air was rare, the deaths of de Rozier and Romain having shown the danger of carrying an open flame aloft with hydrogen or coal gas; but fires might occur on the ground, with severe injury to crew and spectators, particularly during deflation after a flight. John Wise was temporarily blinded and painfully burned when, deflating his hydrogen-filled balloon after a night landing,

... either the lantern, or some other light which had in the meantime been brought to the scene, ignited the explosive mixed atmosphere that was hovering around the balloon, making a report like a park of artillery, throwing me violently back at least ten feet from the place where I was standing, setting fire to the clothes of some, and severely scorching the hands and faces of others. . . . I quickly sprang upon my feet again, and jumped onto the remainder of the balloon which was burning in the car, and which was thus extinguished by tramping it out—the gas that had by the sudden explosion been liberated from the balloon, in the mean time rose rapidly into the air 'like a consuming fire,' with a rushing noise, until, at a considerable height, it was totally consumed like a dying meteor.[12]

The most significant medical phenomena encountered in ballooning, however, related to the problem of altitude sickness, or anoxia. Although oxygen had been isolated by Priestley a few years before the Montgolfier and Charles ascents, and its vital role in human function was suspected, there was no advance awareness that lack of it would impose severe and even fatal handicaps in ascents to high altitude.

Oxygen constitutes one-fifth part of the atmosphere (actually 20·94 per cent), and is essential to all forms of animal life. The percentage of oxygen remains constant for all practical purposes at all altitudes, but since the total air pressure decreases with increasing altitude, the partial pressure of oxygen likewise decreases. Since the earliest measurements of atmospheric pressure were by balancing the weight of the air against that of a column of mercury of equal weight, the standard pressure at sea level is still said to be 760 mm of mercury. Since oxygen constitutes one-fifth of the content of the air, its partial pressure at sea level is 159 mm.

Both figures decrease with altitude. At 18,000 feet the air pressure is 379·4 mm, approximately half, and the partial pressure of oxygen is 79·8 mm. At 33,000 feet the atmospheric pressure is 196·3 mm, and the partial pressure of oxygen is 41·3 mm. At 40,000 feet the respective figures are 140·7 mm and 29·6 mm. It is necessary to point out, however, that in the lungs the partial pressure of oxygen is even less, due to the presence of water vapour (which saturates the lungs) and carbon dioxide. The partial pressure of water vapour is 47 mm at all altitudes, while that of carbon dioxide decreases from 40 mm at sea level to 30 mm at 38,000 feet. These figures, therefore, must be subtracted from the air pressure at any altitude, the partial pressure of oxygen in the lungs being one-fifth of the remainder. With ascent, water vapour and carbon dioxide occupy more and more of the volume of the lungs, until at 50,000 feet they are filled entirely with these gases and even one hundred per cent oxygen at this altitude cannot sustain life. Thus, it appears, oxygen must be under a certain pressure to pass through the lung membranes and into the blood stream.

Regardless of altitude, the tissues of the body require oxygen for their metabolic function, some, such as the brain cells and heart muscle, requiring large amounts and being extremely sensitive to any deficiency. There are numerous cases on record of flyers at high altitude suffering severe brain damage, and even death, when deprived of oxygen for only a few minutes.

Arterial blood carries oxygen from the lungs to the tissues, most of it being taken up by the haemoglobin, the red pigment of the blood corpuscles. The percentage of saturation of arterial blood with oxygen determines whether the tissues are adequately nourished or not. Such is the ability of haemoglobin to combine with oxygen that saturation of arterial blood is maintained above eighty-five per cent until the partial pressure of oxygen in the lungs falls to about sixty mm. When breathing air, this occurs at about 12,000 feet, and when breathing pure oxygen, at about 40,000 feet. These levels, therefore, are the limits to which man can fly breathing air and pure oxygen respectively. Beyond these altitudes, the blood arterial saturation drops sharply, tissue function is impaired, and the individual flyer develops symptoms of *anoxia*. (Because this literally means no oxygen at all, *hypoxia* is a more accurate term, but one less often used.)

The Air Force divides the progress of anoxia into four stages:

Indifferent stage: (breathing air, 0–10,000 feet; breathing one hundred per cent oxygen, 34,000–39,000 feet). The only effect is on night vision; the rods, which are the visual receptors in the retina for dim vision, being so sensitive to anoxia that dark adaptation and night vision can be impaired as low as 5000 feet.

Compensating stage: (breathing air, 10,000–15,000 feet; breathing one hundred per cent oxygen, 39,000–42,500 feet). The entire body responds to the decrease in partial pressure of oxygen, and the fall in arterial oxygen saturation. Breathing becomes faster and deeper; the rate of blood circulation increases, with an increased pulse rate, increased volume of blood pumped by the heart, and a rise in blood pressure.

Disturbance stage: (breathing air, 15,000–20,000 feet; breathing one hundred per cent oxygen, 42,500–44,800 feet). The compensatory measures of the previous stage no longer suffice to maintain an adequate supply of oxygen to the tissues. The individual experiences fatigue, lassitude, sleepiness, dizziness, headache, breathlessness, and an unwarranted sense of well-being resembling alcohol intoxication. Testing will show that vision is impaired, thinking is slow, judgment faulty, and memory poor. Reaction time is delayed. Muscle co-ordination is impaired and fine muscle movements are impossible.

Critical stage: (breathing air, 20,000–23,000 feet; breathing one hundred per cent oxygen, 44,800–45,500 feet). 'This is the stage in which consciousness is lost.' With prolonged anoxia, unconsciousness may result from failure of the heart and circulation. With acute anoxia, this results from injury to the brain. In either case, unless oxygen is promptly administered, unconsciousness is followed by failure of the respiratory centre in the brain, convulsions, and death.

Clearly it is necessary for air crew to be supplied with oxygen at a partial pressure in the lungs of at least sixty mm if they are to perform their duties properly, regardless of the actual altitude at which they are flying. Recognition of this problem, and the development of effective measures to combat it, constitute the earliest and one of the brightest achievements in the history of aviation medicine.

Within a few years of its invention, the balloon was making flights to high altitudes where anoxia was a serious, even a potentially lethal, problem to its operators. It was a time of intense curiosity about natural phenomena, and the savants and scholars of the Age of Reason saw the balloon as an ideal vehicle for carrying them and their instruments to high altitudes, there to investigate the properties of the atmosphere. At this late date, it may seem surprising that the first high-altitude flyers were not prepared for anoxia, for men had previously ascended mountains high enough to bring on its symptoms. Not until the end of the eighteenth century, however, were sportsmen and scientists tackling the Alps. The first ascent of Mont Blanc (15,781 feet), the highest peak in western Europe, occurring in 1786, three years *after* the first balloon flight. De Sassure's classic account of his climb in the following year presents a contemporary picture of 'mountain sickness' a thousand feet below the summit of the peak:

> The rarity of the air gave me more trouble than I could have believed. At last I was obliged to stop for breath every fifteen or sixteen steps; I usually did so standing, leaning on my alpenstock, but about once out of every three times I had to sit down. The need of rest was absolutely unconquerable; if I tried to overcome it, my legs refused to move, I felt the beginning of a faint, and was seized by dizziness. . . . I made different tests to shorten this rest; I tried, for example, not to continue to the end of my strength, and to stop an instant every four or five steps, but I gained nothing; I was obliged, after fifteen or sixteen steps, to take a rest as long as if I had made them

consecutively; and this was very noteworthy, that the greatest distress is not felt until eight or ten seconds after one has stopped walking.[13]

Mountain sickness had been known much earlier in South America, where the Spaniards, forced to cross the Andes in travelling eastward from the Pacific coast, had to climb to 13,000 feet or more in the mountain passes. Acosta, a Jesuit father who travelled in South America at the end of the sixteenth century, was the first to connect the symptoms of *puna* or *soroche* (names used by the local Indians) with the air of high altitude. During an ascent to about 14,500 feet,

> I was suddenly attacked and surprised by an illness so deadly and strange, that I was almost on the point of falling from my horse to the ground. . . . I was seized by such a spasm of panting and vomiting that I thought I should give up the ghost. After vomiting food, phlegm, and bile, one yellow and the other green, I next threw up blood, so that I felt such distress in my stomach that I can say if it had lasted I am sure I would have died. That lasted only three or four hours until we had descended pretty low and had reached a temperature more suited to nature, at which point our companions, about fourteen or fifteen in number, were very much exhausted, one of them asking for confession on the road, thinking they were really going to die, others dismounted and were wracked with vomiting and diarrhoea; I was told that in the past some had lost their lives from this distress.[14]

Others travellers recognized the combination of disabling symptoms that overtook mountain climbers, but the explanations were almost as numerous as the observers. Some Europeans gave credence to native superstitions that mountain sickness was caused by poisoning from 'metallic emanations' from antimony and other minerals in the ground. It soon became obvious that barometric pressure was lower at great altitudes, and some jumped to the conclusion that the lessened pressure permitted hemorrhage from blood vessels. De Sassure, reflecting on his distress during the ascent of Mont Blanc, attributed this to 'the relaxation of the vessels caused by the decrease of the compressing power of air.'[15] One author blamed the whole problem of mountain sickness on that novel phenomenon, electricity, 'which occupies, in the northern hemisphere, the upper part of the body, and in the southern hemisphere, the lower part, and thus tends to draw the blood towards the head in the former, and towards the feet in the second.'[16] Thus, even if aspiring balloonists had consulted the literature, they would not have found help from the authorities. None realized that mountain sickness was caused by a fall in the partial pressure of oxygen in the less-dense air. Most considered that the cause was a lowering of air pressure permitting an expansion of blood vessels—not realizing that the pressure on the body would be equalized internally as well as externally.

As so often happens, the first men to ascend to high altitude were doers, not thinkers, taking off into the unknown with no knowledge of what lay in store. The first significant ascent in the first age of high-altitude ballooning—using the conventional aerostat, fabricated of varnished silk or cotton, or latterly, of rubberized cloth, enclosed in a hempen net from which was suspended an open wickerwork basket—occurred as early as 1803. On 18 July of that year the French aeronaut and physicist Robertson, accompanied by M. Lhoest, rose from Hamburg to experiment in the air with the formation of static electricity on articles of 'brimstone, glass and Spanish wax,' to measure the output of a 'Voltaic pile' of silver and zinc—a primitive wet battery—and to test the flight of birds when released from the balloon.[17] Robertson[18] claimed to have reached an altitude of 7170 metres (23,550 feet). His description of his symptoms at this height will surprise the modern flight surgeon, who must suspect that Robertson had been influenced by theories of the expansion of the body and blood vessels at high altitudes:

Our chests seemed expanded and lacked resilience, my pulse was hurried; that of M. Lhoest was less so; like mine, his lips were swollen, his eyes bloodshot; all the veins were rounded out and stood up in relief on my hands. The blood had rushed to my head so much that I noticed that my hat seemed too small.[19]

Yet the description of the mental effects of anoxia rings true to modern ears:

At this elevation, our state was that of indifference; there the physicist is no longer sensitive to the glory and the passion of discoveries; the very danger which results from the slightest negligence in this journey hardly interests him. . . . We could hardly ward off the sleep which we feared like death. Distrusting my strength, and fearing that my companion would succumb to sleep, I had fastened a cord to my thigh and to his; the ends of this cord were in our hands.[20]

There followed within a year two further scientific flights to high altitude, sponsored by the *Institut de France,* and making use of a war-surplus balloon manufactured at least six years earlier, which had been sent with Napoleon's army to Egypt, but never used there. The chief scientist was Joseph Louis Gay-Lussac, already an experienced investigator of the properties of gases, terrestrial magnetism, hygrometry, etc., and who gave his name to Gay-Lussac's Law.[21] He was assisted in the first ascent on 23 August 1804 by Jean Baptiste Biot, the discoverer of the mineral Biotite. The two young scientists reached only 13,100 feet, where they observed the oscillations of a magnetic needle, tested the properties of a voltaic pile, made temperature and humidity readings, and released and observed the flights of a bee, a linnet, and a pigeon. At this relatively low altitude they experienced no physical hardships, in fact, with an air temperature of 56 degrees F, they were sunburned and had to remove their gloves.

Our pulses were very fast; that of Gay-Lussac, which is ordinarily 62 per minute, was 80; mine, which is usually 89, was 111. This acceleration was then felt by us both in about the same proportion. However, our respiration was not at all affected; we felt no discomfort, and our situation seemed to us extremely agreeable.[22]

Biot allegedly was unnerved by a rough landing, and in any event, Gay-Lussac made the next flight alone on 15 September 1804. By releasing everything he could spare as ballast, he claimed to have attained a maximum altitude of 23,040 feet,[23] where he found the temperature to be 14·9 degrees F. He had two glass flasks, exhausted of their air, and opened one at 21,460 feet, and the second at 21,790 feet. Later laboratory tests showed that the air at high altitude contained the same proportion of constituents as at sea level, including 215 parts per thousand of oxygen.

While occupied with experiments at this enormous elevation, he began, though warmly clad, to suffer from excessive cold, and his hands, by continued exposure, became benumbed. He felt likewise a difficulty in breathing, and his pulse and respiration were much quickened. His throat became parched from inhaling the dry, attenuated air, so that he could hardly swallow a morsel of bread; but he experienced no other direct inconvenience from his situation. He had indeed been affected, through the whole of the day, with a slight headache. . . . but though it continued without abatement, it was not increased by his ascent.[24]

Headache, likewise, is a symptom of anoxia, and it is certain that Gay-Lussac was affected by this condition.[25]

In the light of later knowledge, the aeronauts in this first series of scientific ascents to high altitude had experienced moderate symptoms of anoxia. Probably, through being only briefly at maximum altitude, these did not lead to unconsciousness, and probably also, through the development of mental dullness and apathy so well known as features of anoxia, the aeronauts failed to observe and record the full extent and nature of their symptoms. The next series of scientific ascents would prove that the insidious onset of unconsciousness, and even death, inevitably assailed those who mounted too high.

The British Association, composed of well-to-do private citizens interested in the progress of science, and which had sponsored several earlier scientific ascents to lower altitudes, resolved in the year 1858 to organize four flights from Wolverhampton, a centrally-located town in the English Midlands. After several distressing failures they procured the services of the foremost English aeronaut of the day, Henry Coxwell, a dentist who had made many successful exhibition ascents beginning in the year 1844. Learning that the Committee of the British Association expected to explore the atmosphere at an altitude of five miles, Coxwell insisted that a balloon larger than any yet built would be needed. Within three months—such was Coxwell's skill and energy—he had fabricated at his own expense a balloon of 'American cloth' (cotton), eighty feet high, over fifty-five feet in diameter, and with a volume of 93,000 cubic feet. Coal gas, because of its cheapness and availability, was the chosen lifting medium.

The Association's choice of a scientific observer to accompany Coxwell was James Glaisher, a trained meteorologist with many years of experience leading to a staff appointment at the Royal Observatory in Greenwich. Although Glaisher represents himself as having diffidently offered his services simply because the public and the British Association expected it of him as a member of the Committee, he had probably been yearning to fly for some years—at least from the year 1852, when he had remained glued to his telescope atop the Observatory to follow from beginning to end an ascent to 22,930 feet by Mr Welsh and the aeronaut Green in the latter's 'great *Nassau* balloon.' To fulfil his role, Glaisher provided himself with a portable table holding ten different instruments—hygrometers, thermometers, an aneroid and a mercury barometer, etc., and trained himself to read them all rapidly during flight, and to note their readings (one piece of equipment was 'a lens to read the instruments'[26]).

The first of the high-altitude flights from Wolverhampton with the 'Mammoth' balloon took place on 17 July 1862. It should be noted that a specially light variety of coal gas, rich in hydrogen, had been prepared by the Stafford Road Gas Works, and stored in a gasometer for a flight. As a result, the aeronauts claimed to have reached briefly a maximum altitude of 26,200 feet. They, of course, experienced anoxia, and Glaisher recorded (remember, it was his first balloon ascent!):

At 19,415 feet palpitation of the heart became perceptible, the beating of the chronometer seemed very loud, and my breathing became affected. At 19,435 feet my pulse had accelerated, and it was with increasing difficulty that I could read the instruments; the palpitation of the heart was very perceptible. The hands and lips assumed a dark bluish colour, but not the face. . . . At 21,792 feet I experienced a feeling analogous to sea-sickness, though there was neither pitching nor rolling in the balloon; and through this illness I was unable to watch the instruments long enough to lower the temperature to get a deposit of dew.[27]

The second ascent, from Wolverhampton on 18 August 1862, took

Glaisher and Coxwell only to 23,400 feet, and neither aeronaut mentions any anoxic effects. The third flight, however, which took place from Wolverhampton on 5 September 1862, resulted in a claimed altitude of seven miles (36,960 feet), and nearly led to the deaths of both men.

Again, a specially light gas was manufactured and stored for this flight, and Coxwell 'felt that with still lighter gas I could venture to take Mr Glaisher up to a much higher elevation, and as no symptoms of fainting had been felt previously, I concluded that we might risk a more spirited rise.'[28] Rapidly indeed did the balloon ascend, reaching three miles 25 minutes after takeoff. After 37 minutes they were at four miles' altitude. Glaisher wrote later,

Up to this time I had taken observations with comfort, and experienced no difficulty in breathing, while Mr Coxwell, in consequence of the exertions he had had to make, had breathed with difficulty for some time. Having discharged sand, we ascended still higher; the aspirator became troublesome to work; and I also found a difficulty in seeing clearly . . . about 1 h 52 m or later, I read the dry-bulb thermometer as minus 5 degrees; after this I could not see the column of mercury in the wet-bulb thermometer, nor the hands of the watch, nor the fine divisions on any instruments. I asked Mr Coxwell to help me read the instruments. In consequence however, of the rotatory movement of the balloon, which had continued without ceasing since leaving the earth, the valve-line had become entangled, and he had to leave the car and mount into the ring to readjust it. I then looked at the barometer, and found its reading to be $9\frac{3}{4}$ in, still decreasing fast, implying a height exceeding 29,000 feet.[29] Shortly after I laid my arm upon the table, possessed of its full vigour, but on being desirous of using it I found it powerless—it must have lost its power momentarily; trying to move the other arm I found it powerless also. Then I tried to shake myself, and succeded, but I seemed to have no limbs. In looking at the barometer my head fell over my left shoulder; I struggled and shook my body again, but could not move my arms. Getting my head upright for an instant only, it fell on my right shoulder; then I fell backwards, my back resting on the side of the car and my head on its edge. In this position my eyes were directed to Mr Coxwell in the ring. When I shook my body I seemed to have full power over the muscles of the back, and considerably so over those of the neck, but none over either my arms or my legs. As in the case of the arms, so all muscular power was lost in an instant from my back and neck. I dimly saw Mr Coxwell, and endeavoured to speak, but could not. In an instant, intense darkness overcame me, so that the optic nerve lost power suddenly, but I was still conscious, with as active a brain as at the present moment of writing this. I thought I had been seized with asphyxia, and believed I should experience nothing more, as death would come unless we speedily descended; other thoughts were entering my mind, when I suddenly became unconscious, as on going to sleep.[30]

Glaisher frankly admitted to having been overcome by anoxia, which he described with a clinical accuracy that could hardly be improved on by modern investigators; and he knew that his death had been averted only by a prompt descent from high altitude. By contrast, Coxwell's personal account may be labelled the very first of many to follow in the category of 'I-was-doing-fine-but-everyone-else-was-passing-out':

When Mr Glaisher's troubles commenced, I was absorbed in my own duties, which prevented me from noticing my colleague's uneasiness. I thought that his eyes were dazed by the constant use of the lens and did not perceive that insensibility was approaching. The premonitory symptoms were not thought to be anything more than a desire for a few moments' quiet, and when I really began to apprehend that something was amiss, I looked far up above the balloon for Supreme help, and then found myself springing aloft to do what at this critical juncture seemed necessary. I had previously taken off a thick pair of gloves so as to be better able to manipulate the sand bags, and the moment my unprotected hands rested on the ring, which retained the temperature of the air, I found that they were frost-bitten, but I did manage to bring down the valve line.[31]

Because his hands were frost-bitten (*not* paralysed by anoxia, as stated in some modern accounts), Coxwell had to pull the valve line with his teeth, starting the balloon downwards in the nick of time.

How high did they go? Glaisher offers some arguments, so naïve for a trained scientist as to be considered self-seeking, to prove that the balloon reached 37,000 feet. Arguing that when he was last conscious, the balloon was at 29,000 feet and ascending 1000 feet per minute, and thirteen minutes later when he recovered consciousness it was descending 2000 feet per minute, he assumed by simple extrapolation that the maximum altitude was 37,000 feet. He claimed also that a reading by Coxwell of the aneroid barometer indicated a pressure of seven inches of mercury, corresponding to a 37,000 foot altitude.[32]

There is another rough measure, however, of the maximum altitude reached by Glaisher and Coxwell—their bodily responses to anoxia. In the light of modern knowledge, it would seem impossible for the aeronauts to have greatly exceeded 25,000 feet. I myself have experienced anoxia at 25,000 feet in a pressure chamber, noting at the time the progressive development in myself of symptoms—'aware of slight dizziness, know I am not concentrating so well, disregarding questions on test sheet, offering myself childish excuses for not answering them. Noting developing bluish colour of finger nails, acceleration of heart rate. Distinct feeling of elation and well being towards the end, though I am aware this is abnormal.' After breathing air at 25,000 feet for four minutes and fifteen seconds, attendants in the chamber, noting signs of distress which I myself was not aware of, forced the oxygen mask back on my face. And the Air Force, it will be remembered, considers 20,000 to 23,000 feet to be the 'critical stage':

This is the stage in which consciousness is lost. This may be the result of circulatory failure ('fainter'), or of central nervous system failure ('nonfainter,' unconsciousness with maintenance of blood pressure). The former is more common with prolonged hypoxia, the latter with acute hypoxia. With either type there may be convulsions and eventual failure of the respiratory centre.[33]

In pursuit of more meteorological data, Glaisher made a number of further ascents as late as the year 1866. On 18 April 1863 he and Coxwell reached 24,000 feet on a flight from London to Newhaven, and on 26 June 1863 the pair attained 23,500 feet; but there is no mention of any respiratory or physical problems in Glaisher's account. He in fact believed he had developed a tolerance for high altitudes, writing:

At length I became so acclimatized to the effects of a more rarefied atmosphere, that I could breathe at an elevation of four miles at least above the earth without inconvenience, and I have no doubt that this faculty of acclimatization might be so developed as to have a very important bearing upon the philosophical uses of balloon ascents. At six and seven miles high, I experienced the limit of our power of breathing in the attenuated atmosphere. More frequent experiments would increase this height, I have little doubt, and *artificial appliances might be contrived to continue it higher still.*[34]

On another page he remarks, 'it is not to be supposed that additional frequency of respiration in an attenuated air makes amends for the want of oxygen.'[35] Did Glaisher realize that future high-altitude balloonists would have to carry oxygen to compensate for its deficiency in the atmosphere?

That this was necessary was proved during the next few years by Paul Bert. A physician, a physiologist, the pupil and successor of the great Claude Bernard, and a passionately radical politician, a member of Leon Gambetta's famous but short-lived Grand Ministry of 1881, Bert ended his life in French Indo-China as Resident General, dying there of dysentery. As a physician he was best known in his lifetime for his pioneer studies on skin grafting. His title of 'Father of Aviation Medicine' was conferred posthumously. Most of his studies were made on animals subjected to decreased and increased atmospheric pressures. His monumental work (*La Pression Barometrique. Recherches de Physiologie Experimental:* Paris, Masson, 1878), is in large part a detailed record of individual experiments on sparrows, dogs and cats which today would surely embroil him with the society for the prevention of cruelty to animals. Yet his animal studies led to human experiments on himself and on two young balloonists, Sivel and Crocé-Spinelli, who under his direction made the first high altitude flight with oxygen equipment.

Bert's interest in high altitude physiology led him to assemble all available information on the experiences of balloonists and mountaineers. After reviewing all the theories put forward, he wrote in 1869, 'I cannot repeat too often that these are reasonings, likelihoods, possibilities at most. When shall we have the experimentation which will bring conviction?'[36] He commenced giving the answer shortly afterwards with animal experiments under beli jars which proved that regardless of differences in atmospheric pressure, the *partial pressure* of oxygen was a constant, averaging thirty-five mm of mercury, when death occurred. Even with air enriched with oxygen at the start, the figure of thirty-five mm was still found with the death of the animal.

Having proven that the partial pressure of oxygen was the essential factor in maintaining life in the atmosphere, Bert designed and built the first pressure chamber. Actually his apparatus consisted of two adjacent cylinders of boiler plate, standing $6\frac{1}{2}$ feet high and $3\frac{1}{4}$ feet in diameter, and connected by a door. Portholes permitted a view of experimental subjects inside, and a vacuum receiver—a boiler-like vessel, in which a vacuum could be created—permitted the pressure in the chamber to be suddenly lowered by receiving part of the contained air. A miniature steam engine drove a vacuum pump, but such were its limitations that the lowest pressure Bert could achieve was 170 mm of mercury, equivalent to an altitude of 36,000 feet, and 250 mm, equivalent to 28,000 feet, was more generally used.

Through experiments on large dogs, Bert demonstrated that with decreased pressure, the heart rate increased, respirations accelerated, digestive processes were slowed, intestinal gases expanded, body temperature fell, and a state of apathy and torpor occurred. Bert ran an experiment on himself in one of the big chambers, lowering the pressure to 550 mm (8500 feet) in thirty-three minutes. This was not enough to produce real symptoms of anoxia, and he merely noted a slight increase of the pulse, and 'was forced, by the expansion of the intestinal gases, to open my garments wide.'[37] The next experiments on animals proved the vital importance of oxygen, for with pure oxygen admitted at low pressures, the symptoms of altitude sickness disappeared. Bert, on 20 February 1874, again ran a chamber experiment on himself, reaching a pressure of 408 mm, equivalent to 16,000 feet, and spent nearly an hour and a half above 11,000 feet. He noted abdominal distention and escape of intestinal gas; increase in pulse rate; nausea; dizziness; convulsive trembling of the legs which he could not control; and at 15,000 feet, 'having found that the number of my heart beats for twenty seconds was twenty-eight, I have very great difficulty in multiplying this number by three, and I write in my notebook, "hard to calculate".'[38] But Bert had carried into the chamber with him a large bag 'filled with air extremely rich in oxygen' with rubber tubing which he held in his mouth, and from time to time he inhaled this mixture. Invariably his unpleasant sensations were relieved, and the pulse rate went down.

A few days later, on 10 March 1874, the experiment was repeated on two young scientists, Crocé-Spinelli and Sivel, who, planning to ascend 'to a great height,' had heard of Bert's researches and came to him 'with the purpose of studying upon themselves the disagreeable effects of decompression and the favourable influence of super-oxygenated air.'[39] At 480 mm pressure, equivalent to about 12,000 feet, Crocé-Spinelli noted 'oppression begins to be quite perceptible,'[40] he became lazier, while his face felt hot, but both were gay and talkative. Beyond 20,000 feet vision became dim, and at 23,000 feet, both aeronauts, who had been 'very gay, very talkative and active' to 18,000 feet, were listless and not talking, their faces purple. They had with them a bag of oxygen which they passed back and forth, wasting a good deal of the gas, because the flavour of rubber from the container at first repelled them. Discomfort and nausea improved after oxygen; Crocé-Spinelli's dim vision cleared immediately on taking oxygen at 20,000 feet. Bert, looking in through the porthole, noted that Crocé-Spinelli's purple right ear instantly became normal in colour when he breathed oxygen.

Bert himself in an experiment on 28 March went to 412 mm (16,000 feet) without oxygen and became nauseated and quite uncomfortable, with dimness of vision. At this altitude he began inhaling 'superoxygenated air' continuously, and felt perfectly comfortable, except for the escape of intestinal gas. He continued to a height of 21,000 feet with no discomfort, though noting he could not whistle because of the low density of the air. Hereby he proved that the prodromal symptoms of altitude sickness could be eliminated by breathing oxygen even though the ascent continued. 'Nothing is more conclusive.'[41]

Profiting by their 'pressure chamber course' in Professor Bert's laboratory, Sivel and Crocé-Spinelli, in an ascent on 22 March 1874, took along several bags of oxygen—one mixture containing forty per cent oxygen and sixty per cent nitrogen, the other seventy per cent oxygen and thirty per cent nitrogen. Their balloon, the *Etoile Polaire* of 99,000 cubic feet, attained a maximum height of 24,300 feet during a flight that lasted two hours and forty minutes, being one hour and forty minutes above 16,400 feet. The altitude was only slightly greater than that in their chamber run of 10 March, but both men felt much more uncomfortable, attributing this correctly to the greater physical effort ('when M. Sivel threw out ballast, which prevented him from breathing gas, the fifteen kilogramme bag seemed to him to weigh 100'),[42] the lower temperature (eleven degrees below zero F) and the length of time spent at high altitude. Above 11,800 feet both aeronauts breathed the forty per cent oxygen mixture, and above 19,700 feet, the seventy per cent mixture. At maximum altitude, both kept the rubber tubing in their mouths, but breathed the oxygen only intermittently, clamping the tube shut with their teeth between breaths. Crocé-Spinelli, 'of lymphatico-nervous temperament,' breathed two-thirds of the oxygen, suggesting overventilation due to anxiety. When not breathing oxygen,

He was obliged to sit down on a bag of ballast and make his observations, motionless in that position. During the absorption of oxygen, he felt revived, and after about ten inhalations, he could rise, chat gaily, look at the ground attentively, and make delicate observations. His mind was keen and his memory excellent. To look into the spectroscope, he had to breathe this gas, rightly called *vital*; the lines, at first confused, then became very clear.[43]

It is certain that both the young aeronauts suffered distortion and impairment of judgment at great heights, which they could not evaluate properly because of their impaired awareness. Enthusiastic about the effects of the oxygen—which they did not realize should have been used continuously to maintain normal alertness and function—they were now filled with a 'reckless confidence.'

Chauvinism—the desire of proud and sensitive Frenchmen to salve the wounds of defeat inflicted by the hated Prussians only four years earlier—now led to disaster. 'They say that an Englishman could live and make observations above 8000 metres (26,200 feet); the flag we carry must float higher yet!' Without consulting Bert, who was out of town, Crocé-Spinelli and Sivel prepared to surpass Glaisher's record with only three bags of gold beaters' skin, each of 200 litres (seven cubic feet) capacity, which, because of the decreased pressure at high altitude, contained only 100 litres (three and a half cubic feet) of a sixty-five per cent oxygen : thirty-five per cent nitrogen mixture. They proposed to take a third companion, M. Gaston Tissandier, who would increase the drain on their already inadequate supply. When he heard of their plans Bert wrote in anguish, 'in the lofty elevations where this artificial respiration will be indispensable to you, for three men you should count on a consumption of at least twenty litres per minute; see how soon your supply will be exhausted!'[44] Bound for death or glory, the trio simply decided from Bert's letter to reserve their meagre supply of oxygen until they felt the need of it.

On 15 April 1875 at 11.35 am, they ascended in the balloon *Zenith* from the gas works of La Villette in Paris. Eight thousand metres (26,200 feet) was their goal, and Sivel particularly was determined to come back with a new record. At 1.20 they were at 23,000 feet, and Tissandier, testing the apparatus, wrote 'I breathe oxygen. Excellent effect.' All three were elated, euphoric, noted their rapid pulse rates without drawing the appropriate conclusions, and were determined to go still higher before using their oxygen. Tissandier's hands were cold, 'but without realizing it, the action of taking (a pair of fur gloves) from my pocket demanded an effort which I could no longer make.'[45] In a scrawling hand he wrote:

My hands are icy. I am well. We are well. Vapour on the horizon with little rounded cirrus clouds. We are rising. Crocé is panting. We breathe oxygen. Sivel closes his eyes. Crocé also closes his eyes. I empty the aspirator. Temp. −10 degrees (+14 F.). 1.20. H = 320 mm (22,000 feet). Sivel is drowsy.... 1.25. Temp −11 degrees (+12 F). H = 300 mm (23,500 feet). Sivel throws out ballast. Sivel throws out ballast.[46]

Tissandier remembered that Sivel took a knife and cut the cords of three bags of ballast hanging outside the basket, and the balloon shot upward:

Towards 7500 metres (24,600 feet), the numbness one experiences is extraordinary. The body and mind weaken little by little, gradually, unconsciously, without one's knowledge. One does not suffer at all; on the contrary. One experiences inner joy, as if it were an effect of the inundating flood of light. One becomes indifferent; one no longer thinks of the perilous situation or of the danger; one rises and is happy to rise. Vertigo of the lofty regions is not a vain word. But as far as I can judge by personal impressions, this vertigo appears at the last moment; it immediately precedes annihilation, sudden, unexpected, irresistible. . . .

Soon I wanted to seize the oxygen tube, but could not raise my arm. My mind, however, was still very lucid. I was still looking at the barometer; my eyes were fixed on the needle which soon reached the pressure number of 290, then 280, beyond which it passed.

I wanted to cry out, 'We are at 8000 metres! (26,200 feet). But my tongue was paralysed. Suddenly I closed my eyes and fell inert, entirely losing consciousness. It was about 1.30.[47]

There followed for Tissandier fleeting moments of awareness, memories of his companions unconscious in the bottom of the basket, and as in a nightmare, he felt himself shaken by the arm and heard Crocé-Spinelli cry, 'Throw out some ballast, we are descending.' Tissandier saw him tossing overboard the aspirator, ballast, wraps, etc., and as the balloon ascended once more, he again became unconscious. At 3.30 he finally awoke, to find the balloon falling fast and his two companions dead, 'crouched in the basket, their heads hidden under their travelling rugs... Sivel's face was black, his eyes dull, his mouth open and full of blood. Crocé's eyes were half shut and his mouth bloody.'[48] Like Tissandier, they had been too weak to reach for the oxygen tubes when they felt themselves losing consciousness, and indeed, the three oxygen bags were largely full when the *Zenith* landed 155 miles from Paris at 4 pm.

A primitive recording barometer indicated that the maximum altitude reached during the second ascent was 8600 metres (28,200 feet), certainly high enough to cause death by anoxia. One can only speculate as to why Tissandier did not share the fate of his companions. Possibly it was because he had not exerted himself as much as they, and therefore did not suffer such extreme oxygen deficiency.

The air, like the sea, is pitiless and unforgiving, and takes a terrible revenge on those who recklessly or carelessly measure themselves against it. Other aeronauts had died by falling; with Sivel and Crocé-Spinelli the end was strange and different. 'They leap up, and death seizes them, without a struggle, without suffering, as a prey fallen to it in these icy regions where an eternal silence reigns. Yes, our unhappy friends have had this strange privilege, this fatal honour, of being the first to die in the heavens.'[49] So mourned Paul Bert at their funeral. In the light of later knowledge, he was quite correct in insisting that continuous use of oxygen would have averted the catastrophe; but in the minds of many, who did not know that Bert's advice had been ignored, the tragic outcome discredited his experiments and theories.

Not for another twenty-five years would proud, mercurial Frenchmen again mount to high altitudes in balloons, and meanwhile their enemies across the Rhine were proceeding with characteristic German thoroughness and scientific method to win the altitude record. Again, meteorological research was the stated purpose. Professor Assmann, the guiding spirit of the German Association for the Promotion of Airship Travel, was also the inventor of an accurate instrument for measuring temperatures in the upper air, the aspiration psychrometer, and the high altitude flights made by the Association were designed among other things to calibrate the psychrometer with a view to its use in small unmanned sounding balloons. It was furthermore an age of nationalistic passions and international rivalries, and these made a significant but unacknowledged contribution to the outcome.

In the first ascent by the Association, in the year 1893, no oxygen was used, and at approximately 17,000 feet the aeronauts complained of heart palpitations, shortness of breath, exhaustion, apathy, and trembling of the entire body. On 11 May 1894 the participants (Major

Gross of the Prussian Airship Battalion and the meteorologist, Professor Artur Berson) used compressed oxygen in steel flasks, but were not completely spared the symptoms of altitude sickness, apparently because of the severe cold and the fatigue of being up the entire night before making preparations for the flight. Major Gross later wrote of the flight above 23,000 feet:

The temperature fell to 30 degrees below zero (−22 degrees F.) and we began to freeze. In front of us in the basket lay the heavy furs, but we no longer had the energy to pull them on. We found ourselves in a condition of bodily apathy; only the spirit and the will were strong; the wish to climb a further 1000 metres (3300 feet) animated us. Our lips and our finger nails had turned completely blue, our limbs trembled from cold and weakness. But again and again we were refreshed by the oxygen which we inhaled at short intervals. The thought that we were approaching the sea at an unknown rate of speed forced a rapid decision. I sacrificed the last scrap of ballast that we dared to use to ascend, the balloon broke out of the sea of cloud at 7750 metres altitude (25,400 feet) and was flooded with dazzling sunlight. With a clatter the long icicles broke free from the meshes of the netting. The warmed balloon mounted upward and finally, at 10.40 am, reached the longed-for 8000 metres (26,200 feet). In my log book I find scribbled in a barely legible hand, 'we feel horribly miserable and weak, but still completely alert mentally, we are breathing oxygen.' I had seated myself on the bench, since I was no longer able to stand, in my upper thighs I had a feeling of being frozen, a prickling pain. For a moment Herr Berson permitted his head to sink down on his chest and closed his eyes. I called to him and shook him. I too closed my eyes at times, and a drowsy stupor overcame me. By mustering all our energy and strength we succeeded in obtaining several accurate readings of the instruments, then I seized the valve line, as the balloon seemed inclined to rise further, solely from concern for the approaching sea.[50]

On 4 December 1894 Professor Berson alone reached 30,000 feet. Here:

I checked my condition and found that I could easily go higher, which my reserve of ballast would have permitted. Of course I am breathing oxygen continually, meanwhile experiencing only a mild feeling of the head swimming accompanied by a moderately severe palpitation, but otherwise I am fully capable of observing, reflecting, writing. . . but as soon as I drop the mouthpiece of the tubing, even for a moment, either to work in the basket, or as a physiological experiment, I am seized by very severe palpitations, almost fall over in a faint, and quickly reach out again for the life-giving tube.[51]

Undoubtedly Berson reached a higher altitude by ascending alone, but he ran a terrible risk of dying quickly if he had lost the mouthpiece of the compressed oxygen tube, and had no companion to reinsert it. Similar recklessness and overconfidence marked a solo ascent by another meteorologist, Professor Reinhard Süring, to 26,200 feet on

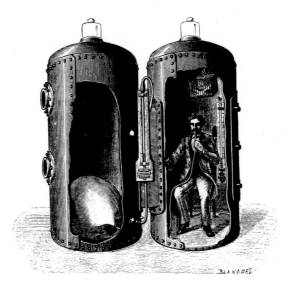

1. Cut-away view of Paul Bert's pressure chamber, 1878. Bert is conducting an experiment on himself, breathing from a bag containing oxygen-enriched air.

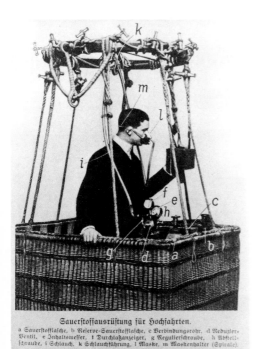

Sauerstoffausrüstung für Hochfahrten.

a Sauerstofflasche, b Reserve-Sauerstofflasche, c Verbindungsrohr, d Reduzier-Ventil, e Inhaltsmesser, f Durchlaßanzeiger, g Regulierschraube, h Abstellschraube, i Schlauch, k Schlauchführung, l Maske, m Maskenhalter (Spirale).

2. German oxygen equipment for high altitude balloon flights of about 1908. The illustration shows oxygen flasks, with reduction valves, flow meter, and contents gauge in basket, and tube leading to a mask covering both nose and mouth.

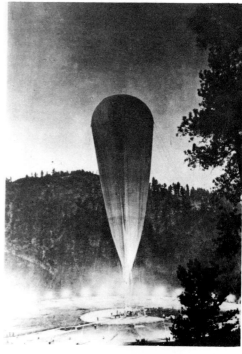

3. Stratosphere balloon *Explorer II* in the Stratobowl near Rapid City, South Dakota, on the morning of 11 November 1935. (Air Force Museum)

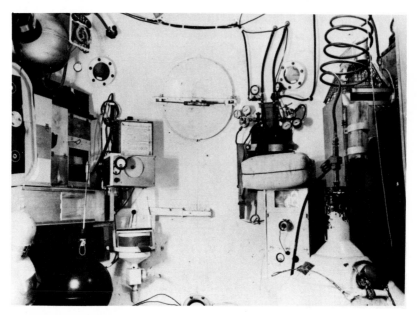

4. Inside the *Explorer II* gondola. Large flask of liquid oxygen and nitrogen at lower right, with evaporating coil. Vertical cabinet to right rear contains bags of sodium hydroxide to remove carbon dioxide and water vapour. (Air Force Museum)

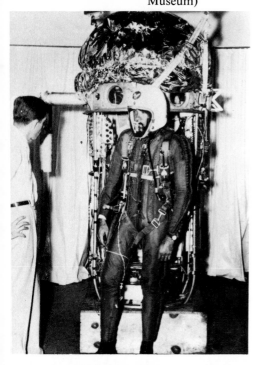

6. Major David B. Simons (MC) in pressure suit just prior to Man High II flight on 20 August 1957. Gondola in rear is minus its metal outer capsule. (Air Force Museum)

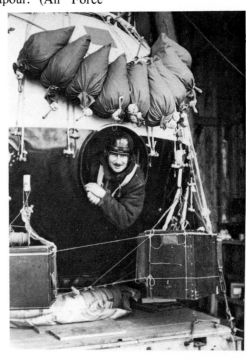

5. Captain A. W. Stevens in the hatchway of the spherical Dowmetal gondola of *Explorer II*. Sandbag ballast above, and batteries below, could be released from inside the gondola (1935). (Air Force Museum)

24 March 1899, a flight prolonged by freezing of the manœuvring valve in the top of the balloon. For two hours and fifteen minutes Süring experienced a temperature below forty degrees below zero F, with a minimum temperature of 54·7 degrees below zero F.

Thirty thousand feet thus appeared to be the ceiling for conventional balloons of about 70,000 cubic feet capacity, even in dangerous one-man attempts. Yet higher ceilings seemed desirable, not only for checking the accuracy of automatic registering apparatus borne aloft by sounding balloons, but also for physiological studies. Considering the extreme expansion of the lifting gas at high altitudes, only a large balloon could be expected to carry two men beyond 30,000 feet; but with the year 1901 the Association saw its ambitions within reach when a huge balloon of nearly 300,000 cubic feet capacity was presented to the society and promptly christened 'Preussen.' Using hydrogen, it was calculated that 39,400 feet could be attained. Whether human beings could tolerate such a height, even with oxygen, remained to be seen.

Part of the answer came from the Viennese physiologist, Hermann von Schrötter, whose name stands second only to Paul Bert's in the developmental history of aviation medicine. A bold and imaginative student of high altitude physiology, who himself made two balloon flights to promote his studies (one to 28,750 feet),[52] von Schrötter instructed Professors Berson and Süring in theory, and learned from them in practice. In a 'pneumatic chamber' in his laboratory in Vienna the physiologist taught the two meteorologists to recognize the effects of the thin air of the heights on pulse, blood pressure and respiration, and accompanied them on a training flight to 24,800 feet. He also supervised the oxygen equipment loaded aboard the 'Preussen,' comprising four steel cylinders each containing 35·3 cubic feet of the gas compressed to 100 atmospheres, with appropriate reducing and control valves. Despite von Schrötter's insistence that face-fitting masks be employed so that the aeronauts would still breathe oxygen even if unconscious, they used rubber tubing terminating in glass-tube mouthpieces.

On 11 July 1901 'Preussen,' filled with cheap illuminating gas, made a trial flight from the Airship Battalion's parade ground at Templehof, later to be the Berlin airport. On 31 July came the real attempt. With Berson and Süring in the oversize wicker basket were meteorological instruments (the recording barometers froze later, both ink and clockwork drive), including aneroid and mercury barometers, mercury thermometer, hygrometer, etc.; food and drink (they took only soda water during the flight, and would have preferred hot tea in thermos flasks), the indispensable oxygen apparatus, and fur flight clothing with fur boots and reindeer-skin jackets, both containing hot water bottles as a heat source. To conserve gas, which otherwise would have been valved off at high altitude, only 192,000 cubic feet of hydrogen was piped into the 300,000 cubic foot balloon. About 8000 pounds of ballast—partly sand, partly iron filings—were carried in seventy or eighty sacks, whose contents—to spare the men exertion at high altitude—could be emptied merely by cutting a cord.

At 10.45 am of a hot, calm day, 'Preussen' rose almost vertically from the Tempelhof parade ground, and within forty minutes had ascended smoothly to 16,000 feet. With oxygen there was no impairment of consciousness, but it was difficult to fight off increasing fatigue. On up to 33,000 feet they continued their observations and recordings, with temperatures dropping from twenty-two to forty below zero F. But they had exceeded the limits of the oxygen equipment with the wasteful pipestem mouthpieces. Indeed, even with tight-fitting masks and one hundred per cent oxygen, it is known today that the arterial blood saturation with oxygen begins to fall beyond 33,000 feet. Thus, at 34,500 feet Berson felt obliged to open the valve to start the descent, as he had noticed Süring losing consciousness. The exertion, slight at low altitude, was too much for him, even with oxygen, and he too collapsed unconscious, while the oxygen tube fell from his mouth. Fortunately Süring soon revived and aroused his companion by putting his own oxygen tube into his mouth. Turning to pull the valve line, Süring felt himself losing consciousness, turned back to grasp his oxygen tube, but it was too late—he joined Berson in unconsciousness. Thirty to forty-five minutes passed before they awakened at 20,000 feet with headache, lassitude, nausea and drowsiness, which they only with difficulty overcame to throw out ballast to check the fast-falling balloon. After a flight of seven and a half hours 'Preussen' landed seventy-five miles south-west of Berlin.

After listing the then-known symptoms of anoxia, Süring went on to cite some of von Schrötter's views:

After the effect of oxygen on these symptoms had been experimentally ascertained, there remained the question of the limits to which man could go without oxygen, in what amount and concentration oxygen should be breathed, and where the upper limit of the use of oxygen lies. Already at 5000 metres (16,400 feet) mild oxygen deficiency is manifested even without exertion, at altitudes of 6000–7000 metres (19,700–23,000 feet) a partial adaptation and acclimatization to the thin air is possible, but at heights of 8000 metres (26,200 feet) nobody can escape disturbances of function without breathing oxygen. Individual tolerance of altitude flying depends not so much on the mechanics of breathing—shallow breaths, for example—but predominantly on the oxygen saturation of the blood. A flow of gas from the steel flasks of 3·5 litres per minute appears to be adequate when one wears a mask, which forces him to breathe, instead of a tube with mouthpiece. Despite an adequate supply of oxygen, this sort of breathing equipment eventually no longer suffices, for in proportion to the general decrease in pressure the partial pressure of the inspired oxygen decreases also, and finally a situation develops where a too-small amount of the gas is delivered to the lungs. Calculations indicate that this will develop at an atmospheric pressure of 116 mm, which corresponds to an altitude of about 15,000 m (49,000 feet), but since a further drop in pressure must be taken into consideration with transfer of the oxygen to the blood, the altitude is further reduced, and the top limit to which one may go in a open balloon basket is now established at 12,500 metres (41,000 feet) (160 mm air pressure). Should one desire to break the present altitude record, von Schrötter recommends a *hermetically sealed gondola* constructed like a diving bell.[53]

Thus, as early as 1901, did the Viennese physiologist foresee the inevitable development of the pressurized gondola, first used thirty years later in a high altitude balloon flight by Auguste Piccard, and embodying the principle of the pressure cabin, which has made the modern air transport industry the giant that it is. Von Schrötter's figures were still being accepted for flying at high altitudes early in World War I, but further research has caused some revisions. Thus, the United States Air Force today insists that oxygen be used on flights above 10,000 feet, while 16,400 feet is in the zone of 'disturbance,' and 19,700–23,000 feet is in the 'critical' zone. But his uppermost limit of 41,000 feet for flight with ordinary oxygen equipment is remarkably close to the accepted maximum today. Using one hundred per cent oxygen and tight-fitting masks, modern pilots can go to 40,000 feet and maintain adequate blood oxygenation. Above this level pressurized breathing equipment must be used.

Thus, the flights of Berson and Süring, and von Schrötter's research on the effect of reduced partial pressures of oxygen at high altitude, heralded the end of the first age of high altitude flight using the conventional balloon with open basket. Small, automatically-instrumented sounding balloons took over the study of the upper atmosphere, making routine flights the year round more cheaply and safely than the early pioneer aeronauts. But before the second age opened, marked by the advent of the pressure gondola, there was one more series of old-fashioned high altitude balloon ascents, definitively proving the limitations of unpressurized equipment. The death of Captain Hawthorne C. Gray, US Army Air Corps, resulted in part from a tragic failure of scientific communication, for he does not seem to have known in detail of the experiences of Berson and Süring, and certainly could not have read the above opinions of von Schrötter on the maximum ceiling attainable with unpressurized oxygen equipment.

Gray, an experienced balloonist who had entered the Army in 1915 and had won second place in the 1926 Gordon Bennett race, is said to have undertaken high altitude flying solely with the aim of breaking the 1901 record of Berson and Süring.[54] For his first attempt, on 9 March 1927, Gray had compressed oxygen piped to a face mask. Due to freezing of the oxygen equipment—possibly from condensed moisture in the tubing—Gray lost consciousness at 27,000 feet, but fortunately for him, the balloon descended by itself after reaching 28,510 feet, and he revived in time to drop ballast before a hard landing.

His next attempt was at a more favourable time of year. On 4 May 1927 Gray rose from the Army Air Corps lighter-than-air base at Scott Field, Illinois, in his conventional hydrogen-inflated balloon. In the open basket he carried 3800 pounds of sand, compressed oxygen in steel flasks, and a radio receiver. What purpose the radio served is not clear, for Gray merely used it to tune in on commercial broadcast stations transmitting entertainment programmes. Had he suffered too intensely from loneliness and isolation in his first solo ascent to high altitude? Did the lightweight box of tubes and resistors provide a needed feeling of human companionship in the lonely heights?

Rising at seven hundred feet per minute, all the time listening to the radio playing the popular music of the jazz age, Gray experienced nothing unusual except for sub-zero cold that penetrated his fur-lined flying suit and frosted his goggles. The oxygen equipment worked perfectly until Gray reached 40,000 feet, where he experienced dizziness. Desirous of reaching 41,000 feet, a height which a French rival had claimed to have attained earlier, Gray checked all his sand bags to make sure they were empty, then dropped an empty oxygen cylinder and slowly rose to 42,470 feet, his maximum elevation, attained an hour and five minutes after takeoff. Here he noted discomfort in his chest as he walked around the open basket once again checking the sand bags. He could not know that even with one hundred per cent oxygen at this height, his arterial blood oxygen saturation would have fallen to eighty-four per cent, a level which would produce 'appreciable handicap' by modern Air Force standards, while with possible leakage of air into his mask, he might experience 'considerable handicap.' The new record appeared to be in the bag, and it was time to start down. The balloon obeyed a pull on the valve line, but to Gray's surprise, accelerated alarmingly in its downward progression. The valve had jammed open, and with no means of slowing his plummeting descent, Gray was forced to jump with his personal parachute. This act deprived him of the record, for he had violated a rule of the *Fédération Aeronautique Internationale* that the aeronaut had to retain control of his machine until the landing.

This must have provided Gray with an irresistible incentive to risk his life in another attempt. Some animal experiments—essentially duplicating those of Paul Bert over fifty years earlier—showed that rats and mice under bell jars became unconscious in air when the pressure was reduced to the equivalent of 25,000–28,000 feet. Gray must have been encouraged by the finding that they did not lose consciousness with pure oxygen until reaching an equivalent altitude of 49,000 feet. (Even with pressurized oxygen masks, humans do not attempt this altitude today.) Gray himself devised improvements in his oxygen equipment—oversize valve wheels which could easily be turned by a man wearing fur-lined gloves; an oxygen mask that evidently covered both nose and mouth, for 'it would supply him oxygen even if he fainted,'[5] and a really significant step forward, a barometrically-regulated diluter, which at lower altitudes afforded Gray a mixture of outside air and pure oxygen, thereby prolonging the usefulness of his oxygen supply at high altitude.

At 2.23 pm on 4 November 1927 Gray ascended from Scott Field for his second attempt on the record. His balloon disappeared into a heavy overcast at 3.10 pm, but a logbook full of entries describes everything that he found worthy of note—almost—until he was found dead in the open balloon basket at Sparta, Tennessee, at 5.20 pm. On his way up he again listened to the radio stations, recording some of the tunes they were playing—'Kashmiri Song,' and 'Sympathy.' At 30,000 feet, with the temperature thirty-five degrees below zero F, his clock stopped at 3.17 pm—the oil had solidified in the extreme cold. Was this, as Kurt Stehling suggests, the ultimate cause of the disaster? Or was it that Gray's keen judgement was blurred, his alert memory dulled and clouded by symptoms of anoxia? He certainly knew he could not count on his timepiece, for the log records, 'clock frozen.' But his radio no longer gave him the time either, for an empty oxygen cylinder released as ballast at 34,000 feet had broken the aerial. His last entries were made at 40,000 feet; the writing was shaky, and once he wrote 'hair' for 'air.' A recording barograph shows, however, that the balloon continued to rise, fluctuating up and down, and finally attained 42,470 feet, exactly the altitude reached on the previous flight. Then, it would appear, Gray valved gas to descend, the curve steepening at 4.28 pm at 39,000 feet. But it was too late—Gray's oxygen was exhausted, and in the clear air of the heights, he died. Was he betrayed by the clock which no longer gave him the data from which to calculate the amount of oxygen remaining? Or was he, from the stupor of developing anoxia, incapable of anticipating disaster? The deteriorating handwriting, the lack of entries even though the barograph shows for some time further spasmodic attempts to control the balloon, would favour the latter hypothesis.[56] Nor did Gray attain the official altitude record he desired. Dead in the basket, he again was not in control of his vehicle at the landing.

Gray's fatal ascent ended the first age of high altitude ballooning. No further records were attempted with the open gondola until its reappearance many years later in connection with the development of pressure and space suits.

Others besides von Schrötter had foreseen the inevitable necessity of the fully enclosed, pressurized gondola for high altitude flight: it remained for an obscure Swiss professor of physics, Auguste Piccard, to exploit this idea in the first true stratosphere balloon, with which he won international fame before going on to his later undersea research in the bathyscaphe, a free deep-diving vessel, of which the 'Trieste' was the ultimate development.

The flights of the second age of high altitude ballooning in the early 1930s, distinguished by the use of the pressurized gondola attached to huge balloons of unconventional design, were undertaken to investigate the newly-discovered cosmic rays at the top of the atmosphere. The existence of these sub-microscopic particles, travelling through space with the energy of millions of electron-volts, had been suspected from about 1900 from their ability to penetrate and to ionize gases in closed vessels. For a decade the source of this penetrating radiation was obscure, and it was the balloon which first provided a definite clue: in 1911 and 1912, the Austrian physicist, Victor F. Hess, whose cosmic ray studies eventually won him a Nobel Prize in 1936, made a number of balloon ascents to as high as 16,400 feet. Up to 2300 feet he found that ionization due to radiation dropped steadily, indicating an emanation from the earth itself, but above this level the ionization steadily increased, being several times the sea level value at 16,400 feet. In 1913, further ascents by W. Kohlhörster to 29,600 feet demonstrated an ionization rate twelve times that at sea level. Obviously the charged particles responsible were arriving from outer space and could best be studied at great altitudes, before their energy was absorbed and dissipated by the shield of the atmosphere. In 1928 the rather clumsy cloud chamber used heretofore to study cosmic rays was supplemented by the Geiger–Müller counter, and cosmic ray research was well started on the study of the primary and secondary particles, the protons, electrons, neutrons and mesons, which led via the cyclotron and the synchrotron to the evolution of atomic theory and the development of the atomic bomb.

Determined to take his equipment aloft to the regions where the protons, the primary particles from outer space, were most abundant,

Piccard had a monster balloon of 500,000 cubic feet capacity, 114 feet in diameter, built by the experienced August Riedinger balloon factory at Augsburg, Germany. Because a very light weight rubberized cotton was used, the total weight of the envelope with cordage was only 1600 pounds. To his later regret, Piccard trusted to an ordinary valve-rope to open the valve in the top of the balloon, while fine lead shot ballast was released from inside the gondola through an air lock. To reduce the stress on the fabric and structure, and to conserve gas, it was planned to have only 100,000 cubic feet of hydrogen in the bag at takeoff. Thus, the image of the stratosphere balloon in the public mind became the tall, elongated bag, with its loose, trailing folds raised over a hundred feet aloft by a small bubble of gas in its crown, towering above the spectators in a windless nighttime or early morning takeoff. Because of the unprecedented size of the bag, and the need to save weight, the conventional netting was dispensed with, and loads were carried by a pair of gracefully-scalloped catenary bands, one circling the upper portion of the balloon for ground handling lines used to hold it during inflation, the lower one for the shroud lines supporting the gondola.

Piccard's gondola set the pattern for those that followed. Two hundred and ten cm (82·6 in) in diameter, fabricated of welded aluminium sheets 3·5 mm thick, it was spherical in shape, to best resist internal pressure, and had two circular entrance hatches and eight portholes 3·15 in in diameter. Empty, the gondola weighed 300 pounds, and with occupants and instruments, 850 pounds. Here, with pressure maintained above that of the surrounding stratosphere, two aeronauts could observe their instruments and surroundings in comfort, free from hampering fur clothing and oxygen masks and tubing. The internal atmosphere was maintained in rather primitive fashion: liquid oxygen in double-walled flasks, boiling at 350 degrees F below zero, maintained the life-giving property of the atmosphere, while carbon dioxide given off by the metabolic processes of the human aeronauts was absorbed by dry sodium hydroxide. In addition, the boiling oxygen maintained adequate pressure in the gondola, and if more pressure were needed, it built up quickly in the sealed cabin after spilling an excess of liquid oxygen on the floor of the gondola. (It will be noted that in contrast to present-day aircraft pressure cabins, where-in a normal environment is maintained by compressing the outside air, Piccard's artificial atmosphere was completely self-sustaining and could have maintained life in space). A valve prevented development of excessive pressure in the gondola. To control the inner temperature of the cabin, one side was painted black to absorb solar heat, the other left bright aluminium, with a small motor-driven propeller being intended to turn it as necessary.[57]

Piccard's first flight attempt in the *FNRS*[58] on 14 September 1930, ended before it began when the balloon had to be deflated due to high winds. On 27 May 1931 he and his assistant, Paul Kipfer, reached an altitude of 51,775 feet in a flight that started at Augsburg, Germany, and ended on the Gurgl Glacier in Switzerland. The two aeronauts were plagued by malfunctions: at the start it was found that due to an accidental deformation of the aluminium shell, a plug could not be driven home; the balloon was at 13,000 feet before the hole could be plugged with an impromptu mixture of vaseline and cotton waste, and the gondola pressurized. The motor designed to turn the gondola was damaged at takeoff, and with the black side turned towards the sun, the interior temperature at one point reached over one hundred degrees F. Worst of all, the valve line was inoperable, having been fouled by a holding line attached to the gondola before takeoff. Fortunately the reserve oxygen supply lasted until evening cooling contracted the gas and brought the balloon down after a flight of more than seventeen hours. Otherwise the two aeronauts might have smothered in their hermetically-sealed prison ten miles in the air just as surely as trapped submariners on the bottom of the sea. But Auguste Piccard had set a new altitude record, far surpassing Captain Gray's figure, and with none of the physiological or medical hazards that had overwhelmed the gallant American. To prove the value of his equipment, Piccard made a second flight, with Max Cosyns, to 53,153 feet on 18 August 1932. Nothing malfunctioned, and he and his companion brought back valuable cosmic ray data.

Auguste Piccard had set the style for stratosphere flight, and had stimulated a competition in Russia and America to surpass his results.

The American entry was a 600,000 cubic foot rubberized fabric balloon christened *Century of Progress* in honour of the exposition by that name being held in Chicago in the year 1933, which sponsored the enterprise. Beneath the balloon was suspended a spherical pressure gondola fabricated of magnesium alloy (Dowmetal). Originally, Auguste Piccard and his twin brother Jean were to handle the balloon in a takeoff from Chicago, but both were obliged to withdraw from the project and Lieutenant Commander Thomas G. W. Settle USN, an experienced balloon pilot who had won the 1932 Gordon Bennett race for the United States, took their place. On the night of 4 August 1933, in a carnival-type atmosphere, Settle ascended alone from Soldier Field with 125,000 cubic feet of hydrogen in the top of the bag. There were doubts about the functioning of the valve line, and when Settle tested the valve at 5000 feet, it stuck open. He landed safely in the

Chicago, Burlington and Quincy railroad yards, but the huge rubberized bag was considerably damaged by souvenir hunters.

On 30 September 1933 three Russian aeronauts in a sealed cabin reached 62,230 feet in the balloon *USSR*.

The *Century of Progress* balloon was returned to the builder, Goodyear Aircraft Co. in Akron, overhauled and repaired with 'some 1800 patches . . . most of them very small ones.'[59] The next attempt, on 20 November 1933, was made in privacy from the giant airship dock in Akron, and as scientific observer Settle was accompanied by Major Chester Fordney USMC, 'keeping it a Navy affair.' The balloon was partly filled with some Navy surplus helium which had been contaminated with air in a gas cell casualty to the new Navy rigid airship *Macon* some months before, and which was too low in purity to warrant its being shipped for repurification. The scientific load included ionization chambers, Geiger–Müller counters and film emulsions for cosmic ray studies, a quartz spectrograph for analysis of sun and sky spectra at high altitude, a Fairchild aerial camera, an Eastman kodak with infra-red filters, a light polarization indicator, air sample bottles, high-frequency radio transmitter and receiver for communication and to test emission and reception of radio signals at high altitude, and plant disease spores to assay their viability at low pressure and temperature. Fruit flies failed to arrive before takeoff, so the possibility of chromosomal mutations due to cosmic irradiation at high altitude could not be tested.

The artificial atmosphere arrangements in the sealed gondola drew on Navy experience with the same problem in submarine operations. In Settle's words:

a. For 'make-up' O_2, we had two open-top thermos jugs of liquid O_2, planned to evaporate off into the gondola at about the anticipated rate of usage of O_2 by our lungs. With some unavoidable leakage of air overboard, through glands, we anticipated that, during the flight, our inboard atmosphere would gradually grow in O_2 richness. The evaporating O_2 also served to maintain inboard atmospheric pressure against leakage and absorption. Should we have needed faster evaporation for breathing or pressure, we could have spilled some liquid O_2 on the deck—but as it turned out, that was not necessary. During our closed hatch period, our O_2 percentage almost doubled (approximately 20% to 40%), which caused no inconvenience, and our inboard pressure fell mildly from about equiv. 13,000 feet altitude to about 15,000 feet equiv.

b. For CO_2 absorption we borrowed from submarine practice—used SS type 'grids' of a Li compound,—which worked well and kept our CO_2 content well down.

c. For H_2O vapour absorption, also borrowed from SS practice,—used silical gel pads, which worked OK and minimized moisture condensation (and freezing) on the gondola wall.[60]

Taking off at 9.30 am only thirty pounds light, with 4100 pounds of lead shot and sand ballast aboard, the *Century of Progress* was held at first to low altitudes, where the wind was less. By 12.45 pm the balloon had ascended to 13,500 feet, the hatches were closed and the high altitude phase began. Between 2.10 and 4.15 pm the craft was at maximum altitude, touching 61,237 feet, and then, as Settle anticipated, the gas cooled as the sun descended, and the balloon started down. Contrary to some published reports, there were no difficulties this time with the valve or valve line. At 26,500 feet the hatches were opened and at 5.50 pm, after valving down, a 'normal rip landing' was made in a marsh near Bridgeton, New Jersey. The flight provided information of the highest value for Professor Arthur H. Compton of the University of Chicago, and for the future of nuclear physics: whereas other physicists had contended that high-energy gamma rays, able to penetrate thickly shielded chambers at sea level, were the primary cosmic emanations, Compton had suspected that the proton particle, or charged hydrogen nucleus, was the real primary. The equipment which Settle carried aloft indicated that at peak altitude, less than one-half per cent of the radiation represented gamma rays, and the great majority of the tracks recorded represented protons. Obviously these constituted the primary radiation from outer space, and the gamma rays were secondary phenomena produced in the atmosphere.[61]

The artificial atmospheric equipment functioned remarkably well, and there were no physiological difficulties. The pressure within the sealed gondola remained between 12,000 and 15,000 feet equivalent, the carbon dioxide concentration being no more than two per cent. With the oxygen level reaching forty per cent, Settle and Fordney experienced no breathing problems when the hatches were opened at the relatively high altitude of 26,500 feet, even though they were working hard in preparation for the imminent landing. Some moisture condensed and froze on the upper interior of the gondola, the outside of which was painted white above and black below.

The Soviet reply came on 30 January 1934 when the 800,000 cubic foot balloon *Ossoaviakhim* climbed to 72,182 feet, but fell out of control, killing the three aeronauts. It seems a fact that in an attempt to win the altitude record at all cost, they had kept no reserve of ballast; rumours persisted that the Soviet dictator, Joseph Stalin, had threatened them with death if they failed.

Captain Orvil A. Anderson of the US Army Air Corps, the pilot on the next high-altitude adventure, believed that in such a case all ballast could safely be released, and a higher altitude attained, if the balloon were open at the bottom, and thus could function as a giant parachute in the descent. Furthermore, Anderson expected that the trapped air inflating the bag would be superheated by the sun, thus increasing the lift still more. But the sponsors of the *Explorer I* flight, the National Geographic Society and the US Army Air Corps, rejected the radical suggestion.[62]

The object was to raise a seven-foot Dowmetal spherical gondola—a 'scientific laboratory' weighing over 3000 pounds—to an altitude of 70,000 feet, and calculations showed that with hydrogen inflation a balloon of 3,000,000 cubic feet would be necessary. This far exceeded in size every aerostat previously built. For the first time the treacherous valve rope was replaced by a pneumatic hose opening the valve by compressed air. For artificial atmosphere, three flasks containing a liquid mixture of forty-five per cent oxygen and fifty-five per cent nitrogen were carried, together with chemicals to remove carbon dioxide and dehumidifying equipment. The relief valve for control of pressure in the sealed gondola was hand operated.[63] Because the balloon, with only 210,000 cubic feet of hydrogen forming a bubble in its crown, would stand 310 feet tall at takeoff, it would be excessively vulnerable to even a light breeze. A deep natural shelter, a hollow in the Black Hills near Rapid City, South Dakota, was used for the takeoff. To this day it retains the name of 'Stratobowl,' and has been the point of departure for subsequent high-altitude balloon flights.

With Major W. E. Kepner, Captain A. W. Stevens, and Anderson aboard, *Explorer I* took off on 10 July 1934 with 70,000 feet as the goal. At 13,000 feet the hatches were closed; the liquid oxygen and dehumidifying equipment worked well and the men were comfortable. At 40,000 feet the balloon was levelled off and cosmic ray and other measurements were made. The gas continued to expand as the balloon went on up to the next level. The lower portion of the bag below the gondola suspension band had been packed inside the balloon when it left the factory; now, as the expanding gas forced down the bottom of the bag, the three men were surprised and alarmed to see it ripped in many places. Some rubber coating the inside of the bag had remained 'tacky' and large portions of the bottom fabric had stuck, producing the tears on expansion. As Anderson started down from the ceiling of 60,613 feet, the tears increased, but did not extend above the gondola suspension band. Finally the whole bottom third of the *Explorer I* tore free. Descending at 600 feet per minute, the aerostat was now a giant parachute—but filled with a mixture of hydrogen and air. Fortunately the three occupants did not have to take their chances in a crash landing: they had individual parachutes. At 18,000 feet they opened the hatches and debated whether to bail out or not. Their minds were made up for them when, at 3000 feet, the hydrogen-air mixture ignited and exploded, shredding the bag completely. Anderson, outside and on top of the gondola, jumped at once. The other two had to struggle out of the hatches and their 'chutes opened barely five hundred feet from the ground.

Though some valuable data had been obtained, it seemed necessary to repeat the attempt, using helium to obviate the explosive danger, and taking steps to ensure that there would be no sticking of the layers of the bag. The *Explorer II* therefore was increased in size to 3,700,000 cubic feet to attain the same ceiling with helium, producing a rubberized bag standing 316 feet high when on the ground with 250,000 cubic feet of helium in its crown, and 192 feet in diameter at its ceiling, where the expanding gas would have distended it to its full spherical form. The Dowmetal gondola was bigger than that of *Explorer I,* being nine feet in diameter, and with more equipment, including instruments and batteries, but excluding ballast, weighed 4497 pounds. Only Stevens and Anderson were scheduled to operate it, Kepner having been detached. The artificial atmosphere equipment was more sophisticated than any used previously. To eliminate the fire risk associated with pure oxygen, fifty-three pounds of a liquefied mixture of forty-six per cent oxygen and fifty-four per cent nitrogen were carried in a double-wall twenty-five litre container. Helium under pressure (gaseous oxygen and nitrogen were both found to condense and dissolve in the liquid nitrogen–oxygen mixture) forced it through an evaporating coil which converted it into a gas. Tests showed that a one-pound pressure of helium would evaporate 5·2 pounds of the nitrogen–oxygen mixture per hour, providing twenty-seven cubic feet of oxygen—more than enough for each man. There was also a reserve container of 32·5 pounds of a liquid fifty per cent oxygen and fifty per cent nitrogen mixture. Any pressure build-up would be relieved by an adjustable valve which the crew set for a pressure of nine pounds per square foot, corresponding to an altitude of 13,000 feet. Dry sodium hydroxide was chosen to absorb carbon dioxide and water vapour, with a fan circulating the gondola atmosphere through a vertical cabinet, containing 15·25 pounds of NaOH pellets in twelve cloth bags. For temperature control the aeronauts again relied on painting the top of the gondola white, and the bottom black.[64]

The first *Explorer II* flight attempt ended in failure on 10 July 1935 when during inflation the top of the balloon ripped open from a tear starting at one end of the ripping panel. This was eliminated in a revision of the design and, on 11 November 1935, Stevens and Anderson at last succeeded in setting a new altitude record of 72,395 feet. The takeoff was from the Stratobowl at 7.01 am, and the balloon ascended rapidly to 16,700 feet. Here, as the two men levelled off the balloon and prepared to close up, they noted symptoms of anoxia and thirstily consumed the hot water carried in three cans for drinking, this step being designed to prevent its freezing. Undoubtedly their water loss was greater than usual with the low vapour pressure of the atmosphere at that height. The hatches were sealed, pressure built up as the air-conditioning equipment went into action, and the men's symptoms disappeared. At 9.30 am the pressure within the gondola had increased to the equivalent of 10,900 feet, with the balloon actually at 27,700 feet. The sylphon-actuated exhaust valve was set to open at a pressure corresponding to 13,500 feet, and this equivalent altitude was maintained throughout the closed-gondola portion of the flight until early in the descent, when the helium pressure over the oxygen–nitrogen mixture suddenly increased, raising the gondola pressure briefly to 10,375 feet. During the five and three-quarter hours that the gondola was sealed—two hours of which were at the balloon's ceiling—the two occupants experienced no discomfort, and there was no evidence of oxygen deficiency or carbon dioxide accumulation. The relative humidity in the enclosed space varied from thirty-three per cent at the start to fifty-five per cent at the end. This caused frost to form on the porthole in the top of the gondola. The internal gondola temperature varied between 43·7 and 10·4 degrees F, the maximum level being at the ceiling in strong sunlight, with low readings during ascent and descent, apparently due to convection loss due to movement of the gondola through the air. The lowest outside temperature was −81 degrees F at 68,000 feet. On the way down the hatches were opened at 17,000 feet and with further ballasting, the balloon landed gently with its two occupants inside the gondola, and quantities of scientific information in their recording spectrographs, Geiger counters and other instruments. Over 15,000 recording photographs were taken of the instruments while in the stratosphere. Of the oxygen and nitrogen loaded at the start of the flight, 31·6 pounds had been evaporated during the sealed-gondola phase.

Stevens and Anderson both hoped for a third flight with the *Explorer II,* in which all ballast would be dropped, the balloon accelerated upward to pass its static ceiling at a rate of ascent of 1000 feet per minute, and the gondola released to float down on a large parachute. An altitude above 85,000 feet might result. But the sponsors replied 'leave well enough alone,' and the 11 November 1935 flight was the last in the second age of high-altitude ballooning. In 1938 the Poles built a 4,400,000 cubic foot bag which, with hydrogen, could have attained more than 90,000 feet. With no shelter like the Stratobowl, their huge balloon collapsed in a light wind during inflation. A second attempt in the following year never came off due to the German invasion of Poland.

The flights of the second age of high-altitude ballooning were significant for their almost uniform success in solving completely the problems which had so overtaxed the early pioneers—some to the point of death—namely anoxia, extreme cold, and low pressure levels incompatible with human existence. To Auguste Piccard must go the chief credit for developing the pressurized, sealed gondola which enabled him and his successors to ascend in comfort beyond the stratosphere—free from the encumbrance of masks, hoses and heavy clothing. With the technology of the day, however, it appeared that the 72,395-foot record of *Explorer II* represented the maximum altitude, barring the use of operating techniques incompatible with good ballooning practice. The huge 3,700,000 cubic foot rubberized fabric bag of the American record holder—made as light as possible—was the largest that could be handled on the ground at takeoff. After the Polish attempt in 1938, no further flights were undertaken with this type of equipment.

Following World War II, however, there came a series of high altitude ascents, many surpassing the record set by Anderson and Stevens. The third age of high altitude ballooning was made possible by the courageous exploitation of a miraculous technological advance—the development of strong, gas-tight, transparent plastic films of incredible thinness and lightness.

At the end of World War II, there was an urgent need for an inexpensive means of reaching high altitude. The jet age had arrived, the space age was around the corner, higher altitudes would be attained by jet- and rocket-powered aircraft than had ever previously been reached by those fitted with piston engines. Airless space was theoretically within reach. What of the cosmic rays, smashing into human tissue unprotected by the atmospheric shield, with their energies of millions of electron-volts? Could men, even in pressure capsules, survive their bombardment?[65] And even with the pressure cabin a reality, the military services insisted that survival equipment be available in the event of failure. Pressure suits, parachutes adapted to high-altitude use, were being developed: how to test them realistically? Lastly, high-altitude meteorology was an unexplored subject: the jet streams, for instance, in the lower stratosphere, were just beginning to be recognized.

Through the inspiration and hard work of a number of individuals, together with the laboratory and production resources of a large industrial firm—General Mills—and the interest and financial support of the Office of Naval Research, a means was found to send a manned balloon thousands of feet higher than Anderson and Stevens' record in the *Explorer II*. During the war years remarkable advances had been made in the manufacture of plastics and plastic films, and General Mills had produced much of the plastic wrapping and water-proofing material used during the conflict. Could not this novel, lightweight substance be employed for balloons? So thought Auguste Piccard's twin brother Jean, now at the University of Minnesota. He conceived the idea of sending a sealed gondola to 100,000 feet for ten hours beneath a cluster of as many as 100 plastic balloons. An engineer, Otto Winzen, presented Piccard's idea to the Office of Naval Research, where it was enthusiastically taken up by Lieutenant George Hoover USN. Thus Project Helios was born. Considerable work was done in 1946–47 on Piccard's idea in a contract with General Mills, which had retained Winzen as engineer-in-charge for high-altitude ballooning, with Piccard as consultant. But after the pressure gondola had been constructed, the manned project was cancelled because of the unreliability of the plastic materials then available. Project Skyhook, involving unmanned balloon flights for cosmic ray and other studies, was activated instead, with the further thought of gaining experience with plastic envelopes and their handling problems.

The first plastic balloon flight, on 25 September 1947, reached 100,000 feet carrying a payload of seventy pounds of instruments. The balloon, seventy feet in diameter and one hundred feet tall, had a potential volume of 206,000 cubic feet, but contained only 2700 cubic feet of gas at takeoff. There were no shroud lines, and of course, no net; instead, the load was carried by plastic straps, called load tapes, worked into the structure as reinforcements and terminating at the bottom in a suspension harness.

Many plastic balloons soared aloft during the next few years in the Navy's Skyhook project, and the Air Force's Moby Dick study of high-altitude winds. It was the day of the flying saucers from outer space, and it was difficult for the layman to believe that the distant, round, shiny objects in the sky were the transparent balloons of General Mills and of Otto Winzen, who presently left to form his own company. Not all the unmanned flights were successfully completed: some of the fragile bags ruptured, and many were whipped to pieces, or literally torn in two, at the turbulent interface between fast-moving jet stream layers. Such incidents convinced the Office of Naval Research that polyethylene film 0·002 in. thick was most suitable for balloons, by reason of its great strength, light weight, ability to be extruded into thin sheets, and the fact that it could be heat-sealed to form relatively good gas-tight seams. Meanwhile, animal experiments tended to show that the cosmic ray danger had been overrated; the only positive finding was a sprinkling of grey hairs in black mice sent to the top of the stratosphere. How would a human be affected? And could human life be trusted to the diaphanous vegetable bags? To one man, more familiar than most with their strength as well as their weakness, the temptation was irresistible: on 3 November 1949 Charles B. Moore, of General Mills, made the first manned flight in a plastic balloon at Minneapolis. He rose only a few thousand feet, but he had proved it could be done.

Though others reached high altitudes with the plastic balloons, the pioneers who set the pace were a close-knit team of Navy men, Lieutenant Commander Malcolm D. Ross USNR and Lieutenant-Commander M. Lee Lewis USN. With the Office of Naval Research initiating in 1955 a manned balloon programme—Project Strato-Lab—the pair ascended on 10 August 1956 to 40,000 feet beneath a polyethylene plastic balloon. They were in an open gondola and breathed oxygen from masks, without pressure suits. Though they studied and photographed jet vapour trails, and carried cosmic ray equipment, the flight really served as a preliminary to a much more ambitious high-altitude attempt with a closed gondola, subsequently designated Strato-Lab I.

In many respects, Ross and Lewis began where Anderson and Stevens had left off a generation earlier. Again the gondola—the souvenir of Project Helios—was painted black below and white above. The artificial atmosphere was maintained in similar fashion: five litres of liquid oxygen could be evaporated through a converter, with the oxygen-enriched atmosphere being pressurized to the equivalent of 17,000 feet. Fans circulated the air through chemicals to absorb carbon dioxide and water vapour. After an initial launching failure at New Brighton, Minnesota, when winds of eight to twelve mph ripped the plastic bag, Strato-Lab I went back to the Stratobowl near Rapid City, South Dakota, whence *Explorer II* had made its earlier takeoff. The biggest difference was in the bag: where *Explorer II*'s 192-foot diameter rubberized bag, with its volume of 3,700,000 cubic feet, weighted 5916 pounds, the plastic Strato-Lab balloon, 128 feet in diameter and 2,000,000 cubic feet in volume, weighed only 595 pounds, including its valves. The *Explorer II* ballast alone—3000 pounds—weighed more than the Strato-Lab balloon and its load. There were lesser differences: where Stevens and Anderson had no back-up system in case of pressurization failure at high altitude, Ross and Lewis wore the then-new MC-3A partial pressure suit with MA-1 helmet and face plate, which, in case of emergency, would automatically inflate with oxygen under pressure. And Strato-Lab I set a fashion that would be followed by later researchers in communication with the ground: electrodes attached to the aeronauts' bodies

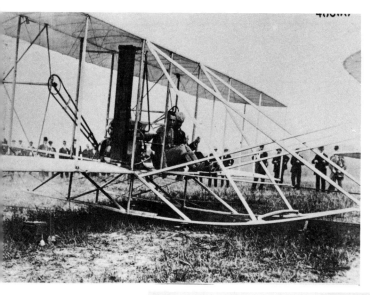

7. The first fatality in powered flight: Lieut. Thomas E. Selfridge (left) about to take off at Fort Myer in the Army Signal Corps Wright 'A' on 17 September 1908. Orville Wright at the controls. (Air Force Museum)

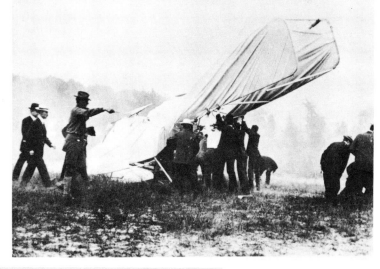

8. A few moments later and the aircraft has crashed. Men on the right of the photograph surround the dying Lieut. Selfridge, while Orville Wright is still trapped under the wreckage. (Air Force Museum)

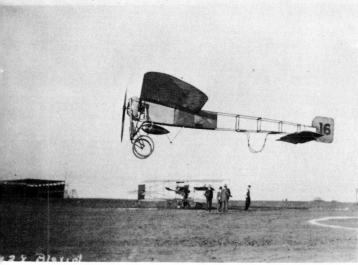

9. A Bleriot monoplane, Type XI, similar to the one in which M. Bleriot first crossed the English Channel on 25 July 1909. Curtiss pusher biplane on the ground. (Air Force Museum)

10. British S.E. 5a fighter in Palestine (1918). (Imperial War Museum)

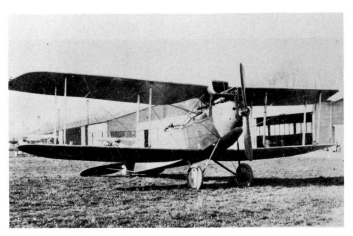

11. Rumpler C-VII. In the photo reconnaissance *Rubild* version with Maybach Mb IVa overcompressed engine, the ceiling was 24,000 feet. (1918). (Imperial War Museum)

12. Oxygen equipment in a British D.H. 4 squadron. Observer's mask being adjusted, Serny Aerodrome 17 February 1918. Undoubtedly of the Dreyer type the mask is supplied from compressed oxygen bottles in the cockpit. (Imperial War Museum)

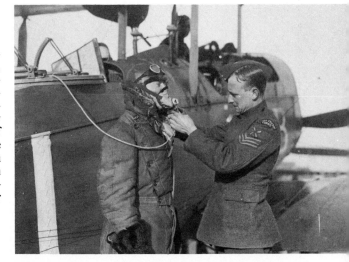

transmitted to monitoring stations on the ground their pulse and respirations, breathing and heart sounds, and electrocardiograms, while an experienced flight surgeon and naval aviator, Captain Norman Lee Barr (MC) USN, followed in a chase plane, constantly monitoring their physiological processes and prepared to direct the aeronauts' activities by radio in case of emergency.

At 6.19 am on the morning of 8 November 1956 Ross and Lewis lifted off from the Stratobowl. The temperature was three degrees above zero. The balloon ascended rapidly, the rate of climb at 6500 feet being five hundred feet per minute. At 10,000 feet the hatches were closed, and the oxygen apparatus turned up full. At 36,500 feet the rate slowed, but picked up after dropping only ten pounds of steel dust. At 55,000 feet there was a pause, but so light was the balloon that five pounds more started it on its way up again. By 8.47 am Ross and Lewis were at 70,500 feet, with a gondola temperature of thirty-eight degrees F and relative humidity of sixty per cent. With the rate of ascent slowed, and cooling diminished, the gondola temperature rose to forty degrees at the ceiling of 76,000 feet. It was a new world's altitude record for manned flight, surpassing by three thousand feet the earlier achievement of Anderson and Stevens. 'A lot of very fine people have passed this way,' murmured Lewis reflectively. At this moment there was a sudden jar, and the gondola sank under their feet like a falling elevator. Fearful that the plastic, rendered brittle by the cold, might have ruptured, the two men strapped themselves into their seats and snapped the face plates into their pressure helmets, while the voice of Dr Barr, far below in the chase plane, boomed out, 'Congratulations! Congratulations on a fine flight!' He had not heard their emergency announcement. At 58,000 feet Ross released 165 pounds of ballast, and the descent slowed. The balloon, mysteriously, was seen to be still intact—only later was it determined that a malfunctioning automatic valve had opened briefly and released part of their helium. At 35,000 feet the rate of descent increased, steadying in the troposphere at 1300 to 1400 feet per minute. Ross and Lewis might have cut the gondola loose from the streaming bag and trusted to the 64-foot cargo 'chute, or have bailed out at a lower altitude with their personal parachutes, but they chose to unballast and ride the gondola down. Away went the rest of their three hundred pounds of ballast, and after the hatches popped at 17,000 feet, they energetically heaved out the oxygen converter, instrument panel, bags of chemical absorbent, the oxygen analyser and air regenerator. A few hundred feet up they strapped themselves in their seats. Still falling at eight hundred feet per minute, the gondola landed hard, but a thick styrofoam pad absorbed the shock and the aeronauts were uninjured. The flight had lasted four hours and four minutes, less than half the anticipated time.[66]

Valuable information had been gained on plastic balloon operations, and in subsequent flights Ross and Lewis turned in flawless performances. On 18 October 1957, in Strato-Lab II, they reached 85,700 feet. On 26 and 27 July 1958 the pair attained 82,000 feet in Strato-Lab III, made a television broadcast from 79,500 feet, and remained 34·7 hours aloft. On 28 and 29 November 1959 a 2,000,000 cubic foot Strato-Lab IV balloon ascended to 81,000 feet, with a 16-inch reflecting telescope and spectrograph mounted atop the gondola for observation of the atmosphere of Venus, unhampered by the envelope of air surrounding the earth. But Malcolm Ross made the flight accompanied by Charles B. Moore, who ten years before had made the first plastic balloon ascent. Only four months earlier, on 6 July, the much-beloved Lee Lewis, then retired and serving as chief flight engineer for Winzen Research, had been killed in a gondola suspended three feet from the ground. A block, used to lift the gondola, had carried away and had catapulted sixty-five feet, striking him in the back.

The 85,700 foot figure still stands as the record for two men in a pressure gondola, and in fact, would seem to be the maximum altitude attainable by more than one man with 'conventional' equipment. With the same size balloon, however, one can always reach a greater height by lightening the payload, and with one man in a small pressure capsule, the Air Force, in its 'Man High' project, surpassed Ross and Lewis in a series of three flights. Previously I have criticized the unacceptable risks involved in one-man flights to great altitude, as illustrated by the tragic fate of Captain Hawthorne Gray, but in the 'Man High' project these were eliminated through a very sophisticated radio communication system whereby the aeronaut's performance was constantly monitored from the ground. Not only were his pulse, respirations, heart beat, etc., continually transmitted, but ground personnel were prepared to control and direct him by radio in case of emergency, while in the event of a high-altitude catastrophe, they could intervene to end the flight by separating the balloon from the capsule, which would then descend by cargo parachute.

A further reason for sending only one man aloft was that the main purpose of 'Man High' was to study the effect on humans of cosmic rays at high altitudes and undoubtedly it was considered better to expose only one man at a time to these hitherto unknown dangers. For several years, as noted above, mice, monkeys, and other animals had been sent aloft in pressure capsules to expose them to cosmic radiation, and in the opinion of Colonel John P. Stapp (whose research with rocket sleds on extreme deceleration—using himself as a test subject—will be covered in a later chapter), the Chief of the Aero Medical Field Laboratory at Holloman Air Force Base, the time had come to send a man aloft. 'As valuable as our animal flights had been, no amount of training will make a scientific observer out of a monkey, though the reverse has sometimes been true.'[67] Stapp chose a volunteer medical officer, Major David G. Simons, as project officer for the manned flights, and experimental subject. 'The animals,' Stapp remarked to Simons, 'did nothing up there but breathe, eat and defecate. They didn't talk on the radio or shift around in an 180-pound mass or fidget in a pressure suit or try to grab scientific observations out of those saucer-sized portholes, or do any of the things you will have to do when you go up.'[68] As test pilot for the project, Stapp named another volunteer, an experienced jet pilot with an intense interest in the medical problems of high-altitude flight, Captain Joseph W. Kittinger Jr USAF.

By January 1956 Otto Winzen had developed a suitable design. The polyethylene balloon, two hundred feet in diameter, would have a potential volume of 3,000,000 cubic feet and be able to ascend to 115,000 feet with a payload of 1000 pounds. Only 150 pounds of ballast would be carried, in the form of droppable batteries (to be lowered by parachute). The one-man capsule was kept as small as possible for the sake of lightness—an aluminum alloy tube, three feet in diameter, capped at each end by hemispherical domes, the whole measuring eight feet in overall height. Inside, in a space further restricted by internally stowed equipment, the aeronaut sat on a nylon mesh net, as he was unable to move about. He was of course wearing the familiar partial pressure suit and helmet, tight and uncomfortable enough even when uninflated, but capable of saving his life by automatically pressurizing with oxygen if the chamber should develop a leak. It was intended that the pressure should be maintained at an equivalent of 25,000 feet, with an adequate partial pressure of oxygen provided by evaporation of a liquid mixture of oxygen sixty per cent, helium twenty per cent (to limit the fire risk), and nitrogen only twenty per cent, to minimize the risk of dysbarism. The emergency back-up system included gaseous oxygen in a 205 cu in high pressure bottle, and a 90 cu in bail-out bottle attached to the aeronaut's parachute harness. A blower system circulated the capsule atmosphere at the rate of twenty-five cubic feet per minute through dry lithium hydroxide, to remove carbon dioxide, and through dry lithium chloride and magnesium perchlorate to absorb water. A novel cooling system was installed—a tank of water, venting to the outside at 112,000 feet, would boil at a temperature of thirty-two degrees F, thereby chilling air blown over it. In the event, this proved inadequate.

Captain Kittinger, acting as project test pilot, flew the Man High I balloon to 96,000 feet on 2 June 1957—a new record. A small failure of a control knob rendered his voice transmitting radio inoperative, and during the flight he had to send laboriously with a Morse code key. Far more seriously, it developed that his oxygen was being exhausted at an alarming rate, forcing a premature end to the flight. Ordered down by Colonel Stapp, Kittinger flabbergasted the control team on the ground by tapping out, 'COME AND GET ME.' Was this the 'breakaway phenomenon' previously reported by some high-altitude jet pilots, and by Ross and Lewis in Strato-Lab I the year before? 'Radio voices of colleagues who were tracking in aircraft and ground vehicles were real, but they, too, seemed far away and remote,' Ross noted. 'It was a sense of being physically—and almost spiritually—completely detached from earth. It was not fear nor depression, probably it was more akin to exhilaration . . . of wanting to fly on and on.'[69]

'Captain Kittinger,' Stapp spoke crisply into the microphone, 'I assume you are only joking. If not, I am *ordering* you to valve as instructed. Right now.' 'VALVING GAS' came the reply, and Kittinger was on his way down, to land safely after a flight of four and a half hours. The oxygen container, designed to meet the aeronaut's needs over a period of forty hours, was empty. Examination showed that an aneroid flow control had been connected up in reverse, permitting the oxygen to discharge overboard instead of into the capsule.

David Simons, the meticulous flight surgeon and scientist directing the Man High project, who had taken balloon and parachute training to qualify himself for his goal of twenty-four hours aloft and an altitude of more than 100,000 feet, made the Man High II flight on 19–20 August 1957. At 9.22 am he rose from the bottom of a 425-foot-deep pit in an open iron mine at Crosby, Minnesota. This time all went well, and Simons was in constant touch by voice radio with Otto Winzen and Colonel Stapp, the ground directing team. Initially inclined to resent the constant queries from the ground, which interrupted his multifarious activities in the capsule and shattered his mood of communion with the profound blue-black infinity outside the gondola windows, Simons came to welcome the warmth of their cheerful presence during the loneliness of the night that followed. On the way up, he was busy and excited as he operated the spectrograph and cameras, or dictated his impressions into a tape recorder. At the ceiling (calculated later to be 101,516 feet), Simons still had 4·2 litres left of his original 5-litre oxygen mixture. Carbon dioxide level of one per cent was well below the permissible three per cent maximum. The capsule pressure was holding at 25,000 feet. Air temperature in the capsule was a comfortable fifty-five degrees. But with the cramped capsule bathed in harsh sunlight and heated internally by Simons himself and all his electrical gear, an ominous temperature climb developed during the afternoon, beyond the capacity of the cooling equipment to deal with. At 4 pm it was seventy-four degrees, at 4.25 an uncomfortable seventy-six. By 6 pm it was seventy-seven, and Simons, confined in the snug, uncomfortable pressure suit, sweating and fatigued, was thinking and acting more sluggishly and apathetically than he realized. Colonel Stapp, on the ground, diagnosed a fall in blood sugar and directed Simons to eat a candy bar. With darkness the capsule and the helium in the balloon both cooled, while a violent thunderstorm moved in beneath the daring aeronaut. Fatigue took its toll, and he dozed, only to awaken to a spectacular and terrifying display of lightning. At 70,000 feet he saw the thunderheads, lit by lightning flickering within them, towering nearly to his altitude. At sunrise, Simons opened a flight meal and savoured cold ham and eggs and canned peaches. Rapidly the sun warmed the helium, and by 8.30 am of 20 August the plastic balloon was at its ceiling, 92,000 feet, slightly below that of the day before. The temperature in the capsule again began to rise, fatigue gnawed away Simons' last reserves, and the limits of battery power and purifying chemicals approached. Dully, Simons read his respirations as 44 per minute, reporting it without comment to those below. They reacted with appropriate alarm, which increased when Simons gave the carbon dioxide content as four per cent. Convinced that Simons was too fatigued and too affected by the high carbon dioxide level to handle the balloon himself, Stapp and Winzen assumed direct control, and Simons' further actions, including the vital valving-down from high altitude and ballasting near the ground, were performed on direct command from the ground. After thirty-two hours and three minutes aloft, Simons came safely to earth in a field near Aberdeen, South Dakota. In the debriefing after the flight, it was recognized that sheer fatigue rather than the high carbon dioxide reading had rendered Simons so inefficient on the morning of 20 August. All concerned had temporarily forgotten that at an equivalent altitude of 25,000 feet, four per cent carbon dioxide had a lower partial pressure than two per cent at sea level.

Man High III, flown by 1st Lieutenant Clifton McClure on 8 October 1958, emphasized the unsolved problem of temperature control which had so plagued Simons during his record flight. Just before takeoff, McClure's personal parachute had come open within the capsule, but he, determined to make the flight, told nobody of this misadventure and at the cost of much effort, succeeded in repacking the 'chute within the cramped confines of the gondola. But in spite of a pack of dry ice on top of the capsule, the internal temperature rose even higher than in the Man High II flight. At 24,000 feet the internal temperature gauge—improperly placed next to the heat-radiating air regenerating equipment—read eighty-nine degrees. At McClure's ceiling, 99,700 feet, the gondola temperature gauge read 118 degrees, and the aeronaut's rectally-measured body temperature was 101·4 degrees. Over McClure's protests, the ground team ordered him to abort the flight. But by the time he had brought the huge plastic balloon to the ground under good control, his rectal temperature had soared to 108·5 degrees, a level that might have been fatal to many men.

In the post-flight analysis, McClure, Simons and Stapp concluded that the effort and the heat developed in packing the 'chute had set off a vicious cycle of events that nearly ended in catastrophe. McClure's perspiration had flooded the water-absorbing potassium hydroxide, which heated up strongly from the chemical reaction. The air blower had circulated the heat. McClure had perspired more, and the temperature of the potassium hydroxide had increased still further. Aggravating the whole problem was the increased warming by the sun and the decreased cooling effect of outside air at great altitudes. While the thermometer might register −80 or −90 degrees F, there were so few molecules in the thin air at great altitude that it conducted heat away relatively slowly.

There remains a series of remarkable *open gondola* high-altitude flights with plastic balloons, taking human beings far above the so-called 'Armstrong Line' at 63,000 feet, where the atmospheric pressure equals the vapour pressure of water at 98·6 degrees F, and the blood and body fluids boil. Only with pressure suits was survival possible, and though these were severely tested, the first series of open gondola flights served still another purpose. In another chapter I shall sketch the problems of bail-out at high altitude: suffice it to state that Air Force medical men had recently become aware of the tendency of the freely falling human body to enter violent flat spins, and this had proved to be an increasingly dangerous problem at greater heights. Yet in high-altitude bail-out, it was necessary for the man to fall to a level of not more than 20,000 feet before opening his 'chute in an atmosphere with sufficient oxygen to sustain life. In the resulting free fall, tests with anthropomorphic dummies had shown that in a descent from 83,000 feet, the body could spin at up to 465 revolutions per minute—not only enough to produce loss of consciousness, but even to cause death. The Excelsior series of experiments was designed to test the novel Beaupré multistage parachute designed to provide stabilized free-fall descent from altitudes greater than twenty miles. The experimental subject and project officer: the courageous Captain Joseph W. Kittinger, Jr USAF, the test pilot of Man High I.

The balloon was a standard plastic creation of General Mills, of 0·002 in. polyethylene, 3,000,000 cubic feet in potential volume, 200 feet in expanded diameter, and 380 feet high from top to bottom in the deflated state. Beneath was a cargo parachute sixty-four feet in diameter. The open gondola, a platform four and half feet in diameter and weighing 800 pounds with equipment, met requirements that would not occur to a layman who might feel that something simple would suffice. A large wet battery hanging outside the gondola powered a quantity of electrical equipment. A liquid oxygen generator with a capacity of five litres provided oxygen for much longer than the estimated ninety to 120 minutes required to reach jump altitude. High frequency and ultra-high frequency radios were carried, and a fantastic array of automatic cameras, mostly designed to take sequential and motion pictures of Kittinger's drop away from the gondola, and the initial opening of the multi-stage parachute. The aeronaut himself was so loaded with gear that his usual weight of 160 pounds was increased to nearly 320! Over several suits of underwear came the vital MC-3 partial pressure suit, with the pressure helmet, then electrically-heated thermal underwear, and on top of this, a heavy winter flying suit. Then electrically-heated socks and gloves, and more socks, gloves and boots. Two parachutes, the back-pack Beaupré under test, and the reserve chest 'chute. Lastly, a 60-pound instrument pack, with bail-out oxygen supply, recorder, batteries and a movie camera. No wonder Kittinger needed two men to help him into the gondola!

At last, on 7 November 1959, came Colonel Stapp's official letter of authorization for the first flight. 'Gentlemen,' he wrote, 'inclosed is your passport to the upper atmosphere. It is good for all flights.'[70] The first ascent, Excelsior I, followed on 16 November 1959. Distracted by the possibility of his helmet blowing off with increased pressure, which would have led to a fatal explosive decompression ('the wet black cloth clamped over nose and mouth'), Kittinger did not notice when he passed the planned bail-out altitude of 60,000 feet. Valving, he checked the ascent at 76,000 feet, and went out of the gondola. Premature release of the Beaupré stabilizing parachute caused it to foul around Kittinger's neck and it failed to deploy properly. He lost consciousness in spinning down, but at 11,000 feet his reserve 'chute opened automatically and saved his life. It must have taken rare courage, together with intense dedication to the mission, for Kittinger to risk his life again in the same way, yet proof of the multi-stage parachute's effectiveness had not been obtained. On 11 December, 1959, in Excelsior II, Kittinger bailed out at 74,700 feet. This time everything functioned perfectly. A final test, Excelsior III, with Kittinger again the experimental subject, took him to 102,800 feet, a new record. Here, as he ascended above 85,000 feet, a striking change took place in the usually ebullient Kittinger. Perhaps it was because the pressurization of his right glove had failed, with resulting swelling and circulation failure, a painful condition which he concealed from the ground-control team; perhaps it was his realization of his utter aloneness in a hostile environment. With the feeling he might not return, Kittinger reported from his ceiling the appearance of the blue-black sky, the view to the horizon, and sombrely added, 'Man will never conquer space. He will learn to live with it, but he will never conquer it.'[71]

Despite his morbid preoccupations, Kittinger jumped successfully and the Beaupré parachute functioned. The right hand, exposed unprotected to a pressure of seven mm of mercury—one one-hundredth of an atmosphere—was numb, swollen to twice its normal size, but returned to its normal appearance and function within three hours. Joseph Kittinger indeed deserved the award of the Harmon Trophy for outstanding accomplishments in aeronautics.

As a dramatic finale, the Navy on 4 May, 1961, sent two men, Commander Malcolm D. Ross USNR and Lieutenant Commander Victor A. Prather (MC) USN, to 113,700 feet in an open gondola. This operation, Strato-Lab V, was intended to test newly-developed full pressurization suits, and also utilized the largest polyethylene balloon to date, one of 10,000,000 cubic foot capacity. As described in the Introduction, Ross and Prather safely completed their flight to high altitude, demonstrating the absolute safety of the full pressure suit, but Prather drowned during recovery operations after the landing. This record still stands today (1973) as the greatest altitude ever attained by a manned balloon.

Thus medical science and engineering technology, working hand in hand, conquered and overcame the hazards of anoxia at high altitude, that remote vastness into which the balloon shouldered its upward way long before any other type of aircraft. Except for Fedossejenko, Vassenko and Oussyskine, the unfortunate occupants of the Soviet *Ossoaviakhim*, who evidently had disregarded all sound principles of ballasting, no man died in high-altitude ballooning after the development of the pressure gondola. The physicians—Paul Bert, David Simons, John Stapp and others working in the general field of aviation medicine—had made their contributions, and they were considerable. But an even larger role had been played by non-medical men, the engineers, the technicians, the inspired men of genius who combined special skills and unconventional imagination with a quick grasp of problems in unrelated fields. First in this group comes the physiologist Hermann von Schrötter, who partly through his own ballooning ventures was the first to evaluate correctly the physiological problems of high altitude, and who was first to propose the only satisfactory answer—the sealed, pressurized cabin. Next, credit goes to the physicist, Auguste Piccard, who had the boldness and imagination to follow von Schrötter's lead, and to trust his life to the first pressure gondola in the stratosphere. Following him, Settle, Anderson, Stevens, Ross, Lewis and Kittinger made their contributions to the safety of balloon flight at high altitude. The fruitful collaboration of medical men with special aviation knowledge, inquisitive and experienced airmen, and engineers with inspired vision would be the means whereby the hazards in other fields of aviation likewise would be overcome.

[1] Whose name lives today in Charles' Law, that gases expand or contract in proportion to their absolute temperature.

[2] James Glaisher, Camille Flammarion, W. de Fonvielle and Gaston Tissandier, *Travels in the Air* (Philadelphia: J. P. Lippincott & Co., 1871), p. 6.

[3] Wingfoot LTA Society Bulletin, vol. 9, no. 4, February 1962, p. 6.

[4] John Jeffries, *A Narrative of the Two Aerial Voyages of Doctor Jeffries with Mons. Blanchard* (London: J. Robson, 1786), p. 48.

[5] Though the guide rope could cause serious damage on the ground in built-up areas, and on this account was not to be used over land at night.

[6] Kriegswissenschaftliche Abteilung der Luftwaffe, *Die deutschen Luftstreitkräfte von ihrer Entstehung bis zum Ende des Weltkrieges 1918. Die Militärluftfahrt bis zum Beginn des Weltkrieges 1914. Anlage-Band* (Berlin: E. S. Mittler und Sohn, 1941), pp. 10–12.

[7] Glaisher, p. xii. A table listing all the balloon flights during the siege of Paris is appended.

[8] Wingfoot LTA Society Bulletin, vol. 10, no. 5, March 1963, p. 4 (Demuyter obituary).

[9] Stabsarzt Dr Flemming, 'Der Arzt im Ballon,' in *Wir Luftschiffer* (Berlin and Vienna: Ullstein & Co., 1909), p. 172.

[10] Glaisher, p. 352.

[11] John Wise, *A System of Aeronautics* (Philadelphia: Joseph A. Speel, 1850), p. 192.

[12] *ibid.*, p. 172.

[13] Paul Bert, *Barometric Pressure. Researches in Experimental Physiology.* Trans. Mary Alice Hitchcock and Fred A. Hitchcock (Columbus, Ohio: College Book Co., 1943), p. 82

[14] *ibid.*, p. 24.

[15] *ibid.*, p. 214

[16] *ibid.*, p. 225

[17] F. Marion, *Wonderful Balloon Ascents* (New York: Charles Scribner & Co., 1870), pp.195–6.

[18] Robertson measured his altitude by reading a standard mercury barometer. A recent table of atmospheric properties *(Flight Surgeon's Manual,* AF Manual 161–1, Department of the Air Force, 17 January 1962, pp. 2–4) indicates that with the barometric readings reported by Robertson, the altitude was only 23,100 feet.

[19] Bert, p. 175.

[20] *ibid.,* p. 176

[21] Which states that when gases combine with one another, they do so in the simplest proportion by volume, and that the volume of any gaseous product formed bears a simple ratio to that of its constituents.

[22] Bert, p. 179.

[23] Modern tables indicate that for the barometer reading reported by Gay-Lussac, 12·95 in., the corresponding altitude would have been 21,400 feet.

[24] Wise, p. 70.

[25] I cannot leave Gay-Lussac without retelling the story of the chair that miraculously fell from Heaven. Among the articles that he threw out on this flight was a roughly-made pine chair, which crashed into a hedge close to a country girl tending a flock of sheep. The young scientist's balloon was of course invisible, and to the simple maiden and her pious friends it was clear that the chair must be of divine origin. The sceptics countered that surely God's workshop would not turn out such a crudely made piece of furniture! and only when news of Gay-Lussac's flight was published in the provinces was the dispute resolved (de Fonvielle and Tissandier in Glaisher, p. 320).

[26] Glaisher, p. 41.

[27] *ibid.,* p. 44.

[28] Henry Coxwell, *My Life and Balloon Experiences,* vol. II (London: W. H. Allen & Co., 1889), p. 138.

[29] Assuming that Glaisher read his barometer correctly, $9\frac{3}{4}$ in. would correspond to an altitude of 27,880 feet, according to modern tables.

[30] Glaisher, pp. 52–3.

[31] Coxwell, II, p. 141.

[32] Seven inches of mercury would equal 35,000 feet, according to modern tables.

[33] *Flight Surgeon's Manual,* AF Manual 161–1, Department of the Air Force, 17 January 1962, pp. 2–13.

[34] Glaisher, p. 9. Author's italics.

[35] Glaisher, p. 21.

[36] Bert, p. 351.

[37] *ibid.,* p. 669.

[38] *ibid.,* p. 698.

[39] *ibid.,* p. 700.

[40] *ibid.,* p. 701.

[41] *ibid.,* p. 704.

[42] *ibid.,* p. 961.

[43] *ibid.,* p. 961.

[44] *ibid.,* p. 963.

[45] *ibid.,* p. 965.

[46] *ibid.,* p. 965.

[47] *ibid.,* p. 967.

[48] *ibid.,* p. 968.

[49] *ibid.,* p. 972.

[50] Professor R. Süring, 'Wissenschaftliche Ballonhochfahrten' in *Wir Luftschiffer* (Berlin u. Wien: Verlag von Ullstein & Co., 1909), p. 52.

[51] *ibid.*, p. 54.

[52] See H. von Schrötter and N. Zuntz, 'Ergebnisse zweier Ballonfahrten zur physiologischen Zwecken,' *Arch. Gen. Physiol.* vol. 92, 479–520, 1902.

[53] Süring, p. 64. Author's italics.

[54] Kurt Stehling and William Beller, *Skyhooks* (New York: Doubleday & Co., Inc., 1962), p. 188.

[55] *ibid.*, p. 195.

[56] Major General Orvil A. Anderson USAF (Ret.), who flew a chase plane on Gray's flight and landed at Sparta, believes that as Gray finished his next to last oxygen flask, he mistakenly dropped the last full cylinder instead of the empty one, leaving himself without oxygen in the stratosphere ('Ballooning in the Stratosphere' in *Air Power Historian*, vol. IV, no. 1, January 1957, p. 3).

[57] See Auguste Piccard, *Earth, Sky and Sea* (New York: Oxford University Press, 1956), pp. 4–7. Also Auguste Piccard, 'Ballooning in the Stratosphere,' *National Geographic*, vol. 63, no. 3, March 1933, p. 353.

[58] The balloon was christened with the initials of the *Fonds National Belge de Recherche Scientifique*, which put up the money for the project.

[59] Letter, Lieutenant Commander T. G. W. Settle to Rear Admiral W. T. Cluverius, 19 August 1933. Settle Papers.

[60] Letter, Settle to author, 8 September 1964.

[61] See A. H. Compton and R. J. Stephenson, 'Cosmic Ray Ionization at High Altitude,' in *Physical Review*, vol. 45, 1 April 1934, p. 441.

[62] See Anderson's 'Ballooning in the Stratosphere,' *Air Power Historian*, vol. IV, no. 1, January 1957, pp. 5–6.

[63] See Captain Albert W. Stevens, 'Exploring the Stratosphere,' *National Geographic*, vol. LXVI, no. 4, October 1934, p. 397.

[64] See 'Medical Problems of National Geographic Society–US Army Air Corps Stratosphere Flight of Nov. 11, 1935,' *Journal of Aviation Medicine*, vol. 7, no. 2, June 1936, p. 55. Also L. D. Bonham, 'Air Conditioning of the Stratosphere Gondola,' *National Geographic Society–US Army Air Corps Stratosphere Flight of 1935 in the Balloon 'Explorer II'* (National Geographic Society, Washington, DC, 1936).

[65] The clinical effect of primary cosmic radiation on humans is still not clearly determined. The high-altitude balloon ascents here described proved that no serious injuries occurred to the human subjects at the altitudes attained. Most cosmic radiation is concentrated in the Van Allen belts, whose minimum distance from earth is greater than the customary orbiting altitude of human astronauts.

[66] Lieut Commanders Malcolm D. Ross USNR and M. Lee Lewis USN, 'To 76,000 feet by Strato-Lab Balloon' *(National Geographic*, vol. 111, no. 2, February 1957), p. 269.

[67] Lieutenant Colonel David G. Simons (MC) USAF, with Don A. Schanche, *Man High* (New York: E. P. Dutton & Co., 1961), p. 73.

[68] Captain Joseph W. Kittinger Jr USAF, with Martin Caidin, *The Long, Lonely Leap* (New York: E. P. Dutton & Co., 1961), p. 73.

[69] Simons, p. 88.

[70] Kittinger, p. 154.

[71] *ibid.*, p. 237.

2

Boxkites, Doves and Dragonflies

For the purpose of this history, the pioneering years of aviation commence approximately with the year 1890 and extend to the outbreak of World War I, when the aeroplane ceased to be a plaything for sportsmen and showmen and commenced serious development as the newest weapon in the arsenal of the contesting powers. Medicine, it must be confessed, ignored the early development of the heavier-than-air machine and made no contributions to the art of aviation during this era; yet, following the premise that any agency causing death or injury to flight personnel is of medical significance, we will find much of interest in the unknown hazards of flight which only today have been finally overcome through increasing knowledge of aerodynamic theory, design and structure.

Though the dream of flying has enthralled mankind since the dawn of history, and forms the basis for many of our most durable fables and legends, only in the nineteenth century was there any attainment of comprehension of the difficulties involved, and what was and what was not possible in overcoming them. Foremost in scientific appreciation of the problem of flight was the Englishman, Sir George Cayley, who as early as 1809 succinctly observed, 'the whole problem is confined within these limits, viz. To make a surface support a given weight by the application of power to the resistance of the air.'[1] Far ahead of his time, this genius, practically unknown until his notebooks were discovered in recent years, made lift and drag calculations on aerofoils, discovered the theory of streamlining, built and flew in the year 1804 an inherently stable glider model, and in the year 1853 constructed a glider which carried his coachman across a valley near his residence at Brompton Hall, Yorkshire—the machine evidently crashing and breaking a leg of its unhappy occupant.

It is frequently claimed that practical aviation was impossible prior to the development of a light-weight prime mover, i.e. the internal combustion engine, first produced by Otto in 1876. It is true that many early experimenters such as Stringfellow, Ader and Maxim, forced to rely on steam engines, experienced failure, but so did others to whom the gasoline engine was available, such as Langley, whose 'aerodrome' twice plunged incontinently from its houseboat catapult to the surface of the Potomac River. Actually, as the historian Charles H. Gibbs-Smith has so brilliantly perceived, the secret of flight lay, not in the light-weight power plant, but in control over the direction of the aerial vehicle.[2] It follows that flight might have been achieved thousands of years ago, and indeed, in my gliding days at Frankfort and Elmira, we wondered more than once that the ancient Egyptians or the Chinese had not discovered the secret. They certainly had the interest, the skill in woodworking and weaving, and a body of scientific knowledge which might have enabled them to achieve the successful glider.

This had to wait until the very end of the nineteenth century, and its development is to the credit of five persistent men who, applying all the scientific knowledge of the day to the problem, and daring to risk their lives in personal experiments aloft, first managed to control a heavier-than-air craft in flight. The first in point of time, and one of the greatest pioneers, was the German, Otto Lilienthal, who with his brother Gustav, between the years 1891 and 1896, built a series of monoplane and biplane gliders which he flew successfully from an artificial hill near Berlin. The fundamental fault of Lilienthal's machines was that they had no movable surfaces and control was uncertainly achieved by the pilot swinging his legs to shift the centre of gravity. This did not suffice to prevent Otto Lilienthal from nosing up and stalling in a flight on 9 August 1896, and in the resulting crash he suffered a fractured spine and other injuries. He died on the following day, his last words being 'sacrifices must be made.'

A similar fate overtook the Englishman, Percy S. Pilcher, who built and flew several gliders of his own design between 1895 and 1899. These likewise he controlled as had Lilienthal (whom he knew and to a degree imitated), but it was the failure of a bamboo strut in the tail assembly of his 'Hawk' glider which caused his fatal crash on 30 September, 1899. More fortunate was the American engineer, Octave Chanute. With a series of 'hang-type' gliders he and his associates made some seven hundred flights in the year 1896. He bequeathed to early aviation the classic wire-braced biplane wing design, an adaptation of the simple Pratt truss so well known to bridge builders. More important, he inspired and encouraged the last and greatest of the indomitable pioneering quintet, the brothers Wilbur and Orville Wright.

Fit to take their place among the handful of men whose ideas have permanently changed the world, the two young men from Dayton learned aerodynamics from experiments in a home-made wind tunnel, tested their ideas in a series of gliders which they flew at secluded Kill Devil Hill in North Carolina in the years 1900, 1901, and 1902, and with these, achieved controlled flight even though their craft was inherently unstable. Unlike earlier experimenters, they rigged a movable horizontal surface ahead of the biplane wings to maintain positive control about the pitch axis; they warped or twisted the flexible wings to maintain control about the roll axis (a problem ignored by most early inventors), and by co-ordination of rudder movement and wing warping, they were able to make banking turns. The triumph of powered flight followed naturally when they fitted a gasoline engine of their own manufacture to a heavier biplane, and made the first controlled flights at Kitty Hawk on 17 December 1903. Yet five years passed before their success was generally acknowledged, and the brothers received the credit they deserved.

In the summer of 1908 Wilbur gave demonstrations in France, astounding the leaders of the embryo European aviation movement with the versatility and performance of his craft, which flew on one occasion for two hours twenty minutes and over a distance of seventy-seven miles. Simultaneously, Orville at home was demonstrating another machine to the US Army at Fort Myer, Virginia. And here, on 17 September 1908, occurred the only serious crash of the brothers' career, and the first death in powered flight, when a propeller failure caused the tail of the 'Flyer' to collapse and the craft dived into the ground from seventy-five feet. Orville suffered broken ribs and a fractured left leg; his companion, Lieutenant Thomas F. Selfridge, US Army, died of a fractured skull.

The accident postponed by a year the United States Army's acceptance of its first aircraft, a Wright Model B delivered at Fort Myer on 28 June 1909. In the same summer Orville triumphantly demonstrated a similar craft in Germany for the benefit of the German Wright Company. This was the height of their fame, for the imitators were fast overtaking them. Not surprisingly, the brothers clung too long to the handicapping features of the models that had brought them fame: chain-driven pusher propellers, wheel-less skid landing gear, seating on the lower wing in the open slipstream, and inherent instability. In 1912 Wilbur died of typhoid fever; three years later Orville retired from the aeroplane building business, to live on for over thirty years as the elder statesman of aviation. Both were deliberate and cautious in all their flying, carefully checking their craft before every ascent, and only once between them experienced a serious crash—caused by an unforseeable structural failure. Both died in bed. Other pioneers might have survived to do likewise had they emulated the Wrights in their respect for the dangers of the air.

In Europe, the first powered flight was made in France in 1906, and in the period between 1909 and 1914, French aircraft, and in particular, French aircraft engines, led the world. The water-cooled V-8 Antoinette engines of 24 and 50 hp appeared in 1906, and two years later the first air-cooled rotary motor, the 7-cylinder Gnome, which delivered 50 hp with a weight of only 167 pounds. It was the Gnome which introduced castor oil as an aviation lubricant, consuming up to half a gallon for every gallon of gasoline. Most of the castor oil, it is true, was hurled out of the exhaust valve by the centrifugal force of the revolving engine, splattering the fuselage and tail surfaces. If the pilot sat behind the engine, his person would absorb its share, and he might suffer from the castor oil's well-known pharmacological effects.

The Gnome-powered Farman biplane was the first European aircraft successfully to compete with the Wright Brothers' product. The light, sturdy wire-braced biplane wing bore four ailerons which moved only downward and which floated horizontally in the slipstream in flight. The pusher engine, mounted behind the pilot, drove a propeller between the long booms supporting the boxkite tail. Twin rudders and elevators aft were supplemented by an elevating plane out forward of the pilot. The undercarriage consisted of a pair of long skids, each bearing a pair of light wheels. There were no brakes. The Farman biplane was the recipient of the ultimate in flattery, in that it was imitated by the German Albatros firm and others, and large numbers ('Boxkites') were produced under license by the British Bristol Company. Of the other biplane types, the most notable was probably the Curtiss, produced in America by a motor-cycle mechanic destined to rival the fame of the Wright Brothers.

The leading monoplanes of the 1909–11 period were likewise French, and reflected the Gallic genius for form, grace and balance, to a degree which makes them aesthetically attractive to this day. Santos-Dumont, the 1906 pioneer, created the tiny *Demoiselle* (dragonfly), whose useful lift was calculated on the basis of his own weight of 110 pounds. Stately and elegant, the *Antoinette,* with its long, slim fuselage and wide, tapering wings, enjoyed an outstanding reputation for performance, largely due to its bold handling by Hubert Latham. Lastly, Louis Bleriot, the determined manufacturer of automobile headlamps, won success and undying fame with his Type XI monoplane when, on 25 July 1909, he crossed the English Channel from Sangatte to Dover. 'No pilot of today, no matter how great, could repeat this exploit in such an aircraft and with such an engine.'[3] The cross-Channel monoplane had a feeble 3-cylinder 25 hp Anzani radial engine, but with the Gnome rotary later fitted, the open-fuselage Bleriot became a popular exhibition and racing craft.

With the rapid progress of aviation in Europe and the United States beginning in 1909, certain trends early became apparent. The leading flyers vied to set records, often being spurred on by cash prizes offered by newspapers or wealthy individuals. In June 1911 forty-three contestants entered a Circuit of Europe race (actually taking them only through France, Belgium, Holland and England), with cash prizes totalling nearly $100,000. Nine contestants finished the course, while three were killed in crashes. ('We are sick of providing black headlines for the newspapers,' complained one of the leading participants).[4] In the same summer, twenty-one contestants set off on a race around Britain. Only four finished, and the two leaders were Frenchmen. On 23 September 1910 a Peruvian pilot, Georges Chavez, made the first crossing of the Alps from Switzerland to Italy. Inexplicably, Chavez never pulled out from his steep glide into the field at Domodossola, and died of his injuries four days later. As a physician, I find myself baffled by this early aeromedical tragedy. Chavez had risen no higher than 8000 feet in crossing the Simplon Pass, and could not have been suffering from anoxia. Although he had warmly clothed himself, it was postulated that he had been too numbed by the cold to flatten his glide in time.

An epic of courage, now forgotten, was Calbraith Perry Rodgers' first crossing of the United States by air in 1911 in the Wright EX biplane 'Vin Fiz.' What with twenty-nine stops and nine serious crashes, it took him forty-nine days to travel the 4231 miles, and only the rudder and the engine drip pan of the original machine reached Long Beach, California. Nor did he win William Randolph Hearst's $50,000 prize, which required that the crossing of the continent be made in thirty days. Four months after his arrival in California, Rodgers stalled and crashed from a low altitude into the surf at Long Beach, and died in a few minutes. Childhood scarlet fever had left Rodgers almost stone deaf, and inability to hear the sounds of flight may have prevented him from realizing that he was losing flying speed.

As always, some saw that the public's fascination with the new marvel of flight could be turned into money, and for a few years, until repetition robbed them of their novelty and glamour, air meets and air races attracted thousands and filled newspaper columns with breathless accounts of the exploits of the daredevil pioneer aviators. The first, and possibly the most colourful, was 'La Grande Semaine d'Aviation de la Champagne' held at Reims, France, from 22 to 29 August 1909. Over thirty aircraft were entered—Wright, Farman and Voisin biplanes, Bleriot and Antoinette monoplanes of different types—competing for height, distance and speed records. The surprise of the meet was the victory in the speed contest of the unknown

American, Glenn Curtiss, in a biplane racer of his own design—thereby winning the Gordon Bennett Trophy. Flying the course at an average speed of 47 mph, Curtiss defeated Bleriot, the cross-Channel victor, in a faster machine, through his superior skill in rounding the pylons. Nobody was killed during the meet, though Bleriot himself suffered a fire in flight—the first on record—when his impromptu rubber-tubing fuel line rotted through, spraying the engine with gasoline. A few days after the meet, on 7 September 1909, Eugene Lefebvre, a French Wright Company pilot who had thrilled the crowds at Reims with his low-altitude flying, was killed when a new machine he was testing nosed into the ground from a low altitude. In six years of powered flying, he was the first pilot to be killed.

The temporary popularity of the air meet led to the formation of several exhibition teams in the United States, those organized by the Wright Brothers, Glenn Curtiss and John Moisant being the most famous. To the dismay of the conservative pioneers from Dayton, their stable of daring but inexperienced young aeronauts—Brookins, Hoxsey, Johnstone, Parmalee, Coffyn and others—promptly commenced a deadly rivalry for the favour of the crowd, each with his repertoire of low-altitude stunts and manœuvres. The boldest of all lasted no more than a few months—Ralph Johnstone dying on 17 November 1910, at Denver, when a wing of his Wright biplane failed under high G loads as he pulled up abruptly near the ground from his steeply-banked 'spiral glide,' and Arch Hoxsey suffering a fractured skull when he stalled in from 500 feet at Los Angeles on 31 December 1910. On the same day John Moisant was killed at New Orleans when his Bleriot undershot in a down-wind landing, stalled and crashed. Lincoln Beachey of the Curtiss team went on from strength to strength until 15 March 1915 when he was killed in the crash of a clean monoplane built to his specifications.

A few years passed, and flying meets lost their attractiveness—the novelty wore off, and too many people found they could enjoy the spectacle from outside the flying grounds without paying admission. One obscure event, however, deserves to be mentioned—the contest for seaplanes held annually at Monaco, in southern France, beginning in 1912. The grand prize winner in this year was an ordinary Farman on floats, powered by the standard 50 hp Gnome; but specialization for racing from the water appeared in the following year with the presentation of a cup by M. Jacques Schneider for the highest speed by a seaplane. The winner was the Frenchman, M. Prevost, flying a Deperdussin monoplane at 61 mph. In 1914, the winner was Great Britain's Howard Pixton in a float-mounted Sopwith Tabloid racer, at a speed of 85·5 mph. In the post-war years, the governments of Great

Britain, Italy and the United States squandered vast sums in pursuit of the absolute world's speed record, rendering M. Schneider's modest trophy the premier racing prize of the era, until it was retired by Great Britain in 1931.

A remarkable feature of the early days of aviation was the success of a considerable number of women pilots, several of whom competed on equal terms with men in the exhibition teams. This was all the more remarkable when it is remembered that women at this time were still living under the restrictions of the Victorian code, were supposed to be fragile, delicate and in need of male protection, and were only beginning their battle for the vote and for equal rights. The first licensed and qualified woman pilot was the French Baroness de Laroche, who trained on a Voisin biplane and received her 'brevet' on 8 March 1910. The second, Mlle Helene Dutrieu of Belgium, was licensed in August 1910. The next were Americans, trainees at John Moisant's school at Hempstead Plains, New York: Harriet Quimby, certified on 2 August 1911, and John's sister Matilde who won her licence on 17 August 1911. Other able and famous women flyers of the early days were Ruth Law and Katherine Stinson, the first woman Wright pilot, who later taught her brothers Eddie and Jack, and her sister Marjorie, to fly.

The year 1909/10 marked not only the development of exhibition flying, but the commencement of military interest in aviation. To many officers the aeroplane had obvious possibilities for reconnaissance in a war of movement—the answer to the question of 'what lay on the other side of the hill.' Individual flying officers experimented with bomb-dropping and carrying machine guns aloft, but were not systematically encouraged. Given the low power of contemporary aircraft engines, this was hardly surprising.

The United States had been the first nation to own a military aeroplane, with the Army's purchase of the Wright B in June 1909; but as with all the Great Powers in the pre-1914 period, funds for development were scarce and progress slow. The enthusiastic young Army officers who dedicated themselves to the future of the air arm, such as Foulois, Lahm, and a certain Second Lieutenant H. H. Arnold, had to battle with the scepticism and apathy of their superiors. Early orders—never for more than seven aircraft of any one type—were divided between the Wright B and C pusher types, and the Curtiss D, which resembled the Reims racer. Unsuitable and dangerous for training, they were gradually superseded by Burgess and Martin tractor biplanes with enclosed fuselages. By 1914, Curtiss was building his J and N trainer types, and the early JN-3s were so highly regarded that many were purchased by Britain for training overseas.

The United States Navy, interested in the aeroplane as an over-water scout, patronized Glenn Curtiss, who had fitted a float under one of his pusher biplanes and flown it off the water at San Diego on 26 January 1911. A few weeks later, on 17 February 1911, Curtiss landed one of these water-borne aircraft alongside the armoured cruiser *Pennsylvania,* was hoisted aboard, and later was put overside and returned to his base.[5] In July 1911 the Navy procured one of Curtiss' 'Triad' amphibious aircraft and assigned Lieutenants Ellyson and Towers to learn to fly it. Later experiments were made with compressed-air catapults and flying boats—a type in which Curtiss held the lead for several years. Some of these were under fire during the Navy's opposed landing at Vera Cruz, Mexico, in April 1914.

As for the major European powers, it must be remembered that several of them already had well-established aeronautical departments based on the airship. With the impassioned partisanship that has characterized the lighter-than-air fraternity since Count Zeppelin's day, the defenders of the vested interest opposed and obstructed the younger and more junior group which believed in the aeroplane. Superficially, there was much to justify their point of view, for no pre-war aeroplane could match the airship, with its range and load-carrying capability, in the reconnaissance role. The competition was particularly one-sided in Germany, whose Army had purchased its first Zeppelin airship in the year 1909 and which by August 1914 had placed in service twelve Zeppelin and two Schütte-Lanz rigid airships, four semi-rigids designed and constructed in its own workshops, and five Parseval non-rigids. By contrast, the aeroplane was viewed by the German War Ministry as a useless toy, and a French one at that. Though Orville Wright demonstrated his biplane at Tempelhof near Berlin in 1909, the German Army did not purchase an aeroplane until the summer of 1910. A year later, however, the handful of Army flyers traded their Wright biplane copies for one of the most striking aircraft of the pre-war period—the so-called 'Taube' or 'dove' monoplane. This tractor machine, with long, enclosed fuselage and spreading wings with gracefully swept-back, flexible tips serving as ailerons, was the most numerous two-seater reconnaissance craft in Germany up to the outbreak of war. The 'dove' form was common to the aircraft of several manufacturers, notably Rumpler. But the German Army through financial encouragement of the industry had developed two powerful and reliable engines for the day—the 100 hp six cylinder in-line water-cooled Mercedes and Argus. By 1913 the new power plants had been installed in sturdy two-seater tractor biplanes—Ago, Aviatik, LVG, and above all, Albatros—whose aircraft were the mainstay of the German air arm early in the war.

The French Army procured over twenty airships before August 1914, most of them small semi-rigids, no two alike, and all distinguished by an enormous number of suspension wires, biplane and triplane control surfaces, open framework bodies, and other drag-producing excrescences. Yet with the aeroplane being a largely French development after 1909, and enjoying popular favour in comparison with the airship which was identified with Germany, the French Army was obliged to take up aviation. Initially, civilian flyers participated in Army manœuvres, and exaggerated praise was heaped on their efforts. Certain trends became definite, with development of sturdy pusher biplanes for reconnaissance with the pilot and observer housed in a nacelle ahead of the wings, such as the Henri and Maurice Farman. A few fast monoplanes with rotary engines were built—predecessors of the single-seater fighters of World War I—the Morane and the Nieuport. Yet the administration of French military aviation was chaotic, and already there was a tendency for officialdom deliberately to deceive the public about the state of French air power—a habit which led to successive crises, culminating in the disaster of 1940.

In England, whose not-so-sure shield after Bleriot's cross-channel flight was still the Royal Navy, a small but professional air force had been created by August 1914. The Royal Flying Corps was established in 1912—initially a unified service comprising both Army and Navy officers—but by 1914 the latter had broken away and were calling themselves the Royal Naval Air Service. The British Army was dissatisfied with the products of commercial aircraft manufacturers, particularly after two different monoplanes (Bristol and Deperdussin) broke up in the air in September 1912, killing their four occupants. This led to a ban on monoplane flying for several months, and played a part in a British prejudice against these potentially faster aircraft which endured for many years. On the other hand, by August 1914, the Government's Royal Aircraft Factory at Farnborough had created an inherently-stable two seater biplane, the BE 2c, which was ideally suited to reconnaissance missions and was ordered in quantity. Unfortunately its stability, low power, and the fact that the pilot sat behind the observer, rendered it grossly unsuited for air fighting, and with the advent in 1915 of the German Fokker monoplane with forward firing machine gun, the RFC reconnaissance squadrons suffered heavy casualties.

The Royal Naval Air Service was especially favoured by the support of the *enfant terrible* of European politics, Winston Churchill, who at the age of 36 had become First Lord of the Admiralty in 1911. Surely the most air-minded cabinet minister in any pre-war nation—'having been thoroughly bitten (in 1912), I continued to fly on every possible occasion when my other duties permitted'—he coined the word 'seaplane' in 1913, and foresaw the use of aircraft as strike weapons as well as for reconnaissance. A Short biplane in the hands of Commander C. R. Samson flew off a ramp over the forecastle of the battleship HMS *Africa* in harbour on 12 January 1912. A year later the obsolete cruiser HMS *Hermes* was commissioned as a seaplane carrier, and her aircraft participated in manœuvres in 1913.

The Italian air force had combat experience even before World War I. When war with Turkey broke out on 29 September 1911 eleven pilots and thirty-one enlisted men sailed with the force dispatched to seize Turkish Libya in North Africa.[6] With them were nine aircraft: two Bleriot monoplanes, three Nieuport monoplanes, two Farman biplanes and two Etrich 'Taubes,' all with 50 hp engines. These initially operated from Tripoli, and further units were based at Benghazi and Derna. The aircraft primarily scouted by day over enemy territory, but also dropped leaflets and crude little 2 kg bombs. The non-rigid airships P 2 and P 3 attempted to make bombing raids from their base at Tripoli, with little success. Rifle fire proved unexpectedly dangerous even at 3000 feet and above, and after one observer was wounded in a Farman, these aircraft were flown solo, as their ceiling with two aboard was only 1800 feet. Remarkably, there was only one death in the flying units in Libya, involving a takeoff crash at Tripoli where the pilot evidently lost control of his low-powered aircraft in a gusty wind.

It cannot be said that medicine made any significant contribution to flying in the period before 1914, and certain it is that the physician was not involved in civil flying, except through dealing with the injuries of flyers who had come to grief. There were no physical standards, and no medical examination was required for licensing, which was the function of the *Fédération Aeronautique Internationale* and of the national flying clubs, acting as private citizens and not on behalf of the government. The military flyers were of course under the same kind of medical supervision as the members of the armed forces generally, but it would be presumptuous to designate as 'flight surgeons' any of the doctors who held sick call at the army posts where flying took place.

One medical officer, Lieutenant Luigi Falchi, played a curious role during the Italian expedition against Libya in 1911. Trained also as an aviator, he was sent to Tripoli as one of the reserve pilots, and assisted his commanding officer, Captain Piazza, in choosing a site for the Tripoli field. Despite his medical training, he apparently was expected to act as a pilot pure and simple, and he received the Bronze Medal of Military Valour for his reconnaissance flights. None the less, he was responsible in February 1912 for the relief of Captain Piazza on medical grounds, after the captain had suffered over a period of weeks from daily attacks of fever, probably malaria.[7]

Thus it is the designers, engineers and other non-medical specialists who deserve the credit for advances in flying safety during this period. The early aircraft were structurally weak and possessed of dangerous flight characteristics, as well as being underpowered, but the pilots themselves were reluctant to admit the built-in hazards of their machines. 'It was seldom the plane, or an unknown quantity in the air, but almost always the pilot, who was blamed for being in error. You *had* to believe that to keep up your morale,' wrote one of the early pioneers, the late General H. H. Arnold.[8]

Aeronautical engineering has progressed along two lines in the succeeding years to make flying safer—in the field of stress analysis and in aerodynamics. From the mechanical point of view, the aeroplane is simply a weight borne aloft by its structure, and this must be strong enough that it does not collapse under the load. Stress analysis consists of accurately calculating the loads on the structure, and selecting properly tested materials to build it. It is relatively easy to design an airframe which will support the weight of the craft and its occupants; but further problems, difficult to foresee, arise when the force of gravity is multiplied, as when the loads on the structure increase during tight turns, aerobatics, or in flying in turbulent air. An airframe strong enough to sustain one G loads will collapse at two or three G. In practice, aircraft are engineered to withstand loads of four to six G, with operating manuals prohibiting aerobatic manœuvres which would impose higher loadings; while aircraft intended for aerobatics will be proof against loads greater than six G, with a correspondingly heavier structure.

In the early days it was customary for the designer to assume that the wings and other structural members would be overloaded equally in all portions, and tests were based on this assumption. Old publicity photographs show men standing shoulder to shoulder on the wings of aircraft to demonstrate their ability to sustain an overload; while testing procedures involved turning the machine upside down, piling sandbags evenly on the under surfaces of the wings, and determining the load which caused structural failure. A more rational approach, developed in wind-tunnel studies in more recent years, is to determine directly the air loads on portions of the structure during manœuvres, and to calculate the necessary strength of the structure accordingly.

The pioneering designers were further handicapped in building structurally sound aircraft by the feebleness of the power plants available to them. Metals such as duralumin, which was commercially available as early as 1910, are stronger for their weight than wood, yet the need to keep the structure very light, plus ease of fabrication, led designers to build flying machines of wood, wire and fabric for many years after the first metal aircraft appeared in 1915. The improved strength of modern aircraft structures derives partly from improvements in power plants, which are now capable of lifting a heavier and more rugged airframe, often entirely made of metal.

Little of this was known, of course, to individual designers in 1909–14, and many of the early fatal accidents were caused by collapse of some part of the aircraft structure, often during violent manœuvres. The death of Lieutenant Selfridge, as noted above, was caused by a structural failure. The third powered flying death, that of the French pioneer, Captain Ferber, on 22 September 1909, illustrated an inherent danger of the pusher type of aircraft: his Voisin dragged a wing-tip and turned over, and he was crushed under the engine. Two of the early fatal crashes occurred when Antoinette monoplanes shed their wings while flying in rough air. The first fatal powered aircraft crash in Britain, which took the life of a popular flyer, the Hon. C. S. Rolls, again involved structural failure: an oversize rear elevator had been fitted to his French-built Wright biplane a few days before the fatal 12 July 1910 with no calculation of the load it would impose on the tail outriggers when deflected. In a spot-landing contest at Bournemouth, Rolls dived over a grandstand, then pulled up abruptly—and the heavy down load on the elevator bent the tail outriggers to such a degree that one of them contacted a propeller and was severed. Johnstone's crash in 1910 was caused by a wing collapse, probably due to excessive G loads in a pull-out.

Even when structural failure did not occur, the early powered aircraft were aerodynamically unsafe. How a plane handles in the air depends on complex interaction between the centre of gravity, centre of lift, line of thrust of the propeller, shape, size and location of control surfaces, wing area and loading, and above all, on the cross-sectional shape of the aerofoil of the wing. Despite the use of a wind tunnel by the Wright brothers, little was known about the most desirable shape of air foils, and thin, flat wing sections, necessitating much wire bracing, were in vogue. In Göttingen, Professor Prandtl was just beginning his research on thick, high-lift aerofoils which some German aircraft used in the latter part of World War I, and which confer on modern aircraft their safe handling characteristics at low speeds. Consequently the 1909–14 aircraft were lethally prone to stall—a condition all the more dangerous because it was not generally understood. The hapless airman merely perceived that his machine was plunging nose-first towards the ground, and that attempts to raise the nose by applying up elevator were ineffective. The reason was that with the speed reduced below a certain point, the smooth air flow over the wing, which created a partial vacuum over the top surface, broke up in eddies and the lift was destroyed. The nose dropped and the machine descended, but would not regain its lift unless the elevators were put *down* to lower the nose still further and regain flying speed. In all too many cases where early accounts describe a fatal, unexplained dive into the ground from low altitude, it is clear that the pilot must unwittingly have lost flying speed and stalled.[9] The fact that exhibition work, and low-powered engines, forced the early airmen to fly close to the ground, aggravated the danger of stalling, as there was insufficient altitude for recovery. Nor could the early birds observe the modern commandment—'watch your airspeed!'—for no air-speed indicator was in use.

The testimony of present-day pilots—offered with all the hindsight of modern aerodynamic knowledge—emphasizes the bravery and determination of the early pioneers who took the first steps with the aerodynamically unsound machines of 1909–14. The greatest amount of comparative information comes from Air Commodore Allen H. Wheeler RAF, in charge of constructing and flying a series of 1910 replicas for the 1965 movie, 'Those Magnificent Men in their Flying Machines.' Powered by modern engines, the Santos-Dumont Demoiselle, Antoinette, Bristol 'Boxkite,' Avro Triplane, Eardley-Billing tractor biplane and Bleriot-type Vickers 22, were built from original drawings, and in material and workmanship resembled the 1910 versions. The Antoinette proved most dangerous of all, being practically uncontrollable about the roll axis even in mild midday turbulence, though its wing warping imitated that in the highly-praised original. One test pilot reported of an experience with the Antoinette, 'it was the most interesting flight an aeroplane had ever taken him for.'[10] So unsuitable was the Antoinette wing section, with its sharply-pointed entry, that Wheeler himself wrote, 'it was in fact the only aeroplane I have ever flown which could quite easily stall one wing while the wheels were still on the ground.'[11] As for Hubert Latham's daring exploits in flying the 1909 original in winds gusting up to 38 mph, Wheeler concluded:

In retrospect one can only assume that Latham's successful flying of the Antoinette was achieved:

(a) by having a very experienced mechanic who was continually checking and adjusting the rigging;

(b) by using what was virtually an irreversible winch form of control on the wing warping:

(c) by always taking off, flying and landing with a very low incidence on his wings;

(d) by being a very brave man.[12]

Wheeler emphasized the ease with which a stall could occur with loss of power in the early aircraft:

At their normal speed, around 38 mph, the drag was just about equivalent to the engine power, which was usually somewhere between 25 and 50 hp. When the power was cut there was, momentarily, the equivalent power (in drag) pulling the aeroplane back. Since the aeroplane was very light indeed it had little inertia to keep it going, so it too stopped very soon after the engine—unless the pilot quickly put it into a dive towards the ground, and even then the most experienced modern pilot would be astonished at the steep angle of glide needed in the old aeroplanes to maintain flying speed. The steep angle is necessary because the aeroplanes are very light, and unless the force of gravity can get a direct pull along the line of flight it will become an enemy instead of a friend.[13]

Commenting on the dangerous lack of lateral control in many of the replicas, Wheeler summed up:

I think one may say that, in the 1910 period, it did not matter inherently which method of lateral control was used, either wing-warping or ailerons, so long as the selected method was properly engineered. Neither was effective by modern standards; both were very dependent on assistance from the rudder if rapid control was needed. Without the use of the rudder, if his aeroplane started to roll over, the pilot could only hold the stick right over and wait—and in some cases, pray.[14]

Early military aircraft, usually being of ordinary commercial manufacture, were prone to all the weaknesses and faults of their civilian contemporaries. In addition, there shortly arose in all countries the fad for what General Arnold called 'demountability'—the requirement that the aircraft be capable of quick assembly and disassembly, so that it might be carried with other army equipment in wagons on the line of march. 'As a result aeroplane competitions were chiefly a test of the ability of the planes to be dismantled and carried up and down hills. The real function of the machines—flying—began to be neglected.'[15] This shortly led to a notorious 1913 crash which killed two popular German Army flyers when their Rumpler 'Taube'—with subdivided wings—lost a surface in flight. 'Demountability' seemingly played a part also in the crashes which preceded the monoplane ban in the British Army in the autumn of 1912: the Royal Aeronautical Club (which, in default of an appropriate government body, officially investigated all crashes in England during this period) found that in the Bristol accident, a quick-release catch had given way, allowing a piece of metal to rip up a wing which lost its covering.

Whereas the public expected the early exhibition flyers to crash to their deaths ('Even after having paid a shilling, one is not entitled to see a man killed,' protested the *Daily Mail*[16]), there was an outcry over the all-too-frequent fatalities involving inexperienced military flyers on these primitive machines. Nor did powerful government departments have to accept without protest whatever the manufacturers chose to give them. As the military aviation services gained in sophistication and experience, and their own engineers in knowledge, they increasingly tended to lay down specifications on ordering from private manufacturers. Flying safety, though not a prime consideration in military aircraft, came in for increasing attention.

The minuscule US Army Signal Corps aviation section suffered particularly heavy and distressing losses, attributable both to their inexperience and the faults of their equipment. Up until 1913, when the Aviation Section established its school at North Island near San Diego, eight out of fourteen qualified Army aviators had been killed in crashes.[17] Their names are commemorated in some of the air bases from which our Air Force operates today—Selfridge, Kelly, Scott, Rockwell, Call, Love, Ellington. The Wright aircraft were most numerous on the casualty list, though the original Curtiss D no. 2 succeeded in killing two officers—Lieutenant George Kelly in a bad landing at San Antonio, Texas, on 10 May 1911 and, after rebuilding, Lieutenant Joseph D. Park in a takeoff accident at Olive, California, on 9 May 1913. In the latter instance the pusher engine fell on the pilot and crushed his skull. There was one fatal crash involving the Wright A—Lieutenant Selfridge's—one in the Wright B, and no less than six in the Wright C, taking the lives of eight pilots and passengers.[18] There is no doubt that many of these accidents were caused by stalls, occurring at low altitude with the engine throttled. With their multiplicity of struts, wires and outriggers, the unstreamlined Wright biplanes had such a high drag that they would quickly lose flying speed and stall with power cut off, unless pointed sharply downward at once. When the aircraft struck the ground, the pilot and passenger, seated in the open on the leading edge of the lower wing, would be thrown to the ground. Orville Wright at least understood the cause, though the Army flyers evidently did not. In the controversy that followed the fatal crash of Lieutenants Eric Ellington and H. M. Kelly on 24 November 1913, in a Wright C, Orville wrote to the colonel 'in charge of aeronautics':

These accidents are the more distressing because they can be avoided. I think I am well within bounds when I say that over ninety per cent of them are due to one and the same cause—'stalling.' 'Stalling' is the term generally used to designate that condition of a flying machine when its speed has dropped to a point where it becomes unmanageable. Recovery is possible only by regaining speed. When in this 'stalled' condition, the machine will dive downward in spite of every effort of the aviator to stop it. Many of these dives would not result seriously if the aviator had but the courage[19] to cause the machine to make an even more fearful dive till it recovers its normal speed. But this usually is not the case. Due to certain peculiar forces acting on the aeroplane in this stalled condition, the machine speeds up, but slowly, although descending at a rapid rate, and normal speed is only recovered after a descent of several hundred feet.[20]

Writing as if he and his brother had invented the perfect aeroplane, Orville Wright continued: 'The model "C" is the best machine and the safest machine we have built, and is capable of manœuvres not possible with any other machine in the service. It is not more liable to "stalling" than other machines.' The answer, he felt, was simple: 'Proper care in observing the angles on the Incidence Indicators' (no airspeed meters were fitted). These, and other 'somewhat casual' responses to the crisis, ended the role of this great pioneer in American military aviation. Faced with the necessity of improving the safety and handling characteristics of the Army's training aircraft, Lieutenant Colonel Samuel Reber, in charge of aeronautics for the Signal Corps, began by hiring Grover Loening, the first aeronautical engineer graduated from Columbia University. On 16 July 1914 Loening reported to the training field at North Island, San Diego, California.

'After examining the planes then in service on the field, I joined at once with the recommendation of several officers that all "pusher" planes be condemned as unsafe. This meant that three or four Wright "C" and two Curtiss pushers were consigned to the scrap heap.'[21] The only aircraft in the establishment considered safe for training were tractor biplanes with the engine forward, in which location it absorbed the initial impact of a crash rather than the pilot and instructor, who were now enclosed in relative safety in the fuselage to the rear. Loening and the Signal Corps persuaded other contractors to build trainers to this formula, and ultimately the Curtiss JN-2 tractor—prototype of the machines in which so many World War I aviators learned to fly—appeared at North Island in 1915.

Thus it required the intervention of government agencies to develop a safe, sound and reliable aircraft with handling characteristics which the average flyer could master. Few indeed were the qualified aeronautical engineers available at this period, and the struggling pioneer aircraft manufacturers could not afford to hire them. Indeed, much basic research was needed to provide the theoretical and practical engineering knowledge essential for training these men. Governments, responding to the potential military value of the aeroplane, created agencies during this period to study aerodynamics and design: in America, the National Advisory Committee for

Aeronautics in 1915, with corresponding facilities in Europe, while certain universities made notable contributions.

Improvements in the state of the art brought their own hazards. It was not enough to eliminate the flimsy pusher biplane with the pilot sitting in the open on the lower wing. Men began to be killed in streamlined, high-speed aircraft through exceeding their structural limitations in high velocity manœuvres. Lincoln Beachey, the great stunt flyer who had made his reputation in the 'Little Looper' biplane which resembled the Curtiss pusher, was ultimately undone by a clean-lined new monoplane with oversize control surfaces for aerobatics. To provide a thrill for the crowds at the Panama Pacific Exposition in San Francisco in March 1915 he attempted to repeat with the monoplane his repertoire of thrills in the biplane pusher: a 1000 foot vertical power dive, then a descent on his back at an angle of 45 degrees, followed by another vertical drop of 500 feet, still with power on. At this point, having attained an estimated velocity of 250 mph and having only 500 feet of altitude left, Beachey abruptly tried to pull out. Both wings collapsed and the wreckage plunged into the bay, drowning the pilot. The monoplane had no airspeed indicator, and the investigators concluded, 'it is our opinion that Mr Beachey misjudged his speed by reason of the fact that his body and face were protected by enclosed fuselage and windshield. In all previous vertical drops, he had used a Curtiss-type biplane (pusher) where he was exposed to the full force of air pressure which aided him in judging his speed.'[22] The monoplane's builder, Warren Eaton, had calculated that in level flight at a speed of 100 mph the factor of safety was 7 to 1, but at 250 mph it was reduced to 1·1 to 1. 'Any over-control would wreck the plane.'

Thus, flight instrumentation, when it came, enhanced flying safety as well as improving aircraft handling. Pure safety equipment was a considerable time in arriving, and was even scorned as effete by some of the more reckless pioneers. Too many died simply for lack of a safety belt: Lieutenant Selfridge, the first victim of powered flight, sustained a fatal skull fracture when thrown head first to the ground. Moisant, thrown from his Bleriot when it turned over, landed on his head with fatal results. One of the early US Navy flyers, Ensign William D. Billingsley, fell to his death in rough air from a Wright float plane at 1600 feet; his passenger, Lieutenant John H. Towers, later to become a vice admiral, saved his life by clinging to a strut. Colonel Sam Cody, the American who made the first flight in Great Britain in May 1908 was killed together with a passenger when one of his monstrous 'Cathedral' biplanes broke up in the air: the centre section of the biplane wing structure landed intact upside down in some trees, and one authority believes that if the two men had been strapped in, they might have survived.[23] Photographs show Cody wearing a high-crowned, reinforced leather head-gear much affected by early flyers, called a 'crash helmet' and designed to protect the skull from injury if the wearer were thrown out on his head. As one authority remarks, 'its chief virtue was to keep the brains from spattering.'[24] Special protective clothing was hardly worn during this era, and seems not to have been necessary for low-altitude flying in warm weather. Old photographs show the airmen of the period wearing street clothing with their cloth caps turned backwards, a sartorial style originated by the Wright brothers. Goggles were customarily omitted, though America's future Chief of the Army Air Forces, 'Hap' Arnold, found good reason to wear them from his earliest flying days: 'I was coming back into the field when a bug hit me in the eye and left one of its transparent wings sticking to my eyeball. The pain was terrific; blinded by tears I could scarcely see to make my landing.'[25]

The parachute, of course, had been long invented and used by ballonists, as described in Chapter 1, but was not yet the life-saving device that it came to be. Yet it might have been so used much earlier, for, as revealed by Charles H. Gibbs-Smith, the free-type pack parachute, opened at will by the wearer with a rip cord, had been invented and demonstrated as early as 1908 by the American balloonist, A. Leo Stevens.[26] In October 1912 F. R. Law made a free drop with a Stevens 'Life-Pack' 'chute from a Wright biplane. 'In my mind,' reported the pilot, 'not as an exhibition stunt, but as a safety factor, it is the greatest move which had yet been made towards aviation safety.' Yet this demonstration was not followed up, and the free, unattached parachute had to be re-invented by others after the end of World War I.

The physician may have been directly involved in some of the later attempts on the altitude record during this period. Nothing better illustrates the rapidity of aircraft and aero engine development than the rise in the maximum attainable height during the space of only a few years. In 1909, Hubert Latham held the record at only 1485 feet, established in an Antoinette monoplane. By 1912, Garros had raised it to 18,400 feet. In 1913, the Frenchman, Legagneux, attained 20,014 feet in a Nieuport with a Le Rhone rotary motor, for the first time using oxygen. This must also have been used by the German pilot, Oelrich, who in 1914, before the war broke out, flew to 25,780 feet in a DFW biplane with 100 hp Mercedes engine. Details unfortunately are lacking.

In the year 1914 aviation was neither an industry, a means of transportation, nor even a military weapon. Daring pioneers had solved the ages-old mystery of flight, but their creations—underpowered, unreliable, fragile, barely able to stay in the air—were of no practical value except to the showman, and were positively unsafe. More knowledge, and more money, were needed to develop the Wright, Farman and Bleriot creations into useful vehicles. With the coming of war, major industrial powers turned their attention to the development of the aeroplane as a military weapon. Engineering and research within four years advanced and altered the boxkites of the pre-1914 era into powerful, swift, and relatively long-ranging weight carriers, fit to explore the skies of the world.

Belatedly, medicine recognized its inevitable involvement in aviation, in that the increasing performance of military aircraft imposed unforeseen physiological and psychological stresses on their crews. Military medical men turned their attention to the problems of the aviator, and a new specialty, aviation medicine, was born.

[1] C. H. Gibbs-Smith, *Sir George Cayley's Aeronautics* (London: HM Stationery Office, 1962), Appendix I, p. 217.

[2] C. H. Gibbs-Smith, *The Aeroplane, an Historical Survey* (London: HM Stationery Office, 1960), p. 37.

[3] Charles Dollfuss, quoted in Gibbs-Smith, *The Aeroplane*, p. 69.

[4] Arch Whitehouse, *The Early Birds* (New York: Doubleday & Co., 1965), p. 223.

[5] On 18 January 1911 Eugene Ely, a Curtiss pilot, had landed a standard wheeled aircraft aboard a platform erected over the after deck of the *Pennsylvania*, and subsequently flew off successfully. Hooks on his undercarriage caught lines attached to sandbags—a primitive arrester gear. Yet this experiment, foreshadowing the aircraft carrier, was not followed up.

[6] Historical Division of the Italian Air Force, *The First War Flights in the World, Libia MCMXI* (Rome, 1953), p. 17.

[7] *The First War Flights in the World*, p. 42.

[8] General H. H. Arnold, *Global Mission* (New York: Harper & Brothers, 1949), p. 20.

[9] In modern aircraft, thanks to the aerofoil section and wing design, the air flow does not break away completely and some lift and controllability remain even below stalling speed. The nose ordinarily does not drop, though the aircraft will descend rapidly in the stalled attitude.

[10] Allen H. Wheeler, *Building Aeroplanes for 'Those Magnificent Men'* (London: Foulis, 1965), p. 33.

[11] *ibid.*, p. 31.

[12] *ibid.*, p. 33.

[13] *ibid.*, p. 67.

[14] *ibid.*, p. 71.

[15] John R. Cuneo, *Winged Mars, vol. 1, The Growth of the German Air Weapon 1870–1914* (Harrisburg: Military Publishing Co., 1942), p. 103.

[16] Quoted in Claude Grahame-White, *The Story of the Aeroplane* (Boston: Small, Maywod & Co., 1911), p. 169.

[17] Grover C. Loening, 'Origin of Air Service Engineering,' *The Air Power Historian,* vol. XI, no. 4, October 1964, p. 93.

[18] 'Mortality in Army Aviation,' *Journal of the American Aviation Historical Society,* vol. 9, no. 2, Summer 1964, p. 109.

[19] and, Mr Wright might have observed, the necessary altitude.

[20] Loening, p. 94.

[21] *ibid.,* p. 96.

[22] E. D. Weeks, 'Lincoln Beachey's Last Ride,' *Journal of the American Aviation Historical Society,* vol. 6, no. 2, Summer 1961, p. 105.

[23] R. Dallas Brett, *History of British Aviation* (London: The Aviation Book Club, (1932)), vol. II, p. 52.

[24] Harry G. Armstrong, *Principles and Practice of Aviation Medicine* (Baltimore: Williams & Wilkins Co., 1939), p. 438.

[25] Arnold, p. 21.

[26] Gibbs-Smith, *The Aeroplane,* p. 167.

3

Untutored Bravery: World War I, 1914–18

Against the titanic backdrop of the drama of World War I, the historic cataclysm in which millions perished and which changed for ever the world in which we live, the scale of effort involved in fighting in the air must appear insignificant by comparison. Yet this first war in the skies not only greatly accelerated the technological development of the flying machine and the aircraft power plant; the lessons of air fighting and strategic bombing in the last two years of the conflict laid the foundation of the air power theory that directed the massive air forces of World War II, and the supersonic, thermonuclear bomb carriers of our own day. Lastly, for the first time, in World War I, the medical science of the day turned its attention to the physical and physiological problems of the flyer, and the modern flight surgeon entered on the scene.

In the summer of 1914 the major European military powers mobilized their air arms along with their mass armies, but the results were ludicrous if not pitiful. On the Western Front the German armies had attached a total of 180 aircraft in thirty field aviation sections; the four squadrons with the British Expeditionary Force included a nominal total of forty-eight planes; the French air force disposed of 136 serviceable aircraft, with about fifteen more added by requisition of civilian machines; and the Belgians owned about twenty-four. In addition, with the dirigible possessing greater range and carrying capacity than the flimsy, underpowered boxkites of the day, the French Army set great store by some five non-rigid airships, and the German Army had five Zeppelins on the Western Front. None of these aircraft were effectively armed, and their intended role was that of reconnaissance in a war of movement. Yet as John Cuneo points out in his scholarly *Winged Mars,*[1] neither the French nor the German doctrine of warfare attached importance to reconnaissance of the enemy: the French Army had for several years been blindly obsessed with the *offensive a l'outrance* as the solution to all military problems, the Germans, since 1871, had held that intelligence of the enemy would be delayed and incomplete, and the commander's offensive decisions could be properly based on hypotheses of the enemy's possible courses of action. Hence, in the colossal blood-lettings on the frontiers that led to the Battle of the Marne in September 1914, the air services made no significant contribution.

Under the more stable conditions of trench warfare, the air arms of the belligerents underwent a gradual expansion. Photography of enemy positions and installations began as a supplement to written observations, and ended by substituting completely for them. Artillery—the smashing weapon of this war, rather than the bomb—found in the aerial observer an invaluable guide to long-range firing. Initially, visual signals corrected the gunners' aim, but presently, primitive wireless sets, with Morse code keys, were carried aloft. The reconnaissance aircraft on both sides carried two people, a pilot in the rear and an observer in front, and were slow, stable, and incapable of self-defence. Speeds of 70 mph or less, ceilings under 10,000 feet, meant that the air crew experienced no serious medical problems except for cold and wind blast in winter.

Fighting in the air was no part of the duties of the pilots and observers of the slow, unarmed Aviatiks, Albatroses, Farmans and BE 2s which flew reconnaissance, took photographs, and ranged the artillery during the first year of the war. True, the firm of Vickers Ltd in England had designed and built before the war the FB 5 'gun bus,' a two-seater pusher biplane with a Lewis gun in the nose commanding a wide field of fire. But the first of these did not reach France until February 1915, and only in July 1915 was the first full squadron of FB 5s sent to the Front. The artillery and reconnaissance squadrons usually had one or two fast single-seaters on their strength. Yet these were not fighter aircraft, as their pilots were unable to fire a machine gun directly forward through the propeller. Therefore, consternation reigned in German two-seater units when, in April 1915, several of them were shot down by a French Morane single seater with a forward-firing machine gun. A few days later, on 19 April, the killer Morane was forced down by engine failure on the German side of the lines. It was found that the pilot was Roland Garros, a famous pre-war French stunt flyer. The secret of his being able to fire through the whirling propeller was simple: triangular steel plates, attached to the propeller, deflected any bullets from his clip-fed Hotchkiss gun that might otherwise strike the spinning blades. German military authorities, alarmed lest their enemies might sweep their aviation from the skies, asked the twenty-four-year-old Dutch designer, Anthony Fokker, to copy the Garros device. Within a few days he came up with something much better: a mechanical synchronizer gear which fired the machine gun when the propeller blades were clear of it.[2] The synchronizer, with a 7·62 mm Parabellum machine gun, was fitted to the Fokker M5K, which thereby became the E I fighter. A few of these were delivered to field aviation sections on the Western Front, and overnight, Leutnants Immelmann and Boelcke became national heroes as they began to shoot down enemy aircraft with the Fokker monoplanes.

The Fokker E II with a 100 hp rotary engine was delivered in quantity beginning in September 1915, and the 'Fokker scourge' was on. So many of the slow, clumsy, unarmed British BE 2c reconnaissance machines were shot down that Royal Flying Corps morale was affected, and in Parliament, Noel Pemberton-Billing, a former Royal Naval Air Service squadron commander, charged that RFC pilots in France were being 'rather murdered than killed.' Lacking a synchronizing gear themselves, the French and British fought back, and by the summer of 1916 had established a measure of equality with the Germans. The British favoured a pusher design, with engine at the rear and a free field of fire forward for a machine gun in the bow of the nacelle. The agile little De Havilland DH 2 single-seater pusher, with a ·303 Lewis in the nose, went to France with No. 24 Squadron in February 1916, and proved superior to the Fokker. The French concentrated on the Nieuport 11, the 'Bèbè,' a tiny, graceful, single-seater tractor biplane already in production, fitting a Lewis machine gun on the top wing to fire forward above the propeller arc.

With these early fighter aircraft came the day of the individual 'ace,' flying alone, preying on lone reconnaissance aircraft, and running up his score to the accompaniment of hysterical adulation by his fellow-countrymen, and a rapid accumulation of all the medals and decorations his nation and its allies could bestow. In Germany, the heroes were Boelcke and Immelmann, in France, Guynemer, Nungesser and Navarre. The Royal Flying Corps, concerned for the morale of the aircrew of the plodding reconnaissance and artillery aircraft, refused to publicize their 'aces,' but the British public came to hear of Albert Ball.

Inevitably, Allied designers developed their own synchronizing gear—the Constantinesco—and a second generation of fighters appeared, each with a single Vickers gun firing through the propeller. By the autumn of 1916 the Fokker had been mastered and the German Air Service discredited, to the point where high-ranking German Army officers complained of their own aviation in the fighting at Verdun and on the Somme. A reorganization took place in the autumn, and for the first time the German fighters were concentrated into units. The first, *Jagdstaffel* 2 under Boelcke, flew its first squadron operation on 17 September 1916. A new machine made its debut that day—the shark-bodied Albatros D I biplane, with two synchronized machine guns firing through the propeller. Again the Allies were caught with inferior aircraft—the British, still using the defenceless BE 2c biplanes which had figured as 'Fokker fodder' a year before, sustaining almost unbearable losses until better machines were available in the spring of 1917.

Not only was aerial fighting becoming more intense, and the control of the air being recognized as indispensable to all aerial operations, but the rapidly advancing performance of fighter aircraft began to impose significant physiological stresses on their pilots. The Fokker E I, with an 80 hp Oberursel rotary, had a maximum speed of 82 mph and a service ceiling of 10,000 feet; the DH 2, with 100 hp Gnome rotary, 93 mph at sea level and a ceiling of 14,000 feet. The Sopwith triplane, however, with a 130 hp Clerget rotary, attained 117 mph at 5000 feet and had a ceiling of 20,500 feet; the Spad S 7 with 180 hp reached 119·5 mph at 6500 feet, and could fight up to 18,000 feet. In other words, these aircraft were attaining altitudes where their pilots were susceptible to anoxia, and more and more as it became apparent that altitude gave a fighter an advantage in combat, patrols were being flown at the higher levels. 'Always above, seldom on the same level, never underneath,' was the motto and guide to air fighting of England's greatest ace, Edward Mannock.

No longer in the last year of the war was air fighting a matter of the lone wolf, the individual 'ace' stalking his prey. All too often, as in the case of Werner Voss, shot down on 23 September 1917 by six pilots of No. 56 Squadron, the 'ace' became a victim of the close-knit team fighting in formation. Larger groups (Germany's greatest fighter pilot, Manfred von Richthofen, started it by combining the forty-eight fighter aircraft of Squadrons *(Jastas)* 4, 6, 10 and 11 into the *Jagdgeschwader* (Wing) No. 1 on 24 June 1917) ruled the skies in the last year of the war. Huge formations battled for air mastery, with tactics agreed on in advance among the flight leaders. Usually the side which disposed of the greatest reserves at higher altitude won. Here is a glimpse of Mannock—the master air tactician—leading the SE 5s of No. 85 Squadron, RFC:

Mannock led a show yesterday and gave us all heart failure. He was leading the bottom flight with three men and found ten Fokkers and played them for fifteen minutes. At any moment it looked as if we were all going to get shot down, but Mannock knew what he was about and kept the top flight up in the sun. He sucked the Huns into where he wanted them and went right under them. They knew there was a flight above up in the sun so only five of them came down. Then Randy and three men came down on them just as they got to Mannock, and instead of their top five getting the cold meat as they expected, Nigger, Mac, Cal, Inglis and myself leaped on them so that our eight below had a picnic with the bottom five Huns. They got two of the bottom ones and Mac got one of the top ones that tried to get down to join the fight below.[3]

The Fokker D VII biplane, a remarkable machine introduced in April 1918, outclassed the British Sopwith Camel and battled on equal terms during the last months of the war with the SE 5s and Spad 13s equipping the British, French and American squadrons. With thick cantilever wings, a 160 hp Mercedes engine, and later a 185 hp high compression BMW, the D VII had phenomenal manœuvrability, particularly at high altitude, and was greatly liked by its pilots. 'The Fokker was a thoroughbred, which responded to the slightest touch of the hand and seemed almost to anticipate the will of its pilot.'[4] Against the eager, brave but inexperienced pilots of the Air Service, American Expeditionary Force, the Fokker D VII in the hands of the veteran German *Jastas* ran up an impressive score.

Much of the dogfighting in the last summer of the war took place at altitudes where anoxia was a problem:

There were five of us and we ran into five Fokkers at fifteen thousand feet. We both started climbing, of course. And they outclimbed us. We climbed up to twenty thousand five hundred and couldn't get any higher. We were practically stalled and these Fokkers went right over our heads and got between us and the lines. They didn't want to dogfight but tried to pick off our rear men. Inglis and Cal were getting a pretty good thrill when we turned back and caught one Hun napping. He half rolled slowly and we got on his tail. Gosh, it's unpleasant fighting at that altitude. The slightest movement exhausts you; your engine has no pep and splutters; it's hard to keep a decent formation, and you lose five hundred feet on a turn. The other Huns came in from above and it didn't take us long to fight down to twelve thousand. We put up the best fight of our lives but these Huns were just too good for us.[5]

It is difficult to ascertain whether oxygen was used by any of the fighters flying high altitude patrols in the last year of the war. Certainly it was not employed in No. 84 Squadron, RFC. The squadron commanding officer, Major Sholto Douglas, recalled:

I found that pushing the Lewis gun back into the fixed position while flying in the open cockpit of the SE 5 at high altitude called for an effort that was almost superhuman. We had no supply of oxygen in those days, and I found that my strength at height fell off considerably. It was difficult enough to change the double drum of ammunition on the Lewis gun without having to man-handle the gun into position for an attack and fly the aeroplane at the same time. There were others who had the same experience, and more often than not we had to dive down to a lower altitude before we could reload.[6]

One British fighter aircraft, the Sopwith Snipe, certainly carried oxygen equipment when it went out to France shortly before the

Armistice. John Milner, formerly of No. 43 Squadron, RAF, recalls that 'though we had oxygen bottles and masks fitted in the Snipe (for patrols at 25,000 feet), the cylinder was a very small one and you'd had it after a few gulps.'[7]

As for strategic bombing, it was Imperial Russia, curiously enough, which developed the first four-engine bomber aircraft, the Sikorsky 'Ilya Mourumetz,' which first flew in January 1914. It was the Germans, however, who evolved the first doctrine of strategic bombing—a doctrine which, incidentally, perished with the Armistice and was not handed down to Hitler's ground-support *Luftwaffe*. Remarkably, where British and French military leaders were hostile to the strategic bombing concept, it was the traditionally hidebound German generals and admirals who gave active support to the building of long-range bombing aircraft designed to burn the enemy's cities, cripple his transportation system, destroy his war industries, and undermine civilian morale. One reason for their attitude was their realization that the Fatherland, arrayed against half the world, could not win in a conventional contest of massed armies. Another was the German monopoly at the start of the war of an impressive weapon of strategic air superiority—the Zeppelin rigid airship. With range, lifting capacity, and endurance far in excess of those of the aeroplanes of 1914, the German Army and Navy airships competed to be the first to bomb London, which was attacked for the first time by the military service's LZ 38 on 31 May 1915. Increasingly overshadowed by improved heavier than air craft, the Army airship service was disbanded in 1917. By contrast, the German Naval Airship Division under its aggressive, single-minded and dedicated Leader of Airships, Fregattenkapitän Peter Strasser, made 177 flights across the North Sea to attack England from 19 January 1915 until Strasser's death aboard his flagship L 70 in the last raid of the war on 5 August 1918. Strasser it was who promised his chief, Vizeadmiral Reinhard Scheer, in August 1916, that 'England can be overcome by means of airships, inasmuch as the country will be deprived of the means of existence through increasingly extensive destruction of cities, factory complexes, dockyards, harbour works with war and merchant ships lying therein, railroads, etc.'[8] No combat organization bore heavier casualties than that which flew the Zeppelins, filled with inflammable hydrogen, against the English defences—about forty per cent of the approximately 1100 flight crew members perished during the war in their flaming ships over England or the North Sea. Yet the results were out of proportion to the effort expended. Bad weather, faulty navigation and the Zeppelin's vulnerability brought to naught Strasser's dream of 'a quick and effective conquest of England.'

Yet the Zeppelins, particularly in the last years of the war, encountered and attempted to solve many aeromedical problems which heavier-than-air flyers of other nations only began to encounter in the 1920s and 1930s—anoxia at high altitude, fatigue, frostbite and cold. A turning point in the Zeppelin war came in the autumn of 1916, when within a space of three months, six airships were shot down over England—five in flames, with all hands killed. Raiding altitudes then were 11,000 to 13,000 feet, but to escape the defending British aircraft, Strasser had his Zeppelins drastically lightened to reach altitudes of 17,000 to 20,000 feet with full war load. Oxygen equipment—compressed gas in 1917, liquid oxygen in 1918—was first carried aboard the raiding airships. Fur-lined flight clothing—often lined with layers of newspapers—afforded some protection against bitter cold down to −30 degrees F. The need to discard every superfluous item of weight for the sake of high altitude prevented electrical heating of flight clothing. Similarly, 'attached' type parachutes for the 20-odd crew members, carried early in 1917, were discarded because of their weight.

Though Strasser persisted, with Scheer's support, in high-altitude raids on the north of England, the German Army aviation authorities turned to large bombing aeroplanes to continue the attack on London. The *Gothaer Waggonfabrik,* beginning in 1916, had developed a large twin-engine biplane bomber with a crew of three, a bomb load of 660 to 1100 pounds, and a range of about 500 miles. In May 1917 thirty Gotha G IVs were assigned to Belgian bases for raiding England. After a series of probing attacks, there followed two daylight raids on London which killed more people than all the Zeppelin bombardments heretofore, and had profound political repercussions. The British were not long in organizing a defence against the daytime attackers, and after September the twin-engine bombers came by night. The daylight raiders were relatively lightly loaded with about 660 pounds of bombs, and attacked from 15,000 feet; with a heavier explosive cargo the nocturnal attackers flew at 10,000 to 12,000 feet. There is evidence that in the daylight raids, at least, Gotha crews wore masks and breathed compressed oxygen from individual flasks.

Supplementing the night-bombing Gothas from the end of September 1917 were a handful of the so-called Giant machines. More farsighted than the Allied powers, the German military authorities from the beginning of the war encouraged the larger industrial firms to build huge bombers with three to six engines, all of which had to be accessible for servicing during flight.[9] Of all the many and varied *Riesenflugzeug* designs, only the Zeppelin-Staaken products entered combat, and these only in small numbers and in what might be termed an operational testing status. The R VI variation most commonly employed was the largest aeroplane to bomb England in either world war, with a span of 138 feet $5\frac{1}{2}$ inches, and a loaded gross weight of 25,269 pounds. An R VI dropped the first 2200 pound bomb on England on February 16/17, 1918. Fifteen thousand feet was an average bombing altitude over London, and some at least of the Staaken Giants carried liquid oxygen equipment.[10] At no time were more than six of these monsters available to the detachment joining the Gothas in night raids on England. On the other hand, though frequently attacked by night fighters, none of them were shot down over England. They were the direct ancestors of the long-range, four-engined strategic bombers with which the Allies, not the Germans, conquered in World War II.

British strategic bombing was a late-war development, although the Royal Naval Air Service possessed as early as December 1915 a 'bloody paralyser' of an aeroplane in the twin-engined Handley-Page 0/100, with a span of exactly 100 feet and a bomb load of nearly 1800 pounds. Originally designed for over-water patrols, the 0/100 in small numbers made night bombing raids in France in the hands of naval crews. The German daylight attacks on London in June and July, 1917, rudely directed the attention of His Majesty's Government to the progressing development of the air weapon and led to the establishment of the Royal Air Force, the first unified air service, in April 1918. The German Gothas also inspired the creation of a comparable strategic force. This, known initially as the 41st Wing and later—and provocatively—as the Independent Force, made attacks on the railroad lines carrying French iron ore from the Lorraine fields into Germany, and on industrial cities such as Mannheim, Cologne, Karlsruhe, Stuttgart, Coblenz and Saarbrücken. Never as large as its leader, the later Marshal of the RAF Lord Trenchard, would have wished, the Independent Force by November 1918 comprised only nine squadrons. Four of these operated single engine De Havilland day bombers—the Royal Flying Corps' idea of an effective craft for short-range strikes across the lines. The remainder flew Handley-Page 0/400s, improved versions of the 0/100 of 1915. At the Armistice a four-engined Handley-Page, the V/1500, with a bomb load of up to thirty 250 pound bombs, was ready, and a wing of these monsters was forming in East Anglia with a view to attacking Berlin.

The day bombers, forced to battle their way through swarms of enemy fighters, suffered heavy casualties, particularly the DH 9s. Equipped with the unreliable, de-rated, 230 hp BHP engine, the DH 9's bombing altitude was no more than 10,000 feet. The Rolls-Royce powered DH 4s of No. 55 Squadron were able to reach 14,000 feet with a bomb load over German cities, yet the squadron lost sixty-nine aircraft in thirteen months of strategic bombing. The DH 9a, with the American 400 hp Liberty engine, had a service ceiling of 16,750 feet with two 230 pound bombs. There is some evidence that these aircraft, particularly the DH 4s of No. 55 Squadron and the DH 9a's of No. 110 Squadron, used oxygen equipment in their long daylight raids. The night-flying Handley-Page 0/400s had a ceiling of not more than 10,000 feet, and usually flew much lower.

French aviation was the first to mount a strategic bombardment campaign in World War I. As early as 23 November 1914 the First Bombardment Group, consisting of eighteen aircraft, was established under the direct control of GHQ to attack rail transportation and industry far to the rear of the German lines. It made its first attacks on Freiburg-im-Breisgau on 4 and 19 December 1914. Three more groups were organized, and through the summer of 1915 daylight raids were made by as many as fifty aircraft at one time on Ludwigshafen, Karlsruhe, Saarbrücken and Dillingen. But the material was not equal to the grandiose plan of destroying German industry by aerial bombardment. Clumsy, pusher-driven Voisin bombers, their tails on latticework booms and the pilot and gunner out in front in an open 'bathtub' nacelle, carried 110 pounds of bombs at a speed of 65 mph, and required forty-five minutes to climb to 9800 feet. In the autumn of 1915 the bombardment aircraft were again placed under control of individual army commands and the strategic campaign was abandoned—probably just in time to escape heavy losses at the hands of German home defence fighters.

As in later wars, it was the photo-reconnaissance aircraft of World War I which flew at the highest altitudes, and which made the utmost demands on their crews. The Germans in the final year of the war possessed in the Rumpler C VII *Rubild* a fast two-seater reconnaissance plane with a service ceiling of 24,000 feet and an endurance of three and a half hours. With a high-compression, high-altitude airship engine, the Maybach Mb IVa of 245 hp, it had a good power output at its ceiling, and its crews were accustomed to making long flights deep into the rear of the Allied lines unmolested by enemy fighters. The *Rubild,* for the sake of lightness, had only the observer's Parabellum machine gun and no forward-firing weapon; but liquid oxygen equipment was carried and the crew's flight suits were electrically heated.

The Allied air services had no craft especially built for high-altitude, long-range photo-reconnaissance, but the Rolls-Royce powered De Havilland DH 4, specially lightened and modified for this work, had a performance not much inferior to that of the *Rubild*. No. 55 Squadron

of the Independent Force possessed two special DH 4 reconnaissance aircraft with larger DH 9a wing panels. No bombs
were carried, only 150 rounds of ammunition for the pilot's Vickers
instead of 750, and two drums for the observer's Lewis instead of six.
An engine-driven generator heated the crew's flight clothing, camera
and guns. A typical photo sortie over German targets involved an
hour's climb, two to three hours above 19,000 feet, and a three-quarter
hour descent. Compressed oxygen was breathed above 15,000 feet. It
was not unusual for the pilot or observer to lose consciousness due to
oxygen failure; in this case the other crew member would fly the
aircraft down with dual control to 14,000 feet. No DH 4 was lost when
19,000 feet was exceeded, and enemy aircraft were often seen 'hanging
on the prop' a thousand to three thousand feet below.[11]

In the air war over the North Sea, the Imperial German Navy
enjoyed an enormous advantage in the great range and endurance of
their Zeppelin airships. In the Sunderland operation by the German
High Seas Fleet two months after the Battle of Jutland, four airships
formed a scouting line from Scotland to Norway, and four more
operated off the British coast from the Firth of Forth to the mouth of
the channel. L 31, a new Zeppelin with a capacity of 2,000,000 cubic
feet of hydrogen, was in the air for twenty hours and fifty-five minutes
on this day, travelling 1167 miles at an average speed of 55.7 mph.
The comparable British scouting aircraft, the seaplane, such as the
Short Type 184, a two-seater biplane mounted on flimsy box-shaped
floats, had a maximum speed of $88\frac{1}{2}$ mph, but an endurance of only
two and three-quarter hours. Nor was the seaplane an effective anti-
Zeppelin weapon: throughout the first six months of 1915, fast
steamers went deep into German waters to send off Sopwith seaplane
fighters. Yet none of these ventures were successful, the frail float-
planes usually breaking up on the water during takeoff attempts.

A regular aircraft carrier was needed that could keep up with the
Fleet, and in July 1917 the first of the breed, HMS *Furious*, came to
the Grand Fleet base at Scapa Flow. Designed after the outbreak of
war as a 'large light cruiser,' she could make 32 knots, and still had a
single 18 inch gun mounted aft. The forward gun had been replaced by
a hangar, with flying-off deck on top, enabling her to handle four Short
184 seaplanes—which took off on wheeled trolleys—and half a dozen
Sopwith Pup fighters. These, too, were intended to land on the water,
but on 2 August 1917, with *Furious* steaming into the wind at 26
knots, her senior aviator, Squadron Commander Dunning, succeeded
in landing aboard after flying around the funnel and superstructure
amidships, and being pulled down to the deck by a party of flying
officers. In a later attempt on 7 August Dunning went over the side and

was drowned. Partly as a result, *Furious,* in November 1917, went back to the yard to have the aft 18 in. gun removed and replaced by a stern hangar with flying-on deck. The midships funnel and super-structure remained, however, and when she rejoined the Fleet in the spring of 1918 it was found that turbulence from these structures made the aft flying-on deck practically useless. None the less, it was from *Furious* that seven Sopwith 2F 1 Camels made the first carrier strike in history on 19 July 1918, bombing the Zeppelin sheds at Tondern and burning the airships L 54 and L 60. Had the war lasted into 1919, it is possible that torpedo-armed Sopwith Cuckoos from *Furious* and other carriers would have gone after the High Seas Fleet at its anchorage in Schillig Roads, anticipating Taranto and Pearl Harbour by more than twenty years.

For another two decades the generals might procure horses for the cavalry, and the admirals lay down battleships for the benefit of the 'gun club.' To Trenchard in England, Mitchell and Moffett in America, Yamamoto in Japan, and Seeckt in Germany, it was obvious that the aeroplane, the plaything of rich sportsmen and the death-defying vehicle of stunt men and barnstormers, had changed permanently the nature of warfare on land and sea. With this conviction they would build for the future war which they knew would prove them right.

Nor would this revolutionary development have been possible without the participation of medicine, both in evaluating the fitness of men to fly, and in aiding them to overcome the physiological problems of life in the air. From the medical experience of World War I have come down to us the earliest use of oxygen in aeroplanes at high altitude, the first awareness of flying fatigue, and the routine use of parachutes to save the lives of air crew. A new medical specialist also appeared—the flight surgeon, the physician who, combining special medical skills with familiarity with aviation, was equipped to meet the physical and emotional needs of flying men.

It must be admitted that the medical man played only a minor role in the early development of air power in World War I. Only with experience could his duties be defined in the selection of candidates for flying, and in maintenance of flying fitness; and few indeed had by the date of the Armistice accumulated the personal knowledge of the new medical specialty of aviation medicine which would qualify them to speak with authority. Most of this knowledge derived from the last two years of the war, the period when expansion of the air services began to strain the manpower and supply resources of all the belligerents, while the swiftly-progressing capabilities of more efficient aircraft imposed greater demands on flight personnel.

Selection of air crew in the early war period was haphazard. To be familiar with horses and horsemanship was an outstanding recommendation: in the forgotten era before the internal combustion engine, the horse was the young man's outlet for aggressive, reckless, exhibitionistic behaviour. The scions of the aristocracy raced, steeple-chased, played polo, and rode to hounds—and gambled on their prowess—as a matter of course. Joining the army, they obtained commissions in the traditional cavalry regiments, continuing the above activities with their own mounts, and on manœuvres, letting themselves go in wild charges with sabre and lance. With some reason, line officers held that the recklessness, the gambling spirit, the 'hands' of the horseman, would qualify him to be a good aeroplane pilot. (The medical service was much slower in discovering the supreme value of motivation compared to flawless physique.) An outstanding example of the cavalryman turned flyer in World War I was Rittmeister Manfred von Richthofen, top-scoring 'ace' with eighty victories.

Indeed, reckless daring was the attitude for the combat aviators of World War I. There were no parachutes for Allied flyers, and only in the last months of the war were their German opponents able to save their lives with the silken umbrella. Structural failure, combat damage, meant certain death. Small wonder that good-luck charms were universally popular. Most dreaded of all was fire in the air—all too common with unprotected fuel tanks and incendiary ammunition. Many pilots were morbidly obsessed with premonitions of going down in flames. Mannock carried a revolver in the air 'to finish myself as soon as I see the first sign of flames . . . that's the way they're going to get me in the end—flames and finish.'[12] And in the end, they did.

Mannock's score of seventy-four victories is all the more remarkable in that he suffered from such severe astigmatism in the left eye as to be virtually blind, and indeed, had been repatriated from Turkey (where the war had found him in 1914 working for a telephone company) 'on grounds of age, apparent bad health, and defective eyesight.'[13] He bluffed his way through the medical examination for the Flying Corps by memorizing the eye charts in a few seconds with his good right eye. Many of the top-scoring pilots of World War I rose to 'acedom' despite physical defects which would have barred them from flight training in a later and stricter age: Guynemer, the French ace with fifty-three victories, suffered from pulmonary tuberculosis; Oswald Boelcke, the pioneer of air fighting tactics in the German air force, with forty victories, was grounded more than once by bouts of asthma; William Thaw, 'the soul of the *Escadrille Lafayette,*' had nor-mal vision in only one eye; Frank Luke, the 'balloon buster,' America's second ranking ace with twenty-one victories, would probably have failed a present-day psychiatric intake examination. Moody, withdrawn, at odds with his squadron mates, he may well have been a psychopathic personality. Yet it has been observed in both world wars that success in air fighting often correlates with the psychopathic traits of exhibitionism, egocentricity, explosive aggressiveness, a taste for violence, and a certain callousness towards others.

In the early period of the war the medical examination for selection of pilots reflected the ingenuity or prejudices of the medical or physiological savants called on to serve their country in this capacity without personal knowledge of aviation. The German Army established a medical section under the Commanding General of the Air Forces as early as 1915, this having charge of the medical testing of all candidates. Among others, a typically Teutonic scheme was designed to test simultaneously the candidate's 'attentiveness, memory, quickness and sureness of movement, capacity to withstand fatigue, timidity, orientation, and discrimination':[14]

The candidate had several tasks to perform, the one chief, the others secondary. In front of him a panorama rolled by which represented a landscape from a perspective of 2000 metres. On this were designated a series of 30 artillery stations. This landscape was mounted on a kymograph drum and thus could be presented continuously. A complete revolution was made every two minutes. The candidate observed this landscape through a sighting apparatus and his task was to 'photograph' the artillery stations as they passed by a midline by pressing a reaction key. This constituted the chief task.

As a secondary task, he had to react to different coloured lights which were flashed on around the central field of vision. For lights on the left, the right key had to be used, for lights on the right, the left key. The key had to be pressed once for a white, twice for a green, and three times for a red light. . . .

As a visual distraction, a sudden flash of light immediately behind the observer was introduced at the beginning of the eighth minute.

At one time the British were alleged to be sending into the Royal Flying Corps men disabled by wounds or injuries received in combat in France and Flanders. This practice eventually became the target of deserved criticism, and a small Medical Research Committee under Major Martin Flack RAMC was set up in London to advise the military heads of the RFC and RNAS on aeromedical matters, while six examining stations were established in England for medical evaluation of all pilot candidates. British examiners placed great stress on cardiovascular performance, particularly in response to exercise. They also utilized the so-called 'Flack bag,' an apparatus which purported to indicate the ceiling to which a candidate could ascend without oxygen. Breathing in and out of a five-litre bag, the subject gradually reduced the partial pressure of oxygen in the container, while the exhaled carbon dioxide was absorbed by a canister of sodium hydroxide. Thus, within twenty or thirty minutes, the man would be breathing air with an oxygen partial pressure equivalent to that at high altitude. 'The length of time that the man was able to keep this up was noted; then a sample of the air in the bag was taken and immediately examined, and the percentage of oxygen in the bag was determined by careful analysis; and in this way it was very simple to determine to what altitude this man would be able to attain.'[15] Sixty-one per cent of the men found fit for flying were able to tolerate an oxygen percentage equivalent to that at 20,000 feet or above; twenty-five per cent were not able to tolerate more than an equivalent of 15,000 feet; and fourteen per cent could not surpass more than 8000 foot conditions. The Flack rebreather test, simulating an ascent at a rate greater than that of which contemporary aircraft were capable, bore no relationship to a man's ability to tolerate anoxia for long periods. It fell into disuse when experience made it clear that all personnel required oxygen above 12,000 feet; but this need was not generally accepted during World War I, and the false results of the Flack test encouraged the belief that young, healthy candidates could fly at the ceiling of contemporary fighter aircraft without oxygen.

The French aviation medical service grew up in an impromptu way through the studies of several physiologists—Professor Josue, interested in the cardiovascular system; Professor Lombard, a specialist in the middle ear and vestibular apparatus; and Dr Garsaux, who investigated the problems of low oxygen partial pressures in a pressure chamber. In January 1918 the French aeromedical service was reorganized, with Professor Nepper in administrative charge. It was he who, together with Dr Jean Camus, devised the notorious test for 'nervous shock' which measured changes in respiration, heart rate and vasomotor response when a revolver was fired close to the candidate's ear:

> For the man whose nervous system is perfectly balanced . . . the discharge of a weapon scarcely upsets their respiratory rhythm, neither do they tremble before or after the shot, and no vasomotor modification is noted in their organism. On the contrary, weaknesses are shown in the graphic of the candidate who will have to be eliminated. . . . When he hears the revolver shot, troubles arise in his respiration, his nervous trembling becomes intensified and a typical vasoconstriction takes place in his organism.[16]

At the Italian Psycho-Physiological Institute in Rome the examination of air service candidates emphasized reaction time—not surprising inasmuch as the director was the famous neurologist, Professor Gradenigo. A feature of the laboratory much admired by visiting Americans was the *carlinga,* a regular aeroplane seat and nacelle, with the control stick and rudder pedals connected to lights that measured the reaction time of the subject under test.

The Americans, coming fresh to the war in 1917, were determined not only to have the biggest air force, but also the best. The formula guiding their medical selection boards was the allegation that of all flying casualties, two per cent were caused by 'the Hun,' eight per cent by 'failure of the engine or the plane,' and ninety per cent by 'failure of the flyer himself,' though further scrutiny indicates that the majority of these failures were pilot error resulting from inadequate training and experience, rather than medical incapacity.[17] Unlike the Allies in Europe, with whom by 1917 it was a case of 'selecting the best of a poor collection,'[18] the American air service could maintain the highest standards in choosing the approximately 20,000 men accepted for wartime aviation. During the summer and autumn of 1917, sixty-seven medical examining units were established in large American cities by order of Lieutenant Colonel Theodore C. Lyster MC, Chief Surgeon, Aviation Section, Signal Corps, United States Army. 20/20 visual acuity in both eyes, normal red/green colour vision, 40/40 hearing in both ears with the watch test, were absolute requirements rigidly adhered to; the candidate's motivation for flying, however, was not considered. Years later, one of Lyster's right-hand men recognized that disproportionate emphasis had been laid on physical perfection alone: Bill Thaw of the *Escadrille Lafayette*, he wrote, had only one functioning eye. Guynemer was 'dying of consumption. I was told at the Front that he would retire and have a haemorrhage, only to return and again become a terror to the enemy.' Leech, a Canadian pilot, flew successfully in combat with a wooden leg—after breaking it in a crash he had to pay for its repair! Yet the psyche, for this influential pioneer, was a thing of mystery. 'With some timidity, I suggest that there is a real danger in the probing of the soul.'[19]

A feature of the American aviation physical examination was the emphasis placed on the function of the vestibular apparatus. This structure, located in the temporal bone of the skull close to the ear, but not part of the hearing apparatus, is made up of three tiny semi-circular canals filled with fluid, and serves to determine motion of the head and its position in relation to the downward pull of gravity, probably by the flow of fluid through the appropriate canal when acted on by changing forces and accelerations. Nowadays it is known that the semi-circular canals, capable of giving a man on the ground a sense of his orientation with respect to the earth, can give false and even misleading information in the air: for example, once stimulated by rapid rotary motion as in a spin, they continue to register rotation after it has stopped. In today's aviation physical examination, the vestibular apparatus receives only secondary attention, befitting its relatively unimportant role in spatial orientation in flight: it should neither be so sensitive as to cause the flyer to develop vertigo or airsickness, nor so insensitive as to provide no information whatever.

In 1917, however, it was of prime importance, for it was the belief of medical men that the vestibular apparatus could orient the flyers in the air as on the ground. Such were the views of an influential member of the medical department, Dr Isaac Jones, an otologist turned flight surgeon, who in a standard text, *Equilibrium and Vertigo,* had written of his conviction that the vestibular canals were essential for orientation in the air and wrote that 'perhaps the ear would be able to tell us whether we were upside down or right side up.'[20] Jones later publicly regretted this statement, after experience had shown that orientation in flight depended very largely on vision, while the vestibular apparatus was of secondary importance. Initially, as Jones remarks, the early examination of inner ear function was both meaningless and misleading: 'One test was to place the candidate on a piano stool and spin him. If he vomited he was rejected. This was not so good, particularly as it was rejecting the normal!'[21] The turning-chair test established by Jones measured the response of all three semi-circular canals, the most important being the test for nystagmus—the jerky motion of the eyes to right or left which indicates the sensitivity of the vestibular canals to rotary motion:

Head 30 degrees forward; turn candidate to the right, eyes closed, 10 times in exactly 20 seconds. The instant the chair is stopped, click the stop-watch; candidate opens his eyes and looks straight ahead at some distant point. There should occur a horizontal nystagmus to the left of 26 seconds duration. Candidate then closes his eyes and is turned to the left; there should occur a horizontal nystagmus to the right of 26 seconds duration. The variation of 8 seconds is allowable.[22]

After the Armistice, a number of American aces were tested at the Medical Research Laboratory, Issoudun, France, with respect to inner ear function. One showed distinctly subnormal responses, another an abnormally prolonged response, while the others fell within normal limits, proving that vestibular function, and accompanying sensitivity to spatial displacement, could vary over a considerable range in successful flyers:

Captain Harold R. Buckley (5 victories), nystagmus 26-26 sec. (noted 'not fit to fly').

'Stovall' (1st Lieutenant Wm. H. Stovall, 7 victories), nystagmus 26–28 sec.

'Steerley' (1st Lieutenant John H. Seerley, 5 victories), nystagmus 29–33 sec.

'Guthrie' (1st Lieutenant Murray K. Guthrie, 6 victories), nystagmus 13–14 sec.

'Luff' (1st Lieutenant Frederick E. Luff, 5 victories), nystagmus 20–20 sec.

'Healy' (1st Lieutenant James A. Healy, 5 victories), nystagmus 22–23 sec.[23]

As for the 'care of the flyer,' that this required the services of a specially trained medical officer was not apparent to the military leaders of the European air forces, and the flight surgeon as we know him today did not appear until late in the war. The resulting wastage of trained manpower was enormous, not only in terms of men killed at the Front or in training because they were fatigued to the point of being unfit to fly, but also in men who were 'flown out' or 'stale' from months of continuous combat duty without interruption, who might have been continued in flying status with appropriate rest leave advised on medical grounds:

It can readily be seen that a skilful flight surgeon would have been very valuable at the aerodrome where Guynemer had his headquarters. That marvellous flyer had shown increasing nervousness and physical unfitness for some time. . . . 'He became nervous, sick and irritable. His comrades, unable to control their captain, telephoned to Paris, informing their old commanding officer, Brocard, that Guynemer was sick and in no condition to fly and imploring him to come back to the aerodrome to take their captain away for a much-needed rest. He arrived about half an hour after Guynemer had left on his last flight.'[24]

This did not prevent learned medical men, themselves unfamiliar with flying, from offering the wartime aviator much solemn advice on health measures which must have caused ribald amusement on airfields from San Diego to Warsaw. In the automobile age, we downgrade physical fitness; our Victorian ancestors made a fetish of it, and the sportsman-athlete was held up as a model for youth. Hence, much of the advice to the aviator emphasized self-restraint, avoidance of excess and quiet diversions. 'Moderation in the Use of Harmful Luxuries,' reads one chapter heading in a small booklet, published in January 1918, for German aviators:

It is generally known that the three so-called luxuries, alcohol, nicotine and coffee, if enjoyed in excess, prove damaging to the nervous system, heart and stomach. Nonetheless, it is precisely these three luxuries, which are specially favoured during this war. . . . In almost all the rowing clubs the boat crews in training for a race are obligated, by word of honour and over their signature, to refrain absolutely from alcoholic indulgence and sexual relations while training for the race and until the regatta is over. . . . How many times more important is the highest effectiveness in war than in a rowing race? . . . Sexual intercourse is to be considered as a further source of

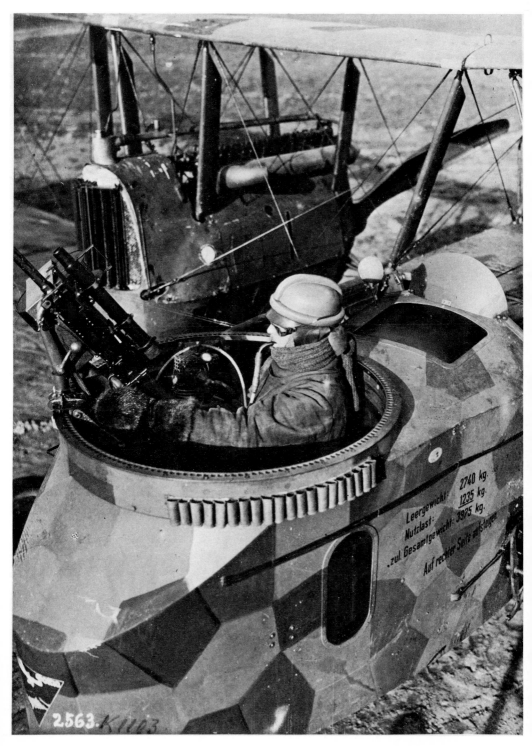

13. Observer in the forward cockpit of a Gotha G-IV German bomber. He wears a crash helmet and holds a pipestem mouthpiece for oxygen in his mouth. The Ahrendt & Heylandt liquid oxygen apparatus is visible fastened to the right side of the cockpit (1917). (National Archives)

14. Observer and pilot in a Handley-Page 0/400, September 1918. Illustrates the exposed situation of flight personnel in the World War I period, particularly when required to stand up in the slip stream as with Lewis gunners. Note fur lined coats, helmets and gauntlets worn to protect against low temperatures and wind blast. (Imperial War Museum)

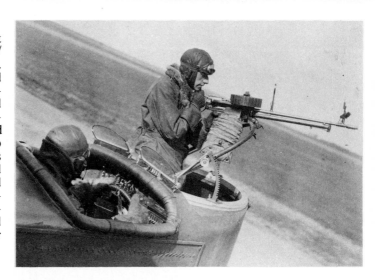

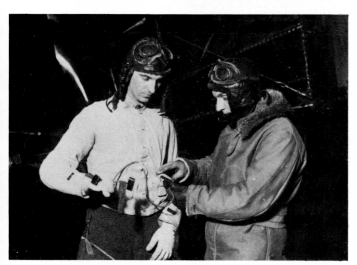

15. Flight crew of an F.E.2b night bombing squadron dressing in electrically heated suits, boots and gloves, January 1918. (Imperial War Museum)

16. The German Heinicke parachute under test at McCook Field, U.S.A. in 1919. Shroud line failed in drop test at 90 mph with 200 lb. lead weight. (Air Force Museum)

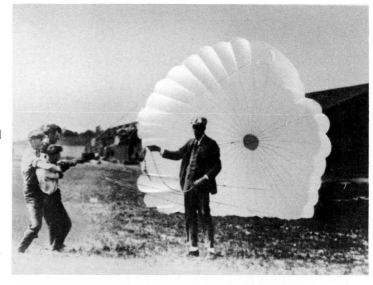

injury. Even though a harmful effect is generally to be feared only through excess, the great danger of infection must be kept in mind.[25]

As for rest periods, the writer recommended:

Hunting, riding, gymnastics and ball games (rounders, strap-ball, football, tennis, etc.), and walks in company are occupations which combine physical effort with mental diversion. . . . Also, a lance should be broken in favour of fishing; it is certainly not true that there is only one occupation duller than fishing, namely to watch someone else fish.[26]

The French authority, Dr Guibert, wrote in May 1917:

Let us speak first of the hygiene of the aviator on the ground. The first thing that would be necessary to him is a great liberty of spirit. He should avoid family attachments and other liaisons too absorbing. He should accustom himself to react against anxieties and unpleasant conditions of all sorts. How can the pilot be a complete master of his apparatus if he is distracted in his mind, and his thought is elsewhere?[27]

And an American authority:

It is now clearly recognized that the aviator's reactions to stimuli are slowed down or disturbed by disease, worry, fatigue, after excess in alcohol, and after other excesses. A delay of a second or part of a second in correcting an error in difficulties in the air or in landing may mean all the difference between a crash and safety. Hence hygienic living is necessary to keep the body and mind in good condition. In addition excellent physical condition permits the body to react with more adequate compensations to altitude and cold.[28]

One notes the Victorian obsession with bowel function extending to contemporary aviation. At the big American advance training school at Issoudun in France in September 1918,

We found that the 575 students, out of the approximate number of 3000 American flyers in France, were as fine a lot of youngsters as one could wish to see; but that, on the whole, their physical condition was bad. Their morale was low, and they had acquired a fatalistic attitude of mind. At that time, there had been about 500 flying hours per day with increasing fatalities, which in August reached the number of 17. There was very little venereal disease, but staleness was common. The men were overeating and under-exercising, constipation being very common.[29]

At the training fields in the United States a non-medical, non-flying officer, his role disguised with an euphemistic title, kept watch over this problem: 'For a period of possibly one or two meals the flyer might be required to fast during purgation or other treatment by the flight surgeon, after which, under the personal supervision of the *nutritional officer,* he might begin to eat again.'[30]

Many strange diagnoses, unknown to today's flight surgeon, were current then to explain the difficulties of the flyer in relation to the novel and frightening world of the air. 'Staleness' was a catch-word describing a condition in experienced flyers, particularly at the Front, which apparently represented chronic anoxia, war neurosis, or a combination of both. 'Fainting in the air' was held to be a frequent cause of air crashes, even at low altitude where anoxia could not be responsible; carbon monoxide from in-line engines with short exhaust stacks certainly was a factor, and at least one documented example represented concealed epilepsy with a grand mal convulsive seizure in the air.[31] Crashes were blamed on bad food and drugs, the fatal accident to the famous Italian flyer, Resnati, in a Caproni bomber at Mineola, allegedly being caused by his taking two aspirins for a cold. Castor oil, used of necessity in rotary engines, was held to produce its characteristic laxative effect on air crew who inhaled the fumes, though this has been denied by some World War I flyers whom the author has questioned on this point.

The flight surgeon, a medical officer with aviation experience attached to flying formations with the special duty of monitoring the health and efficiency of air crew, was an American innovation. The other combatants attached medical men (who had rarely obtained flying experience on their own initiative) to air headquarters as advisers, but the illnesses and injuries of air crew at the Front were referred to physicians at general hospitals in the area. The organization for the care of British flyers in France as late as 1917 emphasizes the small size of the Royal Flying Corps in contrast to the mass armies filling the trenches. Each squadron in the field had a medical orderly attached, but no medical officer. With one Brigade of the RFC attached to each Army, one medical officer was attached to each Brigade and was the first physician to see incapacitated flyers and to decide on their disposition, although he was an Army doctor with no special training in aviation medicine. Beginning in October 1917 the RFC took over a ward of the Army's 24th General Hospital at Etaples in France for the care of unfit flyers; here Captain Dudley Corbett RAMC was in charge. Major James E. Birley RAMC headed the RFC's medical organization in France as chief adviser to the General Officer Commanding. Men considered unfit for further service were sent home to England and invalided out after examination by a medical board. Doctors Birley and Corbett, being inquisitive and interested, learned much about aviation medicine, but the two of them together could hardly give direct attention to the medical problems of the fifty-three squadrons scattered up and down the Front.

American medical officers, studying the aviation facilities of their allies, became convinced of the need for special medical care for their flyers at the Front:

The main thought that Dr Lyster and I brought back with us was that we should not only have a large number of men like Colonel *(sic)* Birley, but that their duties should be just one thing—to determine whether each man was or was not fit to fly. There must be created in the military service an entirely new type of medical officer. He was to do nothing whatever except to be the 'doctor for the pilot'.... This extraordinary creature then needed a military name or title. Colonel Eugene R. Lewis and I were instructed to choose this name. We knew that all military doctors are called Surgeons, so we chose the term 'Flight Surgeon'—the doctor that has to do with flying.[32]

Many of the medical men who had carried out the intake aviation examinations around the country as members of the sixty-seven regional boards were eager to make a further contribution as flight surgeons. After a short, intensive course at the Medical Research Laboratory at Mineola, Long Island, including experience with the Flack rebreather bag and pressure chamber flights up to 35,000 feet equivalent altitude, thirty-two were designated as flight surgeons and assigned to the training fields in the southern and western portions of the United States. Their duties consisted of physical re-examination of trainees every six months, and the medical supervision of all flight personnel. Captain John B. Powers MC outlined the duties involved in a lecture to budding flight surgeons:

He should hold sick call every day. This is for the purpose of keeping in touch with the flyer's physical condition and to enable the flight surgeon to become acquainted with affairs which he might not be able to discover in any other way. Personally, I do not believe the flight surgeon should prescribe or treat except for minor ailments when the patient reports for sick call or in quarters. In regard to those who are sick in the hospital, while the flight surgeon should keep in touch with his men, he should not attempt to treat them there, because of possible conflict with the hospital authorities.

The flight surgeon should make a point of seeing each flyer every day, either on the field, at mess, or in quarters, because he may recognize conditions to which the flyer may pay no attention.

The flight surgeon should keep in intimate touch with the flight commander and with the records of the flying office. He should consider himself as a member of the staff of the flight commander in an advisory capacity, and he must gain the confidence of the flight commander.

The flight surgeon should spend as much time on the flying field as possible, watching for defects in flying, such as bad landings, uncertainties of action, etc., and keep a record of each. For instance, a flyer may start to the ground as if he is going to land, but instead he circles around the field. Still he does not come down although one can see that he expected to do so; but instead he goes around the field again without coming down and repeats this three or four times. When he finally does come down, the flight surgeon should get hold of him, because something of importance in regard to his nervous system, etc., that is just beginning to appear, may be discovered by prompt investigation.[33]

Many of these physicians went through flight training at the wartime fields—Brooks, Carlstrom, Chanute, Kelly, Rockwell and others.[34] Of the wartime flight surgeons, Dr Robert J. Hunter was the first on official orders. The first to be put on flying status was Major William R. Ream MC, and he, too, was the first to die—on 24 August 1918 when he crashed with his Curtiss JN-4 during an Air Service tour of the Middle West.

No flight surgeons as such cared for the men of the Air Service, American Expeditionary Force, in France during the war, though experienced men from the training fields at home would undoubtedly have been sent overseas for the campaigns of 1919. On 30 September 1918 Colonel Wilmer, inspecting the First Pursuit Group, noted that 'at all the aerodromes that we visited at the front, it was noted that the medical men, who were usually exceptionally efficient, did not live in close, constant contact with the flyers as would be the case with flight surgeons.'[35]

By 1917, there was agreement among most medical officers in touch with the problem that oxygen deficiency could impair the performance of air crew above 15,000 feet, and that supplementary oxygen was necessary. Some dissented, notably the researchers at the Italian Psycho-Physiological Institute, which was dominated by the 'acapnia' theory of Professor Angelo Mosso. This physiologist of Turin dogmatically asserted that high-altitude symptoms resulted, not from oxygen deficiency, but from the lowering of carbon dioxide in the alveoli of the lungs by hyperventilation. An American flight surgeon was told by the Italians in December 1917 that:

(1) Oxygen is not necessary for flyers, (2) if given, it should not be pure oxygen, but oxygen 90%, carbon dioxide 10% ... They did not feel that the present heights attained in flying required OXYGEN, and were very definite in their statement that no professors had done as much work on this subject as they had done here in Italy, and that there was no room for argument. (So I did not open any argument.)[36]

Another fallacy was that hyperventilation—forced overbreathing through the mouth—could compensate for low oxygen partial pressures. The German flyers' handbook advised that 'from time to time one may deliberately take several deep breaths. Many flyers have discovered for themselves that through such deep breaths any trace of discomfort can be eliminated. ... Therefore it is advantageous to accustom oneself to breathing with deep inspirations.'[37] Small wonder that many World War I flyers refused to believe that they required oxygen, even when flying above 15,000 feet. It was considered proof of one's masculinity and virility to return from 20,000 feet and boast of 'never having felt better.' These tales reflect on the one hand the fighter pilot's ability to tolerate anoxia for the brief periods that his aircraft could remain at its ceiling, and on the other hand of course, the euphoria which accompanies anoxia and distorts judgment and awareness. An occasional World War I pilot may be found who knew he had had a narrow escape from disaster brought on by anoxia at high altitude. 'I remember how I overshot the field and crashed after a patrol at 19,000 feet,' recalled the late Raymond E. Watts of Naperville, Indiana, formerly flying SE 5a's in No. 84 Squadron, RAF. 'I had a terrific headache when I descended from high altitude, I couldn't think straight, and afterwards realized I had tried to land down-wind. It was oxygen deficiency, of course.'[38] Generally, the medical men, such as Major Birley, found themselves waging an uphill battle to 'popularize' oxygen with the men who needed it most.

As early as 27 March 1917 Birley summed up his experiences, and those of the RFC in the field, with anoxia at high altitude. He observed that the subjective effects of flying at high altitudes varied enormously with the individual; 'a minority of flying officers profess a total ignorance of any symptoms whatever, while others experience them only after they have carried out several flights at high altitudes.'[39] The symptoms included dyspnoea or shortness of breath—'it is usually noticed at about 15,000 feet, and the character of the breathing is described as "gasping" or "panting." It is exaggerated by muscular exertion, such as using the pressure pump, and it is more noticeable in cold weather and cold machines than in warm. Pilots look upon this shortness of breath as something very ordinary, and are not in the least alarmed by it.' Ear complaints such as tinnitus and deafness were said to be exaggerated by high-altitude flying. Fatigue after landing was common: 'It is quite certainly the case that flying at heights over 11,000 to 12,000 feet accelerates the condition, and that the greatest (sic) the height the more lasting is the sense of tiredness.' Other symptoms were blamed on altitude—'fainting and dizziness,' 'nausea and vomiting,' 'pains in one or both ears,' 'frontal headache, 'intense desire to micturate and parched mouth,' 'physical fatigue,' and 'diminished sense of stability.' As Birley remarked, some of these depended on the fall of oxygen pressure, and some on the fall in atmospheric pressure. Many pilots claimed to have become acclimated to high-altitude flying, but 'in my opinion this merely means that they get used to the symptoms thereby induced.'[40] Birley summed up:

I believe that one is justified in concluding that flying at high altitudes (over 15,000 feet) entails additional strain, which will eventually result in a shorter average term of efficiency per pilot; that routine flying above 18,000 feet without artificial aid in a large majority of individuals is not a practical proposition; and that wide benefits are likely to accrue from the adoption of a suitable oxygen apparatus.

The German Navy found its Zeppelin flight crews facing particularly severe demands in the high-altitude raids on England after the autumn of 1916. In 1917 the naval airships began flying at 16,000 feet or above, in 1918 they attained 20,000 feet in flights lasting over twenty hours, of which fourteen hours could be spent above 14,000 feet. No flight surgeons as such guarded the health of the Naval Airship Division, but some of the ground troop doctors took a special interest in the problems of high altitude. One of them, stationed at the Ahlhorn airship base, wrote:

It was interesting for me to observe the crews from the medical aspect during high-altitude flights (5000–6000 metres—16,400–19,700 feet) and extended altitude flights up to eight hours at 6000 metres. Above 4000 metres (13,100 feet) began the well-known altitude symptoms, which manifest themselves as ringing in the ears, dizziness and headache. At greater heights began a marked acceleration of respiration and cardiac activity. Pulse rates of 120 to 150 per minute were by no means uncommon. These serious developments could be controlled only by continuously breathing oxygen from cylinders.[41]

From January to November 1917 the German airships carried gaseous oxygen in cylinders compressed to 150 atmospheres (2200 psi). A sleeve-type reducing valve lowered the pressure, and a needle valve permitted a flow of one, two or four litres per minute depending on the altitude and the number of persons using the apparatus. In most Allied Intelligence accounts of this equipment, the oxygen is described as being delivered to a simple celluloid mask covering both mouth and nose, with an expiratory valve and a valve for drainage of moisture. These valves frequently froze, and for this reason, plus an unwillingness to have the face covered, the airship crews inhaled the gas through a pipe-stem mouthpiece. When four of the eleven Zeppelins participating in the 'Silent Raid' of 19–20 October 1917 were forced down in France, Allied Intelligence officers found on one member of L45's crew a notebook giving specifications of the gaseous oxygen apparatus. The largest oxygen flask, with a volume of 5·5 litres and containing 880 litres of oxygen at atmospheric pressure, weighed thirty-three pounds, the smallest, with a volume of 0·4 litres and a content of sixty-four litres, weighed 8·8 pounds.[42]

Already by then a more efficient apparatus was being introduced, which provided more oxygen for less weight—an important consideration for the hydrogen-filled Zeppelins, for whom high altitude was the only defence. A large, double-walled copper Dewar vacuum flask intended to supply four or five men in one gondola weighed 10·3 kg empty, but held 25·3 kg of the liquefied gas, equal to 12,000 litres of gaseous oxygen; while a smaller edition of the same device, weighing 6·0 kg empty, held 5 kg of liquid oxygen, equal to 4000 litres of the gas. This liquid oxygen device served the Zeppelin crews till the end of the war, and was much better liked than the gaseous oxygen, which was suspected of containing impurities, such as glycerine, that made the men ill. No medical supervision of its use seems to have occurred, the line officers commanding the Zeppelins themselves setting up standing orders that all hands would take oxygen periodically on orders from the control car at altitudes above 16,500 feet. Nobody inhaled the gas continuously, and many bragged of their ability to manage with only a few breaths per hour.

German aeroplane crews made some use of the gaseous oxygen equipment in 1917, but by early 1918 a small Ahrendt & Heylandt liquid oxygen apparatus was being issued. This, with a weight empty of five kg, and seven kg full, provided up to 1800 litres of gaseous oxygen and closely resembled the small apparatus used in the naval airships. The liquid oxygen (actually seventy to eighty per cent oxygen, the remainder being nitrogen) was carried in a spherical double-walled metal flask with charcoal suspended between the walls to absorb residual gas and maintain a more perfect vacuum. Some heat reached the intensely cold liquid oxygen through the walls of the neck of the bottle, sufficient to maintain a head of pressure in the bottle which forced the liquid upwards through a tube into two cylindrical expansion chambers made of copper. Here the liquid gas evaporated, and ascended through coils to a needle flow valve. All this equipment was concealed within a pierced metallic casing designed to protect personnel from frostbite through touching the supercooled evaporating chambers and coils. A rubber bladder served as a regulator, and tubing led off to the pipe-stem mouthpieces of the one or two members of the crew. This equipment was used in some of the Gotha G IV and G V twin-engine bombers which flew at about 15,000 feet with bomb load, and in the Staaken 'Giant' aircraft. Certainly this apparatus served the two-man crew of the high-altitude photographic Rumplers, particularly the *Rubild* with its ceiling of nearly 24,000 feet.

The Heylandt liquid oxygen apparatus provided more of the gas for less weight, compared to compressed gas equipment. Captain Walter M. Boothby MC, later destined to be one of the leading American aeromedical researchers of the 'twenties and 'thirties, reported favourably on the German liquid oxygen apparatus, but his superiors added an adverse endorsement. Much was made of the fact that if the aircraft turned over on the ground the liquid oxygen might spill on the air crew, while live ammunition experiments indicated that if the liquid oxygen made contact with the absorbent charcoal, an intense fire would result. A more serious criticism was that there was no control of the rate at which gaseous oxygen was evolved, and less was produced at high altitude than at sea level. With the needle valve set for two persons, the Ahrendt & Heylandt apparatus produced thirty-one litres per minute at sea level, but only twenty-two litres per minute (measured under standard conditions) at 28,400 feet. This, Allied experimenters felt, might be remedied by an electrical heating coil in the liquid oxygen; a hundred calories of heat could vaporize a litre of liquid air. Another disadvantage was procuring and transporting the liquid oxygen, which was available only in large industrial cities. One Rumpler squadron at Thielt in Belgium received its liquid oxygen containers every four days from Liège, over a hundred miles in the rear. Because the liquid oxygen was constantly evaporating, the contents of the containers boiled off after four days, whether they were used or not.

Boothby's judgement was vindicated by the US Army Air Corps adopting a copy of the German liquid oxygen apparatus about 1923, and the US Air Force uses liquid oxygen today. But American medical men visiting Europe late in 1917 determined to copy one of the Allied gaseous oxygen apparatuses. There were several to choose from.

The 'official' British device was the Siebe-Gorman, manufactured by a firm which had produced diving equipment for over fifty years. The heart of the apparatus was a simple regulator valve with three manual settings; at each setting the amount of oxygen delivered decreased up to 29,750 feet, necessitating a change to the higher setting with ascent. The remainder of the apparatus consisted of one or two oxygen flasks each containing about 500 litres of the gas compressed to 150 atmospheres (2200 psi), a rubber mask covering both nose and mouth (apparently innocent of any valves), and the necessary connecting tubing. The total weight for one person was 24·5 pounds, and 49 pounds for two.

The French Garsaux gaseous oxygen apparatus weighed 11·5 pounds for one person, and 20 pounds for two, and supplied gas for $2\frac{1}{2}$ hours. But it was otherwise severely criticized by AEF investigators because there were no indicators of the quantity of gas remaining in the tanks, or of the rate of flow; there was a rubber diaphragm which cracked and leaked easily; the rate of flow was variable, depending on springs whose tension varied with different conditions of moisture, use, dust and rust; and the mask was clumsy, with inflatable edges which 'balloons out and becomes very hard at high altitudes',[43] while the metal portions of the mask might touch the face and cause frostbite.

Much better liked by both the British and French services was an apparatus designed by a British medical officer, Major George Dreyer, RAMC:

> The best instrument in all Europe today is the Dryer *(sic)* instrument. It is considered so good and valuable that, one by one, as these instruments are slowly produced, they are rushed to the Front by automobile. They are made in Paris by a Major Dreyer,[44] who belongs to the Zone of the Advance of the Royal Flying Corps. The British do not care to have any of the types provided to them from home when they can get the Dreyer instrument.[45]

The chief advantage of the Dreyer apparatus was a cleverly-designed aneroid-controlled regulator, which increased the rate of flow automatically from 0·22 litres per minute at sea level to 2·32 litres per minute at 29,750 feet. Other advantages were: indicators for residual oxygen in the cylinders, a metal diaphragm protected by a metal valve device which delivered a constant flow irrespective of external conditions or continued use; and a mask which was small, light, comfortable, and could not cause frostbite.

Manufacture of the Dreyer apparatus commenced in April 1917 and by 1 December of that year, some forty of fifty examples were in use with the RFC at the Front. Exactly which squadrons used the Dreyer equipment cannot be determined, but it is evident that the high-flying De Havilland DH 4 squadrons were the first to receive it. 'Three DH 4 squadrons are now completely equipped with oxygen apparatus, and use it as a routine in spite of the extra weight entailed and various disadvantages with regard to the present type of mask,'[46] wrote Major Birley in late 1917. 'It should be pointed out that flying at or above 18,000 feet is still the exception rather than the rule. The DH 4 is the only machine that maintains such an altitude for any length of time, although during the last summer one or two Bristol "Fighter" squadrons were carrying out patrols at 17,000 to 19,000 feet of two to two and a half hours' duration.'[47] In June 1918, however, only one Bristol Fighter of No. 88 Squadron was fitted with oxygen equipment. It might appear that some single-seater fighter squadrons were equipped with oxygen apparatus, but the squadron numbers and aircraft types are not stated. Initially, the single seaters were expected to do without: 'The comparative immunity which scout pilots certainly enjoy is largely explained by the fact that they do not maintain great altitudes for very long, and that the actual fighting, with very few exceptions, takes place at 15,000 feet or very much lower.'[48] Even the Dreyer apparatus was not acceptable to many air crew, and Birley admitted, 'the whole question of popularizing oxygen depends on the recognition of the necessity of providing the individual with an apparatus which he prefers to use than do without. And in this connection, too much stress cannot be laid on the mask, because here we are right up against the individual, and the wide use of oxygen resolves itself in the end into the provision of a comfortable mask which pilots will use.'[49] In practice, as indicated by the experience of No. 55 Squadron on high-altitude reconnaissance missions, masks apparently froze and the Dreyer aneroid regulator proved temperamental: 'The crew carried a spare cylinder with a piece of pitot tubing leading to pilot and observer: this was found to be better.'[50]

A summary by Major Birley provides a partial picture of oxygen equipment in use by the RFC at end of 1917:[51]

		Type of Regulator	Cylinder with valve	Duration of supply at 2 litres per minute per person
1. Scout	Pilot	Dreyer (5 lb)	(300 l.) 5 lb	$2\frac{1}{4}$ hr
2. 2-seater fighter	Pilot and	Dreyer (5 lb)	(500 l.) 7 lb	$2\frac{1}{2}$ hr
	Observer			$1\frac{1}{4}$ hr
3. DH 4	Pilot and	Dreyer (5 lb)	(500 l.) 7 lb	4 hr
	Observer			4 hr
4. Long bomber	Pilot and	SG Mark II-2	(500 l. each) 14 lb	8 hr
	Observer	SG Mark II-2	(500 l. each) 14 lb	4 hr each

The standard American oxygen apparatus of World War I was the Dreyer modified for mass production in the United States. On 5 December 1917 the American aero mission in Europe recommended producing $700,000 worth of the Dreyer apparatus, and by 31 May 1918 two hundred sets had been sent to France. By the end of the war 5000 sets of oxygen equipment had been built in the United States, of which 2300 had been shipped overseas.[52] Along with high-pressure oxygen bottles containing 500 litres of oxygen compressed to 150 atmospheres, the American equipment embodied the aneroid-controlled regulator and a rubber mask (without valves) held to the face by a leather apron. This was of course a continuous-flow type of equipment. The mask had an aperture for a microphone for intercommunication with other crew members. The total weight of a single set without cylinders was only four pounds. Each DH 4 aircraft sent from America to France had low-pressure oxygen tubing installed together with holes for mounting the oxygen equipment, and brackets for carrying the oxygen cylinders. There is no record of oxygen being used operationally by any of the eight American squadrons flying American-built DH 4s in France.

With air crew being exposed to very low temperature in open cockpits at altitudes up to 18,000 feet or more, protective flight clothing was the chief defence against cold. This was the day of helmet, goggles, silk scarves, leather coats, long hip boots and fur-lined gloves. The American Air Service flight suit was a one-piece affair, waterproof externally and fur-lined, the preferred animal pelt being that of the Chinese Nuchwang dog. Some 500,000 dog skins were contracted for on behalf of the American Air Service before the Armistice. Muskrat-fur gauntlets and sheepskin-lined leather moccasins extending well up the calf completed the outfit. All services developed electrically-heated suit liners, gloves and socks, but these were rarely used, principally because few aircraft of the day possessed suitable electrical systems. The air crew of the high altitude DH 4s of No. 55 Squadron, RFC, wore electrically-heated flight suits; burns of the fingers were complained of. Frostbite received little attention compared to World War II; the lower incidence reflected shorter flights at lower ceilings than in the later conflict. Cheeks and noses could be frostbitten in winter by the cold blast of the slipstream; whale oil was rubbed on these exposed surfaces, and leather masks covered the entire face, leaving holes only for the mouth and eyes. While goggles were routinely worn to protect the eyes from air blast, some individualistic fighter pilots refused to wear them, claiming better vision without them. The penalty after some weeks of such flying was a chronic irritation and conjunctivitis.

It is curious to find that with the exaggerated attention being given to vestibular function, the problem of equalizing pressure in the middle ear was neglected in World War I. As an aircraft ascends, the excess air pressure within the middle ear cavity normally vents itself without conscious attention, but the Eustachian tubes leading from the middle ear to the throat terminate in a flap valve which will prevent the entrance of air during a descent. Only by voluntary action—swallowing, yawning, sometimes by holding the nose and blowing—can the flap valve be opened to permit the entrance of air. The greater the difference in pressure, the more difficult it becomes to vent the middle ear during the descent. Increasingly severe pain, with inflammation of the ear drum, will be present by the time the flyer reaches the ground—a condition later designated aero-otitis media, signifying an inflammation of the ear caused by flying. The condition is even more prone to occur if the throat and opening of the Eustachian tube are swollen and inflamed, as with a head cold.

The instructions for the US Army Air Service physical examination in World War I fail to mention the Eustachian tubes, whose patency and freedom from chronic disease should be determined in any candidate for flying. With high-altitude flying in low temperatures in the last two years of the war, medical officers in France became aware of the need to instruct aviators in the act of venting the ears, particularly in descent. That flying with a head cold invited acute ear trouble was recognized. Repeated high-altitude flights, particularly with the long dives which were the favourite attack manœuvre of the single-seater fighters of the day, often led to an intractible aero-otitis media that was only relieved by taking the aviator off flying duty. Many suffered premature loss of hearing. This was the case with a significant proportion of World War I Zeppelin crew members, who in the last two years of the conflict were making flights of twelve hours or more above 14,000 feet.

Perhaps the most serious failure of aviation medicine in World War I was the permanent loss from flying duty of many trained men due to flying fatigue and/or war neurosis. Lacking knowledge of flying and the peculiar stresses associated with it, Army and Navy medical officers were unaware of the problem, and no preventive or therapeutic measures were taken to deal with it. No flight surgeons were with the squadrons to note the early symptoms, and to ground a flyer and send him on rest leave. If his condition did not cause him to crash or fall victim to enemy aircraft, the flyer was finally diagnosed as 'stale' and invalided home.

A few medical officers especially interested in aviation became aware of the syndrome and wrote of 'flying fatigue' in terms meaningful to the present-day flight surgeon. The following is by Captain Dudley Corbett, RAMC, in charge of RFC patients at the 24th General Hospital, Etaples, France:

A man first notices that he is beginning to feel generally tired, and that he has lost some of his original keenness. His sleep does not refresh him. He gets occasional headaches. Later he does not get off to sleep quite so well as he did, or he may get off fairly soon, and yet wake up early in the morning. He may lose his appetite. . . . His sleep may be troubled with dreams of flying and fighting, and nightmares of all kinds. He may notice that he is getting irritable, and that he cannot stand the society of his friends 'en masse,' but prefers to go off by himself and read. He probably feels quite fit and keen in the air, but has to force himself to go up. After landing, he may be shaky and feel utterly exhausted. . . . To keep himself going, he may rely on alcohol, although this tendency is rare, but he nearly always smokes too much, for which no one can blame him. He may cease to take trouble about his flying and fighting tactics. Tired pilots have confessed to me that they have got into a frame of mind, when, if they meet any enemy machine, they feel that they must either turn tail or go for it recklessly; they cannot trouble to think about manœuvring. I am not sure that many good pilots have not met their end from sheer carelessness. They become too tired to think.[53]

Dr Corbett recommended regular rest days for all flying personnel at the Front, and rest stations some ten miles from the aerodrome where men could be sent when suffering from flying fatigue, the emotional effects of a crash, or minor physical illness. In practice, it was up to the squadron commanders to 'look out for tired pilots,' the brigade medical officers acting as advisers. At one time RFC flyers were being sent home for duty in England without medical examination, but Major Birley arranged in 1917 for all flying fatigue cases to be sent to the 24th General Hospital for study and treatment. There were also definite policies for leave and rotation which offered some hope of relief to air crew tired out by the fighting in France. Each man received fourteen days' leave in England every three months, and could expect to be reassigned home after five or six months in fighter, long-range reconnaissance, and bomber squadrons, and after seven to nine months in artillery observation squadrons. 'A good artillery pilot will get through, in rough figures, 350 to 450 hours before he goes home; a good scout pilot 150 to 250 or 300 hours.'[54]

The medical effects of acceleration were likewise ignored. Radial acceleration was considered a problem for the designer rather than the air crew; only in 1917, with the development of powerful engines and fighter aircraft able to exceed 100 mph, was it realized that G forces in steep banks, pull-ups from dives, and snap rolls could cause structural failure in the wood and fabric biplanes of the day. Visual disturbances during tight turns were reported as curiosities by an English neurologist, Sir Henry Head, who related of a pilot that 'the sky appeared to be so grey just before he fainted while doing a tight turn at 4·6 G.'[55] In France, Garsaux made a few experiments on dogs in a centrifuge in 1918; these apparently involved negative G forces, for he reported brain haemorrhage and injury.

H. Graeme Anderson, Surgeon Lieutenant, Royal Navy, who spent his four years of wartime duty with the Royal Naval Air Service and who himself learned to fly at one of the training schools, seems to stand alone in his careful attention to the medical effects of linear deceleration, i.e. the aeroplane accident. An article on the subject in the *Journal of the Royal Navy Medical Service* for January 1918 was illustrated with a fascinating and unique series of crash photographs to form a chapter in his aeromedical classic, *The Medical and Surgical Aspects of Aviation*. He presented a series of fifty-eight crashes in six months of flying at one training school in England, involving 4000 flying hours and 9000 flights. In contrast to the high casualty rate at many American schools both in the United States and France, there were only sixteen injured and one killed. Most accidents, including the fatal one, occurred in landing attempts. The causes were listed as 'defect in aeroplane,' 'error of judgment in flying,' 'loss of head,' 'brain fatigue,' 'fear,' 'physical illness,' and 'unavoidable.'[56] Drawing on his experience, Anderson called attention to the frequency with which the head and face were injured by striking the cowling or instrument panel; the likelihood that in a severe crash with a pusher type aeroplane the flight crew would be crushed by the rear-mounted engine falling on them; while in the tractor type machine the forward cockpit (usually occupied by the student) would be demolished, while the rear cockpit usually remained intact. There was a considerable discussion of the value of the safety belt; Anderson held that in pusher machines it should be unfastened just before landing so that in the event of a crash the pilot would be thrown free instead of being buried under the engine.[57] From his own experience Anderson recommended flying to the scene of crashes away from the field. 'An injured aviator should never be dragged out of a crash except in case of fire, but rather the wrecked machine should be cut away from him. In many cases this prevents simple fractures from being converted into compound ones.'[58] Hence the emergency crash kit should contain crowbars, wire cutters, a saw, 'a long stout knife,' a hammer, strong scissors for cutting fabric and a fire extinguisher. In a chapter on 'The Surgery of Aviation,' Anderson drew attention to fractures of the astragulus (one of the bones in the ankle joint), an injury rare in ordinary civil life, but so common in air crashes that he proposed the label of 'aviator's astragulus.' The apparent reason that this lesion was so common then, and is again rare today, is that aeroplanes of the period had a rudder *bar,* which in a crash transmitted impact forces upward through the victim's instep. Often the astragulus bone was split, sometimes crushed, and in one fatal crash 'one astragulus was fractured and shot clean through the skin and free from the body.'[59] Nowadays, of course, the rudder is controlled by pedals, usually toe-actuated.

Anderson, incidentally, was determinedly opposed to a cherished tradition of his day—'before there was much medical interest in or supervision over flying, if a pupil crashed and was apparently uninjured, he was ordered to go up again in another machine almost immediately. This was supposed to prevent loss of nerve or if momentarily lost by the crash to facilitate the immediate recovery of it. The author has seen the results of this method of treatment, and can say emphatically it is a method to be condemned; he is sure that most experienced instructors will agree with him in this.'[60]

Parachutes for the saving of life were used by balloon observers from early in the war, as noted in Chapter 1. For a time in early 1917, following heavy losses over England, the crews of the German naval Zeppelins were issued parachutes. These were of the 'attached' type, similar to those used by the balloonists; but none were used in drops from airships, in an emergency or otherwise. Shortly the parachutes were withdrawn, as each weighed eighteen pounds and the airship commanders realized that high altitude was their best defence against attacking aeroplanes.

The Germans were the only nation to use parachutes in aeroplanes for the saving of life before the end of World War I. Named after its developer, the Heinicke parachute was of the attached type, but with a difference. Observing that the balloon type parachute, attached to the aircraft, tended to foul the tail surfaces, Herr Heinicke packed his 'chute in a sack attached to the aircrew member. As he went over the side, a 50-pound break cord attached to the aircraft, and supposedly long enough to clear the tail surfaces, pulled the canopy out of the bag. The 'chute, made of muslin or silk, had twenty gores and twenty shroud lines around the periphery, and could be spilled on landing by pulling on a central shroud line running to the round vent in the centre. The shroud lines led to a webbing harness which circled the waist, shoulders and thighs. American Air Service investigators after the war dismissed the Heinicke 'chute with the contemptuous remark, 'presents no interesting features, as it failed with a 200-pound weight at 100 miles per hour.'[61] Yet it saved the lives of many German air crew in the desperate last summer of the war, and caused Allied flyers to question why their own governments did not provide them with similar equipment.

Ernst Udet, second highest scoring German World War I ace with sixty-two victories, saved his life by parachute on 29 June 1918 when he was shot up in an attack on a French Breguet:

I received several hits, including one in the machine guns, and another in the tank. Simultaneously, my elevator and aileron control cables must have been shot through, as my Fokker D VII dived out of control. I tried everything possible, both with the throttle and rudder, to bring the aircraft under control but in vain. At about 500 metres (1600 feet) altitude my aircraft was in a vertical dive and could not be brought out of this position. It was high time to get out. I unfastened my safety belt and stood up on my seat and the next moment was blown aft by the terrific air blast. Simultaneously I sustained a heavy jolt and realized that I had become hung up by my parachute harness on the forward tip of the rudder. With my last ounce of strength I broke the tip off and plunged free behind the aircraft, tumbling over and over. I had already assumed that the parachute had failed when suddenly I felt a gentle deceleration and shortly afterwards struck the ground. The parachute had opened only at an altitude of about 80 metres (260 feet). The resulting landing was rather hard and I sprained my left ankle.[62]

Other German flyers died in attempts to escape by parachute from crippled or burning aircraft. On 10 August 1918 Germany's third ranking ace, Erich Loewenhardt, victor in fifty-three air combats, collided with a squadron mate of the Richthofen *Jagdgeschwader* during a dogfight. With the right upper wing of his Fokker D VII shattered by the wheels of Loewenhardt's aircraft, Leutnant Wentz saved his life by jumping with his parachute. But Loewenhardt, abandoning his apparently undamaged aircraft, died when his 'chute failed to open. Probably the static cord broke or was severed without drawing the parachute from its pack.

Among the many ways in which World War I changed our civilization was through the establishment of the science of aviation medicine. Such men as Birley, Corbett, Lyster and Jones had laid a foundation on which others were to build, in further research on anoxia and oxygen equipment, radial and linear acceleration, neuropsychiatry in aviation, parachutes and other protective and safety equipment. Much of this was elaborated further in the period between the wars, with the result that World War II—which marked the coming of age of air power—was fought with sound knowledge of the aeromedical problems assailing the men who manned the fleets of fighters and bombers of the Allied and Axis air forces.

[1] John R. Cuneo, *Winged Mars* (Harrisburg: Military Service Publishing Co., 1947), vol. II, pp. 1–7.

[2] The Fokker synchronizing gear was not the first invented: a Swiss engineer, Franz Schneider, had obtained a patent in 1913 for a similar device, but the German authorities had shown no interest in it.

[3] Elliott White Springs, *War Birds: Diary of an Unknown Aviator* (New York: George H. Doran Co., 1926), p. 232.

[4] Rudolf Stark, *Jagdstaffel Unsere Heimat* (Leipzig: Verlag von K. F. Koehler, 1932), p. 106.

[5] *War Birds*, p. 221.

[6] Sholto Douglas, *Years of Combat* (London: Collins, 1963), p. 217.

[7] John Milner in *Cross & Cockade*, vol. 6, no. 2, Summer 1965, p. 152.

[8] Douglas H. Robinson, *The Zeppelin in Combat* (London: Foulis, 1962), p. xv.

[9] See G. W. Haddow and Peter M. Grosz, *The German Giants* (London: Putnam & Co., Ltd, 1962).

[10] Peter M. Grosz, personal communication.

[11] B. J. Silly, *R.A.F. Quarterly*, March 1931. Courtesy M. C. Armstrong, Silsoe, Bedford, England.

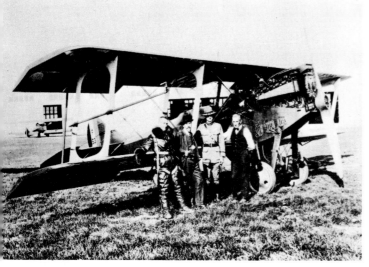

17. The Packard-Le-Pere LUSAC II flown by Major Rudolph Schroeder to a new altitude record of 33,115 feet on 27 February 1920, and by Lieut. John Macready to 34,510 feet on 28 September 1921. Note turbosupercharger on front of engine. Macready is at left. (Air Force Museum)

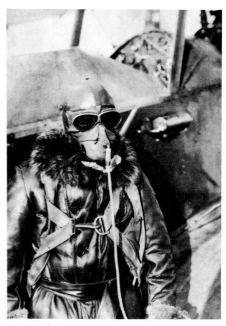

18. Lieut. John A. Macready dressed for a high altitude flight. Oxygen tube leads to pipe-stem mouthpiece; the mask is simply to protect the face from freezing (1921). (Air Force Museum)

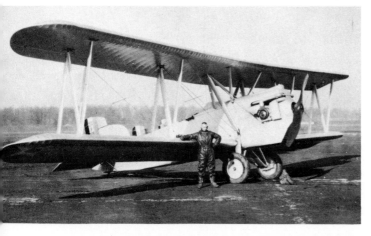

19. Lieut. Macready alongside the XC05-A high altitude aircraft in which he reached a record height of 38,704 feet on 29 January 1926. Note turbo-supercharger on right side of engine. (Air Force Museum)

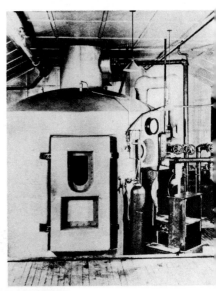

20. The first high altitude chamber at the medical research laboratory at Mineola, New York, 1918. (Edward H. White II Memorial Museum)

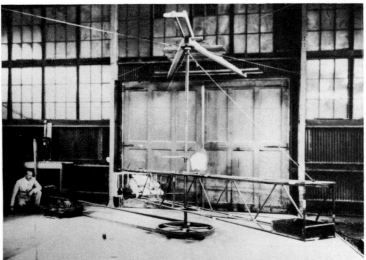

21. The first human centrifuge at the Aero Medical Laboratory, Wright Field, in 1935. (Edward H. White II Memorial Museum)

22. 'The first successful pressure cabin airplane to be flown anywhere in the world.' The U.S. Army Air Corps' pressurized Lockheed XC-35, delivered in 1937. (Air Force Museum)

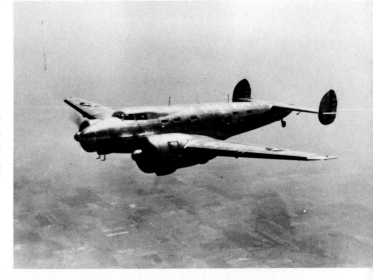

[12] Sholto Douglas, p. 309.

[13] Ira Jones, *King of Air Fighters* (London: Ivor Nicholson & Watson Ltd, 1935), p. 19.

[14] Harry G. Armstrong, *Principles and Practice of Aviation Medicine* (Baltimore: Williams & Wilkins Co., 1939), p. 28.

[15] War Dept., Stencil no. 1092, 'Problems in Aviation from the Point of View of Medical Officers Recently Returned from England, France, and Italy, and Outlining the Immediate Needs of our Service at Home and Abroad,' 20 April 1918, p. 7.

[16] War Dept., Stencil no. 226, 'Psycho-Physiological Examination of Aviators' (translated from *La Nature*, Paris, 6 May 1916), 14 July 1917.

[17] War Dept., Air Service, Division of Military Aeronautics, *Air Service Medical* (Washington: Government Printing Office, 1919), p. 30.

[18] William H. Wilmer, *Aviation Medicine in the AEF* (Washington: Government Printing Office, 1920), p. 248.

[19] Isaac Jones, Discussion, *Journal of Aviation Medicine*, vol. 5, no. 4, December 1934.

[20] Isaac Jones, 'Blind Flying,' *Journal of Aviation Medicine*, vol. 6, no. 4, December 1935, p. 124.

[21] Isaac Jones, *Flying Vistas* (Philadelphia: J. B. Lippincott Co., 1937), p. 94.

[22] *Air Service Medical*, p. 63.

[23] Wilmer, p. 156.

[24] *ibid.*, p. 50.

[25] Der Kommandierende General der Luftstreitkräfte, Sanitäts-Abteilung, *Einflüsse des Fliegens auf dem menschlichen Körper und ärztliche Ratschläge für Flieger*, 2. Auflage, Januar 1918, pp. 18–21.

[26] *ibid.*, p. 23.

[27] War Dept., Chief of Air Service Training, 'Physiology, Physical Inaptitude, Hygiene of the Aviator' (by Doctor Guibert, from Report of Inspection-Générale, French Aviation Schools and Depts., May 1917), vol. I, no. 32, 9 Febuary 1918.

[28] Wilmer, p. 105.

[29] Wilmer, p. 17. The reasons for the notoriously high accident rate at Issoudun were complex. Worn-out, cast-off French aircraft, too rapid progress to tricky *chasse* types, and flying orders coming from non-flying senior officers all played a part (interview 1 May 1965 with Colonel Harold Marshall, 88th Aero Squadron, AEF).

[30] *Air Service Medical*, p. 415.

[31] H. Graeme Anderson, *The Medical and Surgical Aspects of Aviation* (London: Henry Froude and Hodder & Stoughton, 1919), pp. 147–8.

[32] Jones, *Flying Vistas*, p. 209–10.

[33] Wilmer, p. 48.

[34] They were not the first military medical men to fly—as early as 1913, Staff Surgeon H. V. Wells RN, and Captain E. G. R. Lithgow RAMC had voluntarily taken their aviator's certificates in England. In 1916, Colonel Ralph Green became the first American medical officer ordered to fly.

[35] Wilmer, p. 24.

[36] Stencil no. 1092, p. 37. The flight surgeon was Isaac Jones.

[37] *Einflüsse des Fliegens*, p. 12.

[38] Interview with Raymond E. Watts, Dayton, Ohio, 15 June 1963.

[39] Stencil no. 1092, Major James L. Birley RAMC, 'Memorandum on the Effects of High Flying Under Active Service Conditions,' 27 March 1917, p. 14.

[40] Birley in *Bulletin of the Information Service, Air Service, A.E.F.*, vol. IV, No. 182, 23 March 1918, p. 5.

[41] Marine-Stabsarzt der Reserve Dr Nonhoff, 'Bericht über mein Kommando als Trupparzt der III. M.L.T. in Ahlhorn,' in Fritz Strahlmann (ed.), *Zwei deutsche Luftschiffhäfen des Weltkrieges, Ahlhorn u. Wildeshausen* (Oldenburg: Oldenburger Verlagshaus Lindenallee, 1926), p. 92.

[42] Also found aboard one of these airships was a Draeger 'B' type self-contained breathing apparatus, with a half-litre reservoir of oxygen compressed to 150 atmospheres, and a canister of sodium hydroxide to absorb carbon dioxide and water vapour. Though Allied Air Intelligence assumed this was carried to enable the sailmaker to work inside the hydrogen-filled gas cells, I have never heard of such use in my discussions with former German naval airship personnel.

[43] War Department, Stencil no. 654, 17 November 1917.

[44] The small factory where they were made was owned and operated by M. Jacques de Lestang (Jones, *Flying Vistas*, p. 198).

[45] Letter, B. S. Gorrell, SC, Air Service, to Chief Signal Officer, Washington, DC, Paris, 25 September 1917. In *Bulletin of the Information Section, Air Service, A.E.F.*, vol. III, no. 117, 22 April 1918.

[46] Stencil no. 1092, p. 13.

[47] *Bulletin of the Information Section, Air Service, A.E.F.*, vol. IV, no. 182, 6 June 1918, p. 3. (The Order of Battle for the RFC on 31 July 1917, shows Squadrons Nos. 11, 22 and 48 equipped with Bristol Fighters, and Nos. 55, 57, 25 and 18 with DH 4s.)

[48] *ibid.*, p. 3.

[49] Stencil no. 1092, p. 13.

[50] Letter, M. C. Armstrong, 5 May 1965.

[51] Stencil no. 1092, p. 13.

[52] Benedict Crowell, *America's Munitions 1917–18* (Washington: Government Printing Office, 1919), p. 321.

[53] Stencil no. 1092, p. 21.

[54] Stencil no. 1092, p. 10.

[55] William J. White, *A History of the Centrifuge in Aerospace Medicine* (Santa Monica: Douglas Aircraft Company, Inc., 1964), chapter I.

[56] Anderson, p. 142.

[57] Shoulder harness was worn by British, French, American and German fighter pilots in 1917–18. The British Sutton harness 'was made of four stout webbing straps securely fastened to the aircraft, one over each thigh and one over each shoulder. These straps had brass eyelets about $1\frac{1}{2}$ inches apart which made the harness readily adjustable to any size of pilot as he strapped himself in. First, eyelets of the thigh straps at a suitable length were threaded over a cone-shaped pin and then the shoulder straps were similarly threaded on the cone which was positioned in the region of the abdomen. A hole of about $\frac{3}{8}$ in. diameter was drilled through the cone-pin near the top. When all four straps were in position a robust polished-steel split-pin was passed through the hole to secure the straps in position. A stout raw-hide thong was attached to the head of the split-pin. When the thong was pulled out and the split-pin withdrawn the harness fell apart due to the cone shape of the pin on which the eyelets were threaded' (Major W. Geoffrey Moore, *Early Bird* (London: Putnam, 1963), p. 135). Since the object was to hold the pilot firmly in his seat during dogfights, not to prevent injuries in crashes, the shoulder harness was forgotten after the Armistice—only to be revived ten years later as a safety measure.

[58] Anderson, p. 150.

[59] *ibid.*, p. 194.

[60] *ibid.*, p. 105.

[61] US Navy, Bureau of Aeronautics, *Rigid Airship Manual* (Washington: Government Printing Office, 1927), pp. vii–3.

[62] Karl Bodenschatz, *Jagd in Flanderns Himmel* (Munich: Verlag Knorr & Hirth, 1935), p. 110.

4

The Golden Years and the Seed-Time of Aviation Medicine: 1919–38

With affectionate nostalgia, the grown-up boys of my generation recall the years between the wars, the romantic reign of the biplane.[1] This was the time of the barnstormers—the gypsy birdmen flying war-surplus Jennies or shinier Waco 9s or 10s with single-ignition OX-5 engines, who hopped our more reckless seniors out of the local cow-pasture. This was the time of the airmail pilot, forging a new communications link across the vast continent in his open-cockpit Post Office De Havilland. This was the hey-day of the air racers, military and civilian, flashing around the checkered pylons a few feet above the ground. It was the snarling biplane fighter throwing itself about the sky, upside down or right side up—Army Curtiss Hawks and Boeing P-12s glistening in olive drab and orange, Navy F6Cs and F4Bs resplendent in silver and chrome-yellow—and both with the symmetrical red white and blue star in a circle painted large on their wing tips. It was the time of the rigid airship, the most gigantic creation of man ever to leave the earth, moving with slow, silent majesty across the heavens. It was Billy Mitchell leading his Martin bombers to sink battleships off the Virginia Capes, and Admiral Moffett going to his death in the dirigible *Akron* off Barnegat. It was black headlines acclaiming Alcock and Brown, Nungesser and Coli, Charles Lindbergh, Kingsford-Smith and many others, for risking everything to span the ocean in overloaded planes.

This was also the era in which aviation medicine had its true beginnings, with the founding of schools of aviation medicine in the United States Army and Navy and establishment of the Aero Medical Research Laboratory at Wright Field, Ohio. This period saw the evolution of improved oxygen equipment, the free-type parachute, the earliest pressure suits and pressure cabins. 'Blind flying' was as much a medical as a technical accomplishment.

So diverse, so colourful and so rapid were the aeronautical developments of the Golden Years that the historian is hard put to present the events of the period in capsule form. Yet aviation was not then the giant that it has become in our day. In the democracies, all but a handful of visionaries and enthusiasts turned their backs on the aeroplane after the 1918 armistice. Within a few months the air forces of the victorious powers vanished to almost nothing. Governments and men of money saw no future for what had been generally thought of as a weapon of war, now outmoded for ever by treaty. For the remnant of struggling believers, 'the greatest hazard in aviation was starving to death.'[2]

By contrast, the future Axis powers, bent on conquest, had been quick to comprehend the dominant role that air power would play in the next world struggle, and were not only spending large sums on aircraft design and development, but also on publicity campaigns designed to make the citizenry air-minded, and even to get their youth into the air in gliders and light planes.

Germany, the loser in World War I, was denied any semblance of an air force by the Versailles Treaty. Yet the German public was as air-minded as any in the world, and the General Staff, faced with the difficult task of evading treaty restrictions and rebuilding German military power, fully intended to possess a matching air arm when the day of reckoning arrived. Reconstruction of the German Air Force began long before Hitler became chancellor in 1933. Former military aircraft builders, prevented from developing their products at home, simply established factories abroad, financed by secret German Army funds—Dornier in Italy, Rohrbach and Junkers in Sweden. During the French occupation of the Ruhr in 1923, Hans von Seeckt, the Chief of the General Staff, even ordered through a dummy corporation a hundred fighter aircraft from the Fokker factory in Holland. Completed too late for the crisis, the Type XIV biplanes were sent to a flying school at Lipetsk in Russia, maintained by the Red Air Force for training German military airmen. Similarly, the German airline, *Lufthansa,* provided instruction and experience for potential German Air Force bomber pilots and navigators. The Germans threw themselves with particular enthusiasm into gliding. As early as 1920 the first glider meet took place in the Rhön mountains, and by 1922 a glider had stayed aloft for an hour of slope soaring. By the late 1920s, wide-winged German sail planes of advanced aerodynamic design were setting cross-country records, and other countries were beginning to take notice. Hitler and his air minister, World War I ace Hermann Goering, were building on a sound foundation when they secretly prepared for the revival of the German Air Force.

Japan, particularly its younger Army and Navy officers, took up aviation with enthusiasm, and the first flights in the country were made by foreign-trained Army officers in 1910.[3] Following the Armistice the armed services imported foreign instructors and war-surplus aircraft. From the beginning the Japanese Army Air Force was conceived of as a ground-support arm. In the Navy, on the other hand, certain younger officers saw the revolutionary offensive possibilities of the aircraft, and with encouragement from higher authority (though the Imperial Navy also had its 'gun club') laid the foundations for a powerful carrier air arm. The first Japanese carrier was completed in 1923. There followed the two giants, *Akagi* and *Kaga,* which, like *Saratoga* and *Lexington,* were converted from capital ship hulls under the terms of the Washington Treaty.

The aircraft equipping these early Japanese 'flat tops' were entirely of native construction. Though enthusiastic amateurs had turned out a variety of weird prototypes, the government turned to the large industrial firms, such as Kawasaki Shipyard Co. and Mitsubishi Heavy Industries, for its aircraft. For some years the Japanese companies produced copies of foreign machines. For a brief period, alien designers were responsible for home-grown aircraft. Thus, several Kawasaki prototypes were designed by Germany's Claude Dornier and his assistants. Aircraft of completely Japanese design and construction equipped the Emperor's forces during the Manchurian Incident of 1931, the first agression that led to World War II. By 1936, Japan was ahead of her prospective oponents, with the first monoplane fighter for carrier use ('Claude,' to the Allies in the Pacific war), and a long-range twin-engined bomber ('Nell') which reflected the determination of Admiral Isoroku Yamamoto to control the Pacific Ocean with land-based bombers.

Italy, following Mussolini's seizure of power in 1922, created an independent air force and with much bombast, embraced the aeroplane as a symbol of Fascist youth and progressiveness. Even before Hitler employed the technique, Mussolini was using his air force as a weapon of blackmail in his increasingly reckless adventures in Ethiopia and Spain, and by 1939 the Italian *Regia Aeronautica* was conceded to be the leading power in the central Mediterranean.

In the democracies, the attitudes of the leaders towards air power reflected the controlling views of their constituents, who genuinely believed in universal disarmament as a preventative of war. The military services existed on sufferance, and perforce, the airmen, more or less reluctantly, became showmen putting on spectacular displays designed to hold the attention of the public. So meagre and limited were the air forces of Britain and the United States that it is not surprising to find them dominated in this period by a handful of strong personalities.

Thus, the history of the Royal Air Force between the wars is identified with Marshal of the Royal Air Force Lord Trenchard, who served as Chief of the Air Staff from 1919 to 1929. The original exponent (at least on the Allied side) of the long-range strategic bomber force, Trenchard, far from creating the great aerial striking organization he had envisaged in 1918, was hard pressed to prevent his rivals at the Admiralty and the War Office from dismembering the Royal Air Force between them.[4] One expedient was the annual Hendon Air Pageant, in which crack squadrons thrilled the London crowds with low-altitude aerobatics, precision formation flying, and mock air attacks. Another was record-setting with specially-built aircraft. At various times during this period the RAF held the non-stop long distance record, the altitude record, and with three straight victories in the Schneider Trophy race, it held the world's speed record and gained enormously in prestige and in knowledge of high-speed aircraft and high-powered engines. Yet the RAF's operational aircraft during this period tended to repeat the examples of World War I—'redesigning biplanes of the wood era in high strength alloy steel.'[5] Stationary radial engines replaced the World War I rotaries, but the early fighters of the 1920s, such as the Gloster Grebe and Gamecock, were still of wooden construction. Nor did the later Armstrong-Whitworth Siskins and Bristol Bulldogs, all metal in structure but still fabric covered, differ greatly in configuration or performance. In the Gloster Gauntlet and Gladiator the RAF continued to operate biplane fighters through the 1930s and into the monoplane era, while a few of them were in combat in World War II. The bombers likewise were boxy, wire-festooned twin-engined variations of those of the late World War I period—the Vickers Virginia differing little from the Vimy, the Handley-Page Hyderabad resembling the 0/400, and the Hinadini being the Hyderabad with metal framework. Nor was there any move to create a long-range bomber force in England.[6] Most of the RAF's aircraft between the wars were Army Co-operation types—two-seater open-cockpit biplanes such as the Armstrong-Whitworth Atlas and Westland Wapiti—and most of its Squadrons were overseas, maintaining the peace in Iraq and on the North-West Frontier of India.

In the United States it was Brigadier General William Mitchell who placed his stamp indelibly, for better or for worse, on American aviation during this period. Learning to fly in 1916, Mitchell served as Chief of the Air Service of the First Army Group in the St Mihiel and Meuse–Argonne offensives of 1918, and returned to the shores of America with a vision of the aeroplane playing a decisive role in future wars. As Assistant Chief of the Air Service between 1919 and 1925, he employed every publicity device to keep the Army Air Service, and the issue of air power, before the American public.[7]

Beginning as early as October 1919, when seventy-four open-cockpit biplanes flew from New York to San Francisco and return in the first transcontinental reliability test, Mitchell kept the Air Service on the front pages of the newspapers with one spectacular exploit after another. One of these was the first non-stop transcontinental flight, on 2–3 May 1923, from New York to San Diego in twenty-six hours and fifty minutes. The aircraft used was one of two Dutch-built Fokker F-IV monoplanes acquired by the Air Service in 1922, no plane of American design having the necessary load-carrying capacity and range. Another great feat—unaccountably forgotten today—was the first flight around the world by four Douglas 'World Cruiser' biplanes which could be fitted with twin pontoons for over-water flying, or conventional wheeled landing gear. The flight started from Seattle on 6 April 1924 and proceeded westward by short stages, fuel, supplies and spare engines being laid down at each landing place by Air Service advance parties. Two of the aircraft were lost, but the *Chicago* and *New Orleans* returned to Seattle on 28 September 1924, after an elapsed time of 175 days.

By far the most flamboyant of Mitchell's exploits was the series of bombing experiments against warships off the Virginia Capes in 1921. Needing a villain for the drama he was staging for the public, Mitchell chose the Navy, and as early as 1920 he was loudly proclaiming that aeroplanes could sink battleships. His chance came when a number of surrendered German prizes, including the mislabelled 'unsinkable' dreadnought *Ostfriesland,* were placed at his disposal. After sinking with ease a number of smaller vessels, Mitchell's Martin MB-2 bombers sent the big ship to the bottom by dropping their two thousand pound bombs close alongside to burst with a mining effect.

The United States Navy, already air-minded, responded by taking aviation to sea, developing the aircraft carrier in the process. The Army, to Mitchell's chagrin, remained sceptical concerning the aerial weapon. Mitchell had seen a vision of the long-range heavy bomber, bearing large ship-smashing and city-busting missiles, altering the strategic character of the war of trench and blockade. Yet as late as 1927, the Army Air Service counted only seventy-five bombers on hand, sixty-five of which were the survivors of Mitchell's fleet of 130 Martin MB-2s of 1921–22.

The intemperate accusations which led in 1926 to Mitchell's court martial, and the court martial itself, lie outside the scope of this work. But the trial ensured him a permanent place in the hearts of the American public as the martyr and prophet of air power. His devoted disciples—including the late General H. H. Arnold, the World War II Commander-in-Chief of the Army Forces—found increasing public support as they fought to build the strategic bomber force that Mitchell had envisaged.

The United States Navy during the same period found in Rear Admiral William A. Moffett, the first Chief of the Bureau of Aeronautics, its own apostle of air power and literal martyr to the cause. Not that the Navy was hostile to aviation—its General Board as early as 1910 had recorded its interest in naval aircraft development, and two years later Rear Admiral Bradley A. Fiske had obtained a patent on the first torpedo plane. Moffett, hand-picked by his seniors to 'take aviation to sea with the Fleet,' became the first Chief of the Bureau of Aeronautics on 25 July 1921, a post he held through three terms until his death in the crash of the USS *Akron* on 4 April 1933.[8]

Moffett's patient, unwearying and successful efforts laid the foundation for the conquest of Japan through sea–air power in 1941–45. The capital ship of the World War II period was the aircraft carrier, and the concept of the carrier striking force owes much to Moffett and his young assistants during this period. True, the Navy's first 'flat-top,' the *Langley,* had been conceived in 1919, and her conversion from the collier *Jupiter* had taken place during 1920–21. But it was Moffett who saw a unique opportunity in the decision of the Washington Disarmament Conference of 1922 to scrap six large battle cruisers under construction, designed to displace 43,500 tons and to carry eight 16 in. guns at a speed of 33·25 knots. Two of these, USS *Lexington* and USS *Saratoga,* were partially framed and plated, and with 135,000 tons of aircraft carriers allotted by treaty to the United States, Moffett urged the conversion of these vessels to carriers of unprecedented size and power. Completed in 1927, and able to carry over eighty aircraft, 'Lex' and 'Sara' proved to be the cradles of naval attack aviation at sea, training on their broad decks the leaders of World War II's carrier task forces, and serving as guinea-pigs for the elaboration of carrier tactics.

Year by year, Moffett's bureau fostered the development of rugged, powerful aircraft designed to take the beating of arrester-wire landings on carrier decks, and to range the seas further with greater loads of bomb, torpedoes and ammunition. A dramatic—and lethal—Navy innovation was the dive bomber, developed through experiments by the Marine Corps in low-level bombing in their campaigns against bandit forces in Haiti in 1919, and Nicaragua in 1927. Sighting ahead over their engine cowlings, the Marine pilots dived at sixty degrees or more to plant their bombs from low altitude with great accuracy, then pulled up in a climb that stressed both men and machines with high G forces. The accuracy of dive bombing appealed to naval aviators, who were realizing since the Mitchell experiment that level bombers flying at high altitude stood little chance of hitting a vessel manœuvring at high speed. In 1931, Fighting Squadron 1 aboard *Saratoga* was equipped with a built-for-the-purpose dive bomber, the Curtiss F8C-4 'Helldiver,' a sturdy two-seater open cockpit biplane. During later years the type was refined into the Douglas SBD, which decided the crucial Battle of Midway in 1942 by sinking all four of the Japanese carriers present.[9]

All naval aircraft after about 1927 were fitted with air-cooled radial engines in place of the heavy, unreliable, water-cooled power plants left over from World War I. The development of a reliable radial engine, with low weight/horsepower ratio, is one of the major accomplishments of the Bureau of Aeronautics, and did much to place American aviation ahead of the rest of the world. Earlier radial engines had been designed and built in Britain, and a series had been developed in the early 1920s by Charles A. Lawrance and the Wright Aeronautical Corporation of Paterson, New Jersey. These had attracted the attention of the Bureau, and in fact, had been financed in part by the Navy; but when the best brains of the Wright team, headed by Frederick B. Rentschler, resigned to set up the competing Pratt & Whitney Aircraft Company, Moffett assured the new firm of Navy backing.[10] The result was the first of the famous Pratt & Whitney 'Wasps' of 410 hp, which first ran at the end of 1925. Such was the success of the 'Wasp' and later 'Hornet,' and the competing Wright 'Whirlwind' and later 'Cyclone,' that the rival water-cooled power plants as exemplified by the Packard and the Curtiss 'Conqueror' disappeared completely by 1930.

The Bureau of Aeronautics also attempted during this period to implement the naval mission of developing the rigid airship, a type originated by the German Zeppelin Company, not only as a scouting craft for war in the Pacific, but also for ultimate commercial use. Five only were procured, and the programme barely reached the stage of military prototype testing before being abandoned in 1935. In retrospect, the airship, despite its promise as a long-range weight carrier, failed to find acceptance because of its expense in an era of limited budgets; the failure of its proponents to develop a rationale for its employment with the Fleet; and the heavy loss of life in successive disasters.[11] One in particular, the USS *Akron,* flew for only two years and on the night of 3–4 April 1933, in the worst aviation disaster up to that time, went down at sea in a storm off Barnegat, New Jersey. Of the seventy-six persons aboard, all but three died, including Admiral Moffett, who paid with his life for his faith in aviation in general and in the airship in particular.

With some reluctance, Moffett felt compelled to vie with Mitchell for the favour of public opinion through victories in air races such as the international Schneider Cup contest. First offered at Monaco in 1913, the trophy was not in competition during the war years. The post-war contests were not impressive, the entries invariably were biplane flying boats, and the Italians, for instance, won the 1920 race without competition at a speed of 107 mph. In 1923 the American Navy, for the first time in the history of the Schneider rivalry, entered a government-backed team flying the highest performance sea-planes available, and the Schneider races were never the same again. First and second place—at 177·38 and 173·46 mph—went to two Curtiss CR-3s. In 1925 the Army Air Service's Lieutenant Jimmy Doolittle won the Schneider contest for the last time for the United States in a Curtiss R3C-2 at 232·57 mph.

The Italians and the British continued to duel with each other for four more years. By mutual agreement, the contest was now put on an every other year basis, because of the ever-growing complexity and expense of the government-sponsored entries. Aerodynamic design had reached its limit within the contemporary state of the art—both British and Italian technologists having settled on the twin-float monoplane seaplane with thin aerofoil wing of minimal area, large liquid-cooled engine, and fuselage of such slender cross-section that large pilots could not be accommodated in the cockpit. Some of the fuel was carried in the floats.

Two developments just around the corner would have been of great service to the Schneider racers—variable pitch propellers and flaps. As it was, the full power of the big engines could not be used efficiently, for the fixed-pitch propeller had to be a compromise between the flat blade angle necessary for acceleration on takeoff, and the coarse pitch most desirable for speed in the air. With a wing loading of forty pounds per square foot, the landing speed without flaps was a 'hot' 95 mph.[12]

'Blacking out' was becoming a problem in closed-circuit racing. With the high speed Schneider craft developing accelerations of four to six G in turns around the course markers, 'the British pilots had developed a technique of starting their banks far out from the pylons, throttling down as they approached them to avoid blacking out, then whipping around them in a near vertical attitude. Once around, they straightened out rapidly, and opened their throttles wide.'[13]

The British, who had won the 1927 race, now took the 1929 one as well, and when the Italians were not ready in time, they clinched the trophy permanently in 1931. A few days after the 'race,' one of the Supermarine S6-Bs, fitted with a 'sprint' version of the Rolls-Royce 'R' engine producing 2600 hp and guaranteed to run only one hour, set a world's speed record of 407·5 mph.

As with speed records, the military services vied with each other for the altitude mark. In the early 1920s it was the American services that were in the lead. This work was closely connected with efforts by the Army Air Service, the Navy, and the National Advisory Committee on Aeronautics, to develop a reliable supercharger to maintain sea-level horsepower output by compressing the air entering the carburettor at high altitude, so that more oxygen would be available for the combustion of fuel.

The theoretical advantages of such a device for high-altitude flying were obvious, and in the latter part of World War I, some experimental installations had been made but not flown in combat. One of the four-engined German Staaken 'Giants,' the R VI 30/16, carried in its fuselage a centrifugal impeller driven by a Mercedes 120 hp aircraft engine, the supercharger delivering air to the four Mercedes 260 hp D IV engines carried between the wings. With the supercharger increasing engine power at high altitude, the ceiling of 30/16 went up from 12,500 to 19,357 feet. The heavy supercharger installation with the additional engine to drive it could, however, be carried only in a very large machine.

A more practical approach was the turbo-supercharger driven by exhaust gases devised by Professor Rateau of France, which could be fitted to each individual power plant. Some experiments were made with the Rateau compressor during the war. Further supercharger development took place in the United States, but many pitfalls were uncovered.[14] Hot, compressed air delivered to the carburettor caused detonation of the gas–air mixture in the cylinders, until inter-coolers were fitted. Turbine wheels heated to 1500 degrees F and revolving at 20,000 rpm failed until stronger materials were provided. The first American aircraft in squadron service with superchargers were five Curtiss P-5 Hawks with 435 hp liquid-cooled engines, which had a ceiling of 31,900 feet compared to 20,800 feet for the similar P-1C with the same engine unsupercharged.

The first American attempt on the altitude record was made without a supercharger in the autumn of 1918. The pilot was the lanky Major Rudolph W. ('Shorty') Schroeder, and the aircraft was one of thirty LUSAC-11 two-seater fighters manufactured during the last year of the war by the Packard Motor Car Company to the designs of the French Captain G. Le Pere. Schroeder prepared for the flight by fitting high-compression pistons in the 425 hp Liberty engine, with an aneroid-controlled stop which prevented full throttle operation at sea level; primitive oxygen equipment and a heavy fur-lined flying suit with face mask to prevent frostbite. After two previous ascents to 24,000 and 27,000 feet, Schroeder made his record attempt on 18 September 1918. At 20,000 feet his goggles frosted, making it difficult for him to see his instruments. Not until reaching 25,000 feet did he resort to oxygen:

I noticed the sun growing very dim, I could hardly hear my motor run, and I felt very hungry. The trend of my thoughts was that it must be getting late, that evening must be coming on; but I was still climbing. I thought that I might as well stick to it a little longer, for I knew I could reach my ceiling pretty soon, then I should go down, and even though it were dark I could land all right . . . and so I went on talking to myself, and this I thought was a good sign to begin taking oxygen, and I did. . . . As soon as I started to inhale the oxygen the sun grew bright again, my motor began to exhaust so loud that it seemed something must be wrong with it. I was no longer hungry and the day seemed to be a most beautiful one.[15]

Symptoms of anoxia again occurred as Schroeder approached 29,000 feet—in retrospect, he believed he was then running out of oxygen. 'I was beginning to get cross, and I could not understand why I was only 29,000 feet after climbing for so long a time. I remember that the horizon seemed to be very much out of place, but I felt that I was flying correctly and that I was right and the horizon was wrong.'[16] At this point his engine failed, having exhausted its fuel, and Schroeder, lost, broke his propeller in a dead-stick landing on rough ground. His official altitude was 28,900 feet.

Two years later, on 27 February 1920, Schroeder was the first man to exceed 30,000 feet in an aeroplane. Again the craft was the sturdy Le Pere, of which several were available to the Air Service's Engineering Division at Dayton, Ohio. This time, however, it was equipped with a General Electric turbo-supercharger, and with the additional power which it conferred at high altitude, Schroeder managed to reach 33,115 feet after a climb of one hour and forty-seven minutes. Here the main supply of gaseous oxygen ceased. Schroeder switched to his reserve flask. 'Fearing that the emergency supply would become exhausted, he lifted his oil-grimed goggles so that he might see to make an adjustment in the automatic feed, and, deprived entirely of oxygen in that instant of stooping forward, he lost consciousness and fell with his plane, like a plummet, through thin air for six miles.'[17] At low altitude he partially recovered, and with his eyes blinded by ice, made a safe landing. With the same machine Lieutenant John A. Macready 'won the icicle crown,' as Schroeder put it, on 28 September 1921, with an ascent to 34,510 feet. A photograph of Macready about to take off on this day shows him 'clad in several suits of woollen underwear, his regulation army uniform, a knitted woollen garment, and a suit of leather heavily padded with down and feathers. Fur-lined gloves, fleece-lined moccasins over the boots, and goggles treated with an antifreeze gelatine complete the costume.'[18]

The altitude record passed to France in 1923, when Sadi-Lecointe reached 36,567 feet in a supercharged Nieuport-Delage 29 C 1. Then, in 1925, the Engineering Division returned to its high-altitude investigations, the basic aim being to explore the military possibilities of vertical photography being then carried on at these levels by Lieutenant Albert W. Stevens. The aircraft was a 'one-only,' the XC05-A, a two-seater corps observation craft fitted by the Engineering Division with thick-section two-bay wings 55 feet 6 inches in span for better performance at high altitude. In place of the gaseous oxygen with the regulator, which pilots usually turned on at 16,000 to 17,000 feet, the pilot was now to breathe liquid oxygen, better liked because it was free of impurities and moisture, which with the gaseous oxygen tended to condense in tubing and block it by freezing. Flasks of compressed oxygen were still carried for emergency use. In other respects the situation was unchanged: still the native Liberty power plant with turbo-supercharger; still the open cockpit; still the bulky flying suit with heavy underclothing. Electrically-heated clothing was under consideration, but was still believed to be too unreliable. A felt lining to the cockpit kept out draughts, and some of the heat of the engine was conveyed to the cockpit through an asbestos-covered tube. This was little enough to ward off the chill of high altitude, which Macready—again the pilot—found to extend below minus eighty degrees F at 37,000 feet.

With a rear cockpit full of recording barographs, Macready made a series of flights from Dayton between January and April 1926 to altitudes in excess of 37,000 feet. On 29 January 1926 he reached a record altitude of 38,704 feet, a height that was not exceeded for a year and a half. Cold and anoxia made the greatest demands on the pilot—anoxia because Macready was still using the inefficient pipe-stem mouthpiece, which could not possibly maintain normal blood oxygen levels at this height:

> In practically all extreme altitude attempts, the plane reaches its limit about the time the pilot grits his teeth in anticipation of pushing further upward. One isn't thinking as clearly as usual at this height, and it takes some time to convince oneself that the plane's ceiling has actually been reached. I usually remain at this altitude for some half-hour, endeavouring to make adjustments or change the functioning of the supercharger, coaxing the plane higher. . . . The plane wallows about as in a trough, but will not lift its nose an additional foot.[19]

Mitchell by now was no longer the Assistant Chief of the Air Service, and the Army Air Service set no more altitude records. It was now the turn of the Navy, which in 1927 began to explore the possibilities of a turbo-supercharger newly developed by the NACA.

The machine was a tiny single-seater biplane mounted on a single float, the Wright F3W-1 'Apache,' designed as a fighter to operate off battleships' catapults, but never put into production. The original engine was a Pratt & Whitney 375 hp 'Wasp.' Piloted by Lieutenant C. C. Champion, the 'Apache' seaplane reached 33,455 feet on 5 May 1927 and 37,995 feet on 4 July. A few days later, on 27 July, with the float replaced by wheels, Champion attained 38,419 feet over his base at the US Naval Air Station, Anacostia, Maryland.

When the land plane record fell two years later on 8 May 1929, it was to another Navy flyer, Lieutenant Apollo Soucek,[20] in the same Wright 'Apache' with a bigger 450 hp engine. The altitude record was now 39,140 feet. Later in the month, on 26 May, Neuenhofen in a Junkers W 34 monoplane with Bristol Jupiter engine attained 41,783 feet at Dessau, Germany. A year later, on 4 June 1930, Soucek reached 43,166 feet in the same 'Apache' biplane. An oxygen mask, covering nose and mouth, was used by the successful pilot. None the less he suffered some impairment of function at maximum altitude, as might be expected, for without positive pressure breathing, the ambient pressure at this height would not suffice to maintain normal blood oxygenation. It was the last United States altitude mark in this period, and nearly the last in an open-cockpit aircraft.

There were a few more records, demonstrating that the pilot had reached his limits with the open cockpit and oxygen at ambient pressures. On 16 September 1932 Captain Cyril F. Unwin RAF reached 43,976 feet; on 28 September 1933 Lemoine of France attained 44,822 feet. On 28 September 1934 Italy's Commendatore Donati achieved 47,358 feet. This flight was apparently made with ordinary oxygen apparatus,[21] and stressed the flyer beyond the limits of his ability to compensate:

If Donati had been breathing normally at this altitude, he would have had only 12 mm Hg oxygen partial pressure in his lungs. ... This would have resulted in an arterial oxygen saturation of only about seven per cent which would have produced almost immediate death. As a consequence he must have had a respiratory centre which was very sensitive to oxygen want and which caused him to greatly overventilate with a consequent marked increase of alveolar oxygen and decrease of alveolar carbon dioxide. Even then he must have been semi-comatose and close to the point of death.

Reports indicate that Donati, upon landing, suffered a nervous and physical reaction which left him practically unconscious and it was necessary to lift him from the cockpit of the aeroplane. At that time his pulse was 105 and remained at about 100 for some time. After twenty-four hours, during most of which time Donati slept, he was reported to be again in normal physical condition.[22]

The last attempts on the altitude record involved a new and

promising development—breathing oxygen under pressure in a pressurized suit. The garment devised by the Royal Air Force, made of rubberized fabric, ballooned out under a pressure of two and half psi so that the wearer could barely move his limbs within the stiffened envelope, while his vision was much restricted by the face plate. Yet this innovation, which would have provided an equivalent pressure of 41,500 feet in a vacuum, enabled Squadron Leader F. R. D. Swain, on 28 September 1936, to attain 49,967 feet. The aircraft, especially built for the attempt, was a large sixty-six-foot span monoplane, the Bristol 138A, with a wing loading of only 9·57 pounds per square foot, and powered by a 460 hp Bristol Pegasus engine. This was fitted with a two-stage supercharger which, as ultimately developed for World War II aircraft, shifted automatically from low to 'high blower' at 16,000 feet to provide more oxygen at higher altitude. When Lieutenant Colonel Mario Pezzi of Italy flew to 51,348 feet on 8 May 1937 the Bristol was modified and brought out again on 30 June 1937 and Flight Lieutenant M. J. Adam pushed it to 53,937 feet. In a Caproni 151 Pezzi, on 22 October 1938, attained 56,046 feet, and there the record stood during the war years.

Best remembered by newspaper readers of the period were the long-distance flights, which simultaneously demonstrated the improved performance of aircraft and engines and pioneered the present-day long distance and transoceanic air routes. Almost all these feats were gruelling tests of courage, determination and resistance to fatigue of air crew flying in open cockpits at low altitude, often in very bad weather, and—what is often forgotten—staging through primitive grass-covered fields with no rest or maintenance facilities, where the flight crews themselves had to do all the work on the aircraft.

1919 was a year of adventure, with skilled and daring wartime flyers and large aircraft manufacturers vying with each other to be first across the Atlantic. Spurring on the contestants was the London *Daily Mail* prize of ten thousand pounds for the first non-stop Atlantic flight, initially offered in 1913.

It was the United States Navy, however, ineligible for the *Daily Mail* prize, which won the honour of making the first aerial crossing from America to Europe. The Armistice found the Americans with four large flying boats under construction, the NCs 1 to 4, designed for anti-submarine patrol in European waters. To publicize the Navy and naval aviation, Assistant Secretary Franklin D. Roosevelt proposed that the 'Nancies' should fly the Atlantic. On 16 May 1919 three of them got away from Trepassey, Newfoundland, but only the NC 4 made it to Horta in the Azores, the other two being forced down at sea without loss of life. On 27 May the NC 4 arrived in Lisbon to complete the first transatlantic crossing, going on to Plymouth in England on 31 May. Her triumph was won despite the hardships of flying in open cockpits, with only the simplest instruments, with unreliable engines, and with no efficient weather forecasting service.[23]

Between 14 and 15 June 1919 the Britishers, John Alcock and Arthur Whitten-Brown, made the first non-stop Atlantic crossing to win the Daily Mail prize. Their Vickers-Vimy, built as a twin-engined bomber, made the 1890 miles to western Ireland in fifteen hours and fifty-seven minutes, crash-landing in a bog without injury to the two flyers. Good fortune as well as skill brought them through mid-Atlantic storms, in which they fell 4000 feet in a 'graveyard spiral' inside a cumulus cloud, and subsequently were nearly forced down by airframe and carburettor icing.[24]

None tried to follow them eastward for another seven years, but the first westward crossing of the Atlantic was made a month later, between 2 and 6 July by a large rigid airship, the British R 34, a copy of a captured wartime Zeppelin. With thirty souls aboard (including a stowaway) she made it from East Fortune, Scotland, to Mineola, Long Island, in 108 hours 12 minutes, and the return flight to Pulham in Norfolk with thirty-two aboard in 75 hours 3 minutes. The triumph of the R 34, carrying a large number of persons in relative comfort, and with safety apparently assured by her five engines and reliance on gas as a lifting medium, seemed to forecast the dominance of the large rigid airship in transoceanic flying. This impression was reinforced when the next transatlantic crossing was made by another airship, the LZ 126 *Los Angeles* built for the US Navy by the Zeppelin Company, from Friedrichshafen to Lakehurst 12–15 October 1924. During the eighty-one-hour flight, the thirty-two persons on board enjoyed regular hot meals from the galley, and some of them slept in the five passenger cabins abaft the control car. The Zeppelin Company followed up this success by launching a still larger craft, the *Graf Zeppelin,* which had sleeping accommodation for twenty passengers. Yet despite the 'Graf's' successful international career between 1928 and 1937, only one other airship ever flew the Atlantic in regular passenger service—the Zeppelin *Hindenburg*—and with her fiery destruction at Lakehurst on 6 May 1937 the life of the long-range passenger airship came to an end.

The year 1927 brought a series of spectacular transatlantic flights. In May 1919 a New York hotel man, Raymond Orteig, had offered a $25,000 prize for the first non-stop flight between New York and Paris, but attempts to fly the 3600 miles had to wait on improvements in aircraft design, and above all, on the development of reliable, air-cooled radial engines in place of the undependable water-cooled war surplus power plants previously available. Even so, their aircraft contending for the Orteig prize had to be grossly overloaded with fuel to stand a chance of going the distance, and the excessive gross weight led to several fiery takeoff crashes.

To many of the prospective contestants it appeared that only a large aircraft, multi-engined for safety, could succeed in reaching Paris. The first to make the attempt, the Sikorsky S-35 biplane, powered by three Gnome-Rhone Jupiter engines, carried two pilots in a fully-enclosed cockpit, and a radioman and a mechanic in an enclosed cabin. On 21 September 1926, loaded with seven and a half tons of fuel and oil, it failed to lift off the runway at Roosevelt Field, Long Island, crashed and burned. Two crew members died. And on 8 May 1927 the French World War I ace, Charles Nungesser, with François Coli, departed Paris for New York in a single-engined biplane, the *Oiseau Blanc,* only to disappear for ever in the Atlantic.

It was at this point that an unknown airmail pilot, backed by a syndicate of St Louis business men, won the prize in a single-engined monoplane devoid of radio and safety equipment. From the point of view of aviation medicine, Charles Lindbergh's thirty-three-and-a-half-hour solo flight from Roosevelt Field to Le Bourget in the *Spirit of St Louis* on 20–21 May 1927 is most remarkable for his success in resisting fatigue. Rejecting the use of stimulants, he suffered such drowsiness—and quite possibly carbon monoxide intoxication—as to nearly lose control of his aircraft on several occasions over the ocean.[25] On touching down in the dark at Le Bourget he in fact had not slept for sixty-three hours.[26]

The first attempt to cross a portion of the Pacific was made by the US Navy. Two big PN-9 twin-engined flying boats, each with a crew of five, lifted off the surface of San Francisco Bay on the afternoon of 21 August 1925, their destination Honolulu. Five and a half hours later the PN-9 No. 3 was down at sea with a broken fuel line, but the PN-9 No. 1, piloted by Naval Aviator No. 2, Commander John Rodgers, continued on for twenty-five and a half hours, only to run out of fuel prematurely a mere 220 miles from his destination. With his radio out of commission, Rodgers was unable to make contact, but sailed his crippled flying boat to within fifteen miles of the island of Kauai, where he was picked up by a submarine on 10 September.

Three years passed before the first crossing of the Pacific, when the Australian Charles Kingsford-Smith and three companions made it from Oakland, California, to Brisbane, Australia, in the three-engined Fokker monoplane *Southern Cross.* Starting on 31 May 1928 Kingsford-Smith flew via Honolulu and the Fijis, making the 7916-mile flight in eighty-six hours and twenty-nine minutes' flying time. It was not until 15 October 1931 that Clyde Pangborn and Hugh

Herndon made the 4500 mile non-stop flight from Japan to the United States in a Bellanca monoplane. To increase range and speed, they released the landing gear after takeoff, and had to belly-land at their destination.

For five years after the US Army's 175-day world flight of 1924, no attempts were made to girdle the globe by air.[27] Then, in the twenty-one days between 15 August and 4 September 1929 another aircraft circled the earth with only four stops, at Friedrichshafen, Tokyo, Los Angeles and Lakehurst. The craft was Dr Hugo Eckener's demonstration passenger airship *Graf Zeppelin,* and it made the 21,255 mile journey in a total flying time of three hundred hours and twenty minutes, at an average speed of 70·6 mph. Furthermore, the airship carried a crew of forty-one, and up to twenty passengers in her sleeping cabins. The publicity given to this voyage influenced commercial aviation planners for years.

There followed a series of world flights which progressively lowered the record and held the attention of the public until World War II made such aerial journeys commonplace. Between 23 June and 1 July 1931 the superbly prepared team of Wiley Post, pilot, and Harold Gatty, navigator, circled the earth at an average speed of 140 mph with thirteen stops in Newfoundland, England, Germany, Russia, Siberia, Alaska, Canada and the United States. The aircraft, one of the cleanest and fastest of its day, was the Lockheed Vega *Winnie Mae,* with smooth, circular, monocoque plywood fuselage and cantilever wooden wing. A 450 hp Pratt & Whitney Wasp engine in a NACA cowling gave it a maximum speed of 180 mph. Another advance was a controllable-pitch propeller, enabling the pilot to select settings of the blades for optimum efficiency at takeoff and while cruising. Medically, the gruelling flight, with a minimum of sleep, was remarkable for Post's method of dealing with the fatigue problem: 'To train himself for the long hours at the controls, Post practised never sleeping the same hours on any two days of the week. He always said that breaking himself of the habit of regular sleep was far more difficult than piloting an aeroplane around the world.'[28] Even more remarkable was the fact that this great pilot had learned to fly after losing his left eye in an oil-well drilling accident.

Two years later, between 15 and 22 July 1933, Post and the *Winnie Mae* set a new record for flying around the world—alone. This feat was made possible by an automatic, gyro-controlled device without which present-day long-distance flying would make impossible demands on the physical endurance of the human mechanism—the Sperry automatic pilot. Unerringly holding the fleet blue and white Lockheed on course and altitude through the skies above the northern hemisphere, the mechanical guidance system enabled Post to relax, even briefly to sleep in the cockpit.

The last great world flight of the period was a truly professional achievement by a team whose capabilities heralded those of the crew of the modern multi-engined transport airliner. A specially-built Lockheed monoplane, powered by twin 1100 hp Pratt & Whitney engines, made the circuit between 10 and 14 July 1938. Its crew comprised millionaire Howard Hughes as pilot, a co-pilot-navigator, radio engineer, navigator and flight engineer. With autopilot, three radios, blind flying instruments and advanced navigational equipment, they were able to determine their position at all times even when cruising blind at 10,000 to 15,000 feet, and were in almost unbroken radio contact with the ground. The average air speed was 206·7 mph.

In the early years of the period 1919–39 the military had led the way in pioneering new developments in airframe and power plant design, and it was the advanced military aircraft which set the records and made the long-distance flights. After 1925 the opposite tended more and more to be true, and all the long-distance flights mentioned above after this date were by civilian aircraft. Particularly in commercial transport aircraft, civil aviation was far ahead of the military, with all-metal stressed-skin construction, retractable landing gear, flaps, controllable-pitch propellers, de-icing equipment, enclosed cockpits, radio navigational aids, and blind-flying instrumentation. How far the US Army Air Corps had fallen behind was shown in the so-called 'Air Mail Scandal' of 1934.

Charging fraud and collusion between the large airlines and the outgoing postmaster-general, Walter F. Brown, the Roosevelt administration cancelled airmail contracts with the commercial airlines and ordered the Army Air Corps to fly the mail. Their operations, between 19 February and 7 May 1934, showed that inexperienced Army pilots, flying slow, open-cockpit biplanes with inadequate radio and instrumentation, were unequal to the task. True, the Boeing P-12 pursuit planes, Douglas O-38E and Curtiss A-12 observation craft, and Curtiss B-2 and Keystone B-6 bombers had their airmail facilities improvised. But these shortcomings, plus bad weather, caused the deaths of twelve Air Corps personnel during the airmail operations.[29]

With the recognition of the need for air preparedness, and for more appropriations, the military services borrowed from civilian practice, and procured in the last years of the period the fast all-metal monoplanes which entered the lists against the Axis at the outbreak of World War II.

The rapid progress in design and technical knowledge, leading to greatly enhanced aircraft performance during this period, was matched by a growth of medical information. By providing accurate data on an experimental basis, aviation medicine clarified many of the problems posed by increased aircraft performance and enabled the human operator to keep pace with the machine.

Despite budgetary cutbacks, the United States air services continued to manifest their wartime concern for the 'care of the flyer,' while other countries did not have medical men assigned to duty with flying formations.[30] The medical research laboratory established in 1918 at Hazelehurst Field, Mineola, Long Island, was continued in operation after the Armistice, not only as a centre for further clinical investigation, but also to continue its wartime function of training officers of the medical corps of the regular Army to be flight surgeons. Lieutenant Louis H. Bauer (MC) was ordered to command the laboratory in January 1919 and over the next six years created the curriculum and the professional foundation of the first formal school of aviation medicine. Beginning in May 1919 students were sent to Mineola in groups of five to fifteen for a two-month course in ophthalmology, otology, physiology, cardiovascular disease, psychology, neuropsychiatry and physics (in these early days more attention was given to the physical examination of the prospective flyer than to the theory of aeromedical problems). In March 1921 the school building burned to the ground, but was rebuilt, and in November 1922, its name was changed to 'The School of Aviation Medicine.' Various alterations in the curriculum were made, the course being extended to three months in 1920. A Department of Aviation Medicine took over the teaching responsibilities of the Department of Cardiology, and with the passage of time, taught physiology, roentgenology, protective devices and the organization of the aviation medicine service with the squadrons. Various courses were established for reserve medical officers, and for enlisted flight surgeons' assistants. In 1926 the school moved to Brooks Field, a large training field at San Antonio, Texas, and in 1931 to the new flight training centre at Randolph Field. Here, of course, flight training was possible for the embryo flight surgeons, but such instruction was on a voluntary and informal basis and the medical man who went on to solo flying was an exception.

Not until 1939 did the United States Navy establish its own school of aviation medicine and research centre at Pensacola, Florida, the naval flight training headquarters. Prior to this time naval medical officers had been sent to the Army school. Four Navy physicians attended courses at Mineola between February and June 1922 subsequently proceeding to Pensacola for flight training. Two years passed before the Chiefs of the Bureaux of Aeronautics and of

Medicine and Surgery agreed on the qualifications for naval flight surgeons, which stipulated that trainees must complete the course at the Army School of Aviation Medicine and subsequently serve satisfactorily for three months with a naval aviation unit. The medical officer was required to make flights in aircraft only in accordance with his own desires, or in emergencies. Up to December 1926 twenty-four naval officers graduated from the Army School of Aviation Medicine.

The actual function of the Medical Research Laboratory at Mineola illustrates the connection between teaching and research in the new specialty of aviation medicine. All teaching schools have naturally engaged in research, but within a few years a division of labour took place, with the School of Aviation Medicine at Randolph Field being expected to devote twenty per cent of its efforts to research, and the individual flight surgeon in the field expending a proportion of ten per cent.[31] The main portion of the research mission was undertaken at the Army Air Service's Aero Medical Laboratory, located at Wright Field, Dayton, Ohio. Growing from the need of the near-by Engineering Division at Wright Field for medical guidance in the design of advanced experimental aircraft and personal flight equipment, the laboratory evolved from the medical projects implemented by Lieutenant Colonel Malcolm C. Grow (MC), the flight surgeon at Patterson Field, and opened its doors on 15 September 1934. Part of its original equipment was the old pressure chamber from the Mineola laboratory, procured by Captain Harry G. Armstrong (MC), and with this and other apparatus, Captain Armstrong, who served as Director until September 1940, conducted theoretical and practical investigations into many new aspects of aviation medicine. These included the evolution of the concept of 'aero-otitis media,' the pathological changes in the middle ear caused by differences of barometric pressure; the significance of rate of ascent, duration and frequency of exposure in the development of symptoms of anoxia; the first studies in America of the effect of acceleration in a centrifuge on human beings; the pathology of altitude sickness (anoxia) as observed in the pressure chamber; the limits of high flying with one hundred per cent oxygen (unpressurized, of course); and a new aeromedical disease entity, labelled by Armstrong 'aero-embolism,' but today cited in standard texts as 'dysbarism' or 'decompression sickness.' Armstrong demonstrated experimentally the vaporization of body fluids at about 63,000 feet—a level now designated the 'Armstrong Line' in his honour—and pointed to the dangers of 'explosive decompression' of sealed, pressurized enclosures even before any practical experience had been gained with them.[32]

Other countries were slow to catch up with the American lead in aviation medicine research. As late as 1939 the Royal Air Force's Physiological Laboratory 'had been housed in a hut at Hendon airfield,'[33] and the large RAF Institute of Aviation Medicine at Farnborough was created in response to wartime necessity. One nation which did not hesitate to spend large sums of money for research in this field was Nazi Germany, which realized early that the high-performance aircraft which technology could now create for the next war could not be operated without corresponding advances in medical knowledge and equipment. As early as 1934 the *Luftfahrtmedizinisches Forschungsinstitut* at Berlin-Tempelhof possessed the largest human centrifuge in the world, and *Luftwaffe* medical officers were investigating problems of oxygen supply at high altitude in aircraft flights as well as in pressure chambers.

In peacetime, of course, the life of a flight surgeon tended to be routine, with periodic physical examinations, daily sick call, and appearance on the station flight line comprising his usual activities. Periodic manœuvres introduced unusual situations, sent squadrons away from their comfortable permanent bases to what approximated to wartime conditions, and made demands on the ingenuity and improvising ability of everyone concerned, including the flight surgeon. So discovered Major I. B. March (MC), a flight surgeon attached to Selfridge Field, Michigan, who participated in winter manœuvres (all aircraft carried the insignia of a polar bear standing on a cake of ice) in February, 1935, in the vicinity of Grand Forks, North Dakota. The aircraft were the most advanced of their type and of their day, but the fighters, Boeing P-12s, were biplanes with open cockpits. The attack aircraft, Curtiss A-12 'Shrike' low-wing monoplanes, had introduced the trailing edge flap to Army aviation, but the pilot's cockpit was fully open and the gunner's, in the rear, only partly enclosed. The Douglas O-43 observation aircraft, parasol high-wing monoplanes of strikingly graceful form, had sliding glazed canopies completely enclosing both cockpits, and the three-place Martin B-10 bombers were likewise enclosed.

Riding in the rear cockpit of an A-12 without face mask with the ground temperature at twenty-five degrees F, Major March froze his lips and the edges of his nostrils slightly, and other air crew suffered frozen faces. Working around the aircraft in ground temperatures as low as six above zero F, and sometimes in snow as deep as fifty inches, the flight crews suffered even more, tiring rapidly from their arduous exertions while wearing heavy leather flying suits and moccasins. The combination ski and wheel landing gears needed for winter operations gave particular trouble; 'irritability and shortness of temper was evident.'[34] 'White-out,' a phenomenon with which Arctic flyers became all too familiar during the war years, caused the crash of a P-12 fighter from 250 feet while attempting to land on a frozen lake; the pilot lost his horizon with the sun glaring on the snow-covered landscape, but escaped with cuts and amnesia. Major March learned that the cargo aircraft accompanying the travelling squadrons were no more suitable for medical purposes than 'the use of trucks as ambulances in World War I,' and submitted a plea for a specially-fitted ambulance plane.

Initially, the flight surgeon had been a military physician, and aviation medicine a creation of the armed services. Now, in the 'twenties, the specialty put on civilian clothes. Until the year 1926, there had been no federal regulation of civil aviation (though some states had passed laws), and there had been no registration or certification of aircraft, nor examination of pilots, either with respect to their professional ability, or their physical qualifications. All this was changed by the Air Commerce Act of 1926, which provided for the licensing of aircraft and examination and rating of airmen. By the end of the year, the Aeronautics Branch of the Department of Commerce was being organized to administer the act, and the first medical director was none other than Major Louis H. Bauer, the former Commandant of the School of Aviation Medicine, who resigned his commission in November 1926 to accept the post. It was Dr Bauer's task to draw up the physical standards for airmen, and these tended to follow those of the military services, with progressively stricter requirements for the three classes—private pilots, industrial pilots and transport pilots (later classes were limited commercial and student pilots). Initially, the medical examinations were to be given annually, but in 1934 student and private pilots were scheduled for examination only every two years. On 21 February 1927, Dr Bauer announced the appointment of thirty-nine civilian medical examiners located in different cities, who were officially designated to perform examinations of pilots. All were interested in aviation medicine, many of them flew themselves and some had been trained as flight surgeons during World War I.

Dr Bauer resigned as medical director in 1930, but his system, of having medical examinations for civilian pilots performed by designated physicians, has survived despite changes in the governmental agency—it became the Civil Aeronautics Administration in 1938, the Federal Aviation Agency in 1959 and the Federal Aviation Administration of the Department of Transportation in 1967—and pressures to modify the high standards which he initiated. Such efforts have been resisted at the political level by the Aero Medical Association, founded in December 1928 to represent physicians interested in aviation medicine. Undoubtedly the

Association was correct in successfully opposing attempts of the administrative agency in 1934, and again in 1945, to permit flight physical examinations to be done by any physician, instead of by designated examiners. When it appeared in 1945 that even osteopaths and chiropractors would be permited to perform such examinations, Dr Bauer resigned his appointment as CAA medical examiner in protest. On the other hand, in retrospect the Aero Medical Association took too narrow a view in insisting through the years on the maintenance of the high physical standards set in 1927. Undoubtedly their members were unconsciously influenced by their earlier experiences with the rigid requirements of the military services. The gradual liberalization of standards at the instigation of administrative officials, particularly where private flying is undertaken for pleasure, is now seen to have in no way compromised safety. Even the Aero Medical Association has accepted these changes 'because of the increased safety factors in private and sport aircraft, and the ease with which they can be flown after brief instruction.'[35] The majority of general aviation accidents today are still caused by weather and bad judgment, not by physical defects.

The Aero Medical Association promptly became the parent of the first periodical devoted to the specialty, the *Journal of Aviation Medicine* (now the *Journal of Aerospace Medicine*). The first issue appeared in March 1930 and until 1943 it appeared quarterly, carrying many historic articles constituting milestones in the scientific advancement of aviation medicine. Other countries followed suit, with *Luftfahrtmedizin* appearing in Germany in 1936, and *Rivista Medicina Aeronautica* in Italy in 1938.

The revival of scientific interest in aviation medicine also led to the publication during this period of the first textbooks on the subject. Dr Louis H. Bauer in 1926 published the earliest, *Aviation Medicine,* reflecting to a large degree the experiences of World War I and laying special emphasis on the physical examination of the flyer. An epochal event was the appearance in 1939 of the first edition of Armstrong's *Principles and Practice of Aviation Medicine,* with its wealth of research material originating in the activities of the author and his associates in the laboratory at Wright Field, Ohio.

Progress in oxygen equipment came only at the end of the twenty-year period between the wars, and then, only because the increased performance of the high-powered monoplanes then under development permitted routine operations above 20,000 feet. In the ten years after World War I, flights to high altitude were limited to experimental and record-breaking attempts, and the simplest type of oxygen equipment sufficed.

Despite the theoretical advantages of the Dreyer apparatus of World War I, it did not long survive. Sceptical of the need for oxygen at high altitude, the pilots of the day, rugged individualists to a man, refused to accept an uncomfortable mask that covered both the mouth and the nose. Above all, the barometrically-controlled regulator valve proved unequal to the rigours of service use: 'repeated and extended tests showed that these regulators were unreliable, due to their complicated and delicate construction, and that they were unable to compensate for the different requirements of individuals at rest and during exercise.'[36] By 1923 the wheel had turned full circle: the oxygen tube led to a simple pipe-stem held between the teeth (jaws clenched on it might well ache after half an hour).[37] Gaseous oxygen had been abandoned because of the impurities it contained, particularly moisture, which froze and blocked the tubing. Liquid oxygen was now carried in an apparatus resembling the German Heylandt equipment of World War I. The flow of oxygen was of course continuous, in proportion to the rate at which the liquid vaporized, and a regulator was not necessary. The rate of oxygen production of course bore no relationship to the pilot's requirements, which increased with altitude and with physical exertion. Most of the gas in fact was wasted, but this was of little consequence, considering that such flights as Macready's high-altitude attempts lasted only two to three hours. Yet the equipment was extremely simple, positive, and reliable, and the supplemental oxygen it provided enabled flyers in open cockpits to retain a useful degree of consciousness up to 38,000 feet.

Not until thirteen years later, in 1936, was an attempt made to develop more efficient oxygen equipment for longer flights at high altitude. Liquid oxygen was abandoned, because of difficulties in procuring and storing it in the field in wartime, because the amount remaining in the container could not be measured, and because its rate of flow could not be controlled. Gaseous oxygen was now made available, compressed to 1800 psi in alloy cylinders containing from 4·25 to 212 cubic feet of oxygen. Simple regulators indicated the pressure in the cylinders, and provided for manual control of the necessary rate of flow in terms of altitude. With settings for 20,000, 25,000, 30,000 and 35,000 feet on the dial, personnel were instructed to use the next highest setting for heavy manual work, such as operating a flexible machine gun.

By 1938 an acceptable mask had been developed by Doctors W. M. Boothby, W. R. Lovelace and A. H. Bulbulian of the Mayo Clinic.[38] Initially covering the nose only, the B-L-B mask was shortly modified to cover the mouth also. Light in weight, made of thin moulded rubber, it was not uncomfortable to wear, and with the introduction of enclosed cockpits, it would not be torn off by the slipstream. Its most ingenious feature was a rebreather bag which conserved much of the continuously flowing oxygen, which previously had been wasted while the pipe-stem user exhaled. The flyer inhaled oxygen from the rubber bag attached to the lower portion of the mask; he exhaled into the bag, which distended. Initially, the exhaled air was from the upper respiratory passages and relatively rich in oxygen; as the bag pressure rose, however, the last part of the exhaled air, high in carbon dioxide content, was vented through a pair of sponge-rubber ports. With a low rate of oxygen flow at low altitudes, some air was inhaled through the ports along with the oxygen piped into the bag, providing some conservation of the gas by diluting it. Again, the B-L-B mask was used with the manually-adjusted regulator.

Such was the equipment with which the United States Army Air Forces and Navy entered World War II—the 1800 psi high-pressure gaseous oxygen system, the A-8A manually-controlled regulator and the Type A-8 mask, which was simply the B-L-B covering the nose and mouth. The shortcomings of this apparatus during high-altitude flying in World War II will appear in the next chapter.

Von Schrötter's 1901 prophecy, that 41,000 feet would be the upper limit that man could attain with pure oxygen,[39] does not seem to have been known in the English-speaking countries, but by the 1930s accurate information was available on maximum altitude tolerance with oxygen at ambient pressures. The critical factor here, which determined the preservation of normal bodily function, was the oxygen saturation of arterial blood. Armstrong in 1939 discovered that above 33,000 feet with one hundred per cent oxygen, there was a sharp decrease in the arterial oxygen saturation, and at 40,000 feet this fell to eighty-eight per cent. 'Flights at 25,000 feet must be considered as definitely hazardous and 30,000 feet should be the absolute allowable limit of high flying in any except the most unusual circumstances. In no instance should anyone ever be allowed to fly above 40,000 feet.'[40]

One obvious remedy was to maintain an oxygen partial pressure above that of the ambient air by enclosing the flyer in a container, which could be filled either with air or oxygen under pressure. During the early 1930s a number of technical solutions along these lines were proposed, and at the time it could not be foreseen which of these would achieve eventual acceptance. These were listed by Armstrong in an early article[41] as follows:

(1) *The oxygen compartment:* Actually an unpressurized enclosure in which the partial pressure of oxygen would be increased during ascent by releasing pure oxygen into the cabin. Not only would this procedure have been wasteful of oxygen, but the maximum altitude for

the oxygen compartment could not be greater than 37,000 feet. As far as is known, only one oxygen compartment aircraft was ever built—the experimental German Junkers Ju 88 V1 of 1941. Here the partial pressure of oxygen was held constant, with carbon dioxide absorbed by alkali cartridges, moisture by dehydrating cartridges, and odours by filters. The ceiling with this equipment was considered to be 41,000 feet. The aircraft was disliked by its crew, as the pressure changes were extreme and unpleasant, and the high concentration of oxygen constituted such a fire hazard that smoking was forbidden.[42]

(2) *The oxygen-pressure compartment:* Here the partial pressure of oxygen would be increased both by pressurization of the enclosure and by enriching its atmosphere with added oxygen. The successful high-altitude balloon flights of Piccard and his successors, described at length in Chapter 1, represented this approach. It has found no application in aviation otherwise, but the manned space capsules of today are oxygen-pressure compartments.

(3) *The pressure compartment:* A sealed, pressurized enclosure in which the partial pressure of oxygen would be maintained by compressing the outside air to approximately sea-level values. Armstrong saw this as the most promising solution for high-altitude passenger flying, but was unduly apprehensive about the theoretical effects of explosive decompression. These, he felt, would include ruptured ear drums, severe sinus pain, marked expansion of intestinal gas with resulting displacement of the heart and lungs, and generalized shock.

Several pressure cabin designs were under development when Armstrong published his paper—indeed, the earliest had appeared in the year 1920. This was fitted by the Engineering Division, McCook Field, Dayton, Ohio, in a USD-9A aircraft, an American-built version of the British De Havilland DH 9A powered by a 400 hp Liberty engine.[43] Macready, who flew this aircraft, related that the cabin was

A round affair, about as big as a good-sized barrel, constructed of steel, and practically air-tight when the door was closed. A hole, six inches in diameter, was cut in the top of the cabin and one of the same size in the left side. Both were closed with heavy plate glass, through which the vision was not particularly clear. The cabin was entered on the right side, through a round, steel door, twenty-two inches in diameter, which closed and locked from the inside. It was almost necessary to use a shoehorn to get through this opening, and I felt, as I locked myself in for the first test, as if I were about to go over Niagara Falls in a barrel. Pressure was built up within the cabin by means of a small, wind-driven compressor. A valve operated by the pilot for relieving the pressure was at the top of the cabin. After the aeroplane had climbed a few hundred feet, the pressure within the cabin began to build up faster than the relief valve could let it escape. I tried to get the door open to permit an equalization of pressure with the outside air, but found this inside pressure so great that it was impossible for me to move the door inward, much less open it. As the pressure was rapidly increasing, I faced the prospect of finding myself trapped. I throttled the engine and glided back to McCook Field as slowly as possible, in order that the small propeller operating the wind-driven pump would decrease its revolutions and thus cut down the amount of air being forced into the cabin.[44]

This aircraft was deservedly unpopular with the McCook Field test pilots, and made no real high-altitude ascents. The instrument panel was placed, not in the cockpit, but on the trailing edge of the upper wing centre section. On its first flight—8 June 1921 with Art Smith at the controls—the interior cabin pressure registered 7000 feet *below* sea level when the aircraft was flying at 3000 feet, and the temperature in the cabin reached 150° F due to compression and heating of the incoming air.

The first successful pressure cabin aeroplane was the German Junkers Ju 49, a wide-winged cantilever monoplane with a Junkers L-88 engine with two-stage supercharger, built in 1928. The designer, Muttray, enclosed the pilot in a removable cabin with portholes, separate from the structure, the top of which protruded above the decking of the metal fuselage. In 1932 this aircraft reached 32,800 feet, and 41,000 feet in 1936.

A much more ambitious project was the Lockheed XC-35 sub-stratosphere aeroplane, the true ancestor of all modern pressurized airliners. The Army Air Corps initiated a study of the physiological and engineering requirements for the pressurized cabin on 29 April 1935 and on 19 December 1935 placed a contract, incorporating appropriate specifications, with the Lockheed Aircraft Company. The aircraft was accepted in the spring of 1937. Basically, it was the commercial, twin-tailed, low-wing 10E Electra transport, but the circular-section fuselage, with a normal cockpit enclosure and small windows, incorporated a pressure cabin with an operating pressure differential of 9·5 psi, higher than in any cabins until the jet age. Two 550 hp Pratt & Whitney turbo-supercharged engines were substituted for the usual 450 hp power plants, and the cabin compressors were driven directly off the engines. The XC-35 had a service ceiling of 32,000 feet, and carried its crew of five in comfort without oxygen equipment. The award of the Collier Trophy for 1938 to the Army Air Corps for the development of 'the first successful pressure cabin aeroplane to be flown anywhere in the world' was well deserved, and stimulated similar developments by other commercial air transport builders in collaboration with commercial airlines.

The pressure suit provided another answer to the problem of oxygen supply at very high altitude. The few developed experimentally during this period were not practical, however, being inspired by the inflatable deep-sea diver's suit of rubberized fabric—in fact, the developers of one pressure suit in England were Messrs Siebe, Gorman & Co., Ltd, the leading British manufacturers of diving gear. While the diving suit, with external water pressure balanced by internal air pressure, was flexible and permitted considerable activity and movement, the rubberized aviator's suit, with an excess of internal pressure, swelled out rigidly like a balloon, effectively limiting the use of the limbs. None the less, several pioneers wore them in flights to altitudes which would have been unattainable without pressurization.

The first model to be worn in flight was evolved by Wiley Post, a great scientist as well as an airman, with the collaboration of the Goodrich Rubber Company and the United States Army Air Corps. The project was classified at the time and only recently has complete information come to light.[45] Post designed two suits which had to be discarded, the first rupturing in a static pressure test, unoccupied, on 21 June 1934. The third suit, with flexible joints at knees and elbows, was a one-piece affair entered through the neck opening, which was covered with a metal helmet resembling that of a deep-sea diving dress. This was attached by passing a series of wing-nuts through two superimposed yokes of flat metal. Oxygen (generated in a liquid air apparatus) entered the left side of the helmet, flowing across the face plate to prevent its fogging with the wearer's breath, and a hand-set pressure gauge and regulator below the left knee vented the suit and controlled the pressure. Post subsequently wore this suit in a series of high-altitude record attempts in the world-circling Lockheed Vega *Winnie Mae,* fitted with a 450 hp Pratt & Whitney 'Wasp' engine with two-stage supercharger. He is said to have reached 40,000 feet over Chicago on 5 September 1934 and, unofficially, 50,000 feet over Bartlesville, Oklahoma, on 3 December 1934. On 15 March 1935, with his cruising speed of 170 mph boosted to 279·36 mph by a following jet stream, Post flew from Burbank, California, to Cleveland at 30,000 to 40,000 feet. The flight was terminated when he ran out of liquid oxygen. Post made several attempts on the transcontinental speed record during 1935, flying at high altitude and wearing the pressure suit, but each time he was forced down by mechanical failure.

The Royal Air Force pressure suit, used in high-altitude attempts in 1936 and 1937, was a rubberized fabric garment similar to Wiley Post's, but the helmet, with a large window, was likewise made of fabric. Pressure within the suit was automatically maintained at a differential of $2\frac{1}{2}$ psi. Oxygen was piped into the suit, the atmosphere within being circulated through a soda-lime canister to absorb water vapour and carbon dioxide.

A German suit developed for the *Luftwaffe* during the mid-thirties by the *Drägerwerke* of Lübeck (again a manufacturer of diving equipment) suffered from the usual disadvantages. It was unwieldly and when inflated the wearer 'always tipped to the left.' He had to deflate the suit to shift position. An early model leaked so much oxygen as to constitute a fire hazard, and ventilation was needed in the pilot's compartment. The *Luftwaffe* experimented with a similar pressurized 'escape suit' for high-altitude bail-out, in which the wearer could not sit down when it was inflated.[46] Not until late in World War II did the partial pressure suit evolve, a skin-tight garment of open weave non-stretch nylon, with capstans running down the arms and legs to tighten the suit over the extremities, and bladders within the suit and helmet to create counterpressure over the head and trunk.

Not the least of the technical miracles of aviation in the period between the wars was the development of instrument flying, or as it was initially called, 'blind flying.' Here is an ideal example of the fruitful collaboration of the inquiring flight surgeon, himself familiar at first hand with the problems of flying, with the scientifically-minded airman. The former contributed his knowledge of the misleading attitude information which the human flyer, in the absence of visual points of reference, derives from his own senses; the latter brought to the partnership his experience of flying in clouds, and his awareness of the capability of instruments, particularly gyroscope-driven ones, to provide a constant, reliable indication of the aircraft's attitude in space.

Man, the terrestrial biped, orients and positions himself in relation to the earth's surface through two systems: the vestibular apparatus, or semi-circular canals, of the inner ear, which can determine motion of the head and its position in relation to the downward pull of gravity; and the so-called kinaesthetic senses, which transmit position information from bones, joints, tendons and muscles. Vision is useful but not essential on the ground, as shown by the fact that the normal person has no difficulty walking or remaining upright even when blindfolded.

In the air, however, orientation is entirely dependent on vision, whereby in ordinary flying the pilot positions himself and the aircraft by sight of the horizon or the ground below. The vestibular apparatus and the kinaesthetic senses, reliable indications of the 'downward' direction of the earth when man is on the ground, fail to give such precise information in the air. The movements of the aircraft, in turns and other manœuvres, or in turbulent air, produce accelerations in other directions than directly downward. The kinaesthetic and vestibular apparatus, however, still respond to these acceleration forces as though they indicated the 'downward' direction of the familiar gravitational forces on the ground. During a properly banked turn a blindfolded passenger is unaware of the change of direction, or of the fact that the wings are tilted; he may believe that the nose is being pulled up because of the increased G forces. Worse still, the semi-circular canals, once stimulated by rapid rotary motion as in a spin, continue to register motion after it has stopped.

As set forth in the preceding chapter, American otolaryngologists during World War I devoted much attention to the vestibular apparatus and its ability to provide the flyer with attitude information. Yet the results of all this research were disappointing and negative: the semi-circular canals could not precisely determine the flyer's attitude in space, in fact their information was disastrously misleading. In time Isaac Jones, who once had hoped that 'perhaps the ear would be able to tell us whether we were upside down or right side up,' came to realize that too many flyers were dying what he called 'Ear Deaths,' spiralling down through fog or cloud to a fatal crash while their vestibular apparatus failed to indicate the true attitude of their machines.[47]

In the reaction of disillusionment which followed, most flight surgeons lost interest in the sensory role of the vestibular canals. One who did not was Major David A. Myers (MC), who continued to use the rotating Baranay chair in his work with flyers, making a particular point of spinning them blindfolded to demonstrate the illusions which they might experience from vestibular stimuli. Slow turns, for instance, could not be perceived, while the flyer who was spun fast and quickly stopped would be convinced he was turning in the opposite direction, and still turning after the motion was stopped. This was the mechanism of the 'Ear Death'—the fog-bound pilot, believing himself turning in one direction, would move the controls to tighten the actual turn in the opposite direction, and the 'graveyard spiral' would be the outcome.

Most of Major Myers' young flyers probably regarded the blindfolded demonstration in the turning chair as an interesting trick, but Major William C. Ocker, who had learned to fly during World War I, came back the day after the demonstration with a turn indicator in a box. The device, gyroscopically-actuated, had been developed in the year 1917 by the American inventor of the gyro-compass, Elmer Sperry, and his son Lawrence, who in July 1914 demonstrated a gyro-stabilized automatic pilot and with it won a 25,000-franc prize for aircraft safety.[48] The turn indicator, whose hand showed whether the aircraft's nose was turning to right or left, and by its degree of movement indicated the rate, was fitted in most large military aircraft by 1924 or 1925, and in itself offered the key to successful blind flying.[49] Yet pilots caught in cloud or fog were not trained to believe the instrument and preferred to obey their own physical sensations.

Ocker was willing to believe the instrument, and quickly demonstrated to his and Myer's complete satisfaction that he could accurately determine the direction and rate of turn of the Baranay chair every time by reading the turn indicator. This discovery led to the establishment of instrument flying instruction in the military services, and very shortly thereafter, on the commercial airlines. Sperry it was who developed in the early 1930s two more gyro-driven instruments of prime importance to this day in IFR flying—the directional gyro, impervious to the accelerations which cause constant movement of the magnetic compass; and the artificial horizon, which, with a small aircraft silhouette on its face, constantly indicates to the pilot the attitude of his machine—nose up or down, wings level or banked.[50]

One old problem received considerable attention during this period, and was largely eliminated—that of carbon monoxide poisoning of the air crew. This colourless, odourless gas is always present in the exhaust of any internal combustion engine, with one to seven per cent in the exhaust gases of aeroplane engines, depending on whether they are delivering maximum takeoff and climb power with rich mixture, or cruise power with lean mixture.

Diluted further with air, it might seem that the low concentration of carbon monoxide that reaches the pilot or passenger in cockpit or cabin is insignificant, but there is a unique reason for very small concentrations being poisonous: the haemoglobin of the blood, which picks up oxygen in the lungs and transports it to the tissues, is much more ready to combine with carbon monoxide—in a ratio of 250 to one. This means that a low concentration of carbon monoxide will saturate a large proportion of the blood haemoglobin, rendering it incapable of transporting the indispensable and life-giving oxygen. Forced to get along with the lesser amounts of oxygen which the tissues now receive, the individual now develops such symptoms as severe headache, weakness, dizziness, nausea, vomiting, coma, convulsions and death. Actually these dangerous symptoms result from the tissues being starved of oxygen, rather than from any toxic reaction from the carbon monoxide. At higher altitudes, with the partial pressure of oxygen being lowered, the symptoms of carbon monoxide poisoning come on even more rapidly.

Prevention of carbon monoxide poisoning is an engineering matter; exhaust systems have been designed to lead the fumes away from the pilot, openings from the slipstream into the fuselage have been closed, and above all, engines moved out into the wings are less likely to poison crew members and passengers than those in the nose of the fuselage.

During the period between the wars, carbon monoxide poisoning was shown to be particularly frequent in the open-cockpit biplanes of the period with a single engine in the nose. Furthermore, it was proven that certain types of aircraft, due to peculiarities of airflow around the cockpits, exposed their pilots to a much higher concentration of carbon monoxide than others.

Writing in the *Journal of Aviation Medicine*, Dr Charles H. Gorman suggested that 'doubtless, great numbers of fatal unexplained aeroplane accidents have been caused as a result of a toxic condition of the pilot which rendered him incapable of operating his plane properly.'[51] He wrote of carbon monoxide poisoning causing the two pilots of a tri-motored transport to land a hundred miles off their route; the six passengers thought they were intoxicated. A mail pilot who could not explain having landed in a cow pasture was grounded: 'it was alleged that his mind was failing and a person with mental deficiency had no business operating an aeroplane.'[52] Leaky heaters passing exhaust gases through the cockpit or pilot's compartment were highly dangerous; in one such case a mail pilot flying from the West Coast to New York City turned on the heater at 16,000 feet, remembered nothing beyond Winslow, Arizona, and made a forced landing at Wink, Texas. Here he had to be assisted from the cockpit by the emergency field attendant, who thought he was drunk. In another open-cockpit mail ship (not identified) a canvas boot was left off the tail wheel aperture in the rear of the fuselage. The pilot suffered severe headache and confusion during a flight from Kansas City to Columbus, Ohio. Subsequently he experienced extreme fatigue, weakness, and dizziness, with marked anaemia, and was out of work for three months. Carbon monoxide from the slipstream, it was found, was entering the rear fuselage through the tail wheel opening and passing forward in relatively high concentrations to the cockpit. One major hazard for the pilot were the individual 'bayonet' type exhaust stacks on the early radial engines, each cylinder venting directly into the pilot's face. Shortly, collector rings were fitted to discharge the exhaust at a single point low down on the engine, and usually on the side towards which the propeller was turning downward. The closed cockpit mitigated but did not eliminate the carbon monoxide hazard. Multi-engined aircraft with power plants in the wings were unlikely to expose their flight crews to the gas. The problem ended only with the advent of the jet engine, whose exhaust contains only infinitesimal percentages of carbon monoxide.

Other new problems were anticipated by researchers during this period, even though they did not present themselves operationally until several years later. Thus, between 1934 and 1939, Armstrong[53] was able to demonstrate, by pressure-chamber experiments, involving animals and humans, that with decreased atmospheric pressure, dissolved nitrogen came out of solution in the blood stream in the form of bubbles. Depending on the location where the bubbles accumulated, the victim might experience headache, confusion, or paralysis due to blockage of blood vessels in the brain or spinal cord; burning or choking sensations in the chest, caused by bubbles in the lung circulation; pain in joints from bubbles in the joint fluid; or severe itching, from blockage of vessels under the skin. True, Armstrong was following in the footsteps of Paul Bert and J. B. S. Haldane, who years previously had studied 'the bends,' a serious and often fatal condition in compressed-air workers and deep-sea divers, and had found the problem caused by nitrogen bubbles blocking the blood vessels. Yet Armstrong was able to predict that in aviation, symptoms of aero-embolism would not appear below 30,000 feet, and that half the nitrogen dissolved in the blood and body tissues could be eliminated by breathing pure oxygen for half an hour before takeoff—values generally borne out by military experience in World War II.

The effect on flight crew of radial acceleration in aircraft manœuvres also began to receive attention, as speeds increased and G forces correspondingly rose.

The aeroplane in straight and level flight is constantly subject to the force of gravity, which under these circumstances acts on the pilot in a positive sense, i.e. from head to foot. Since much higher head-to-foot forces may be encountered in manœuvres, or in turbulent air, the normal force of gravity is designated one G.

Whenever an aeroplane (or a moving object of any kind) deviates from a straight course, it does so in response to *centripetal* force in the direction of the turn, while an equal and opposite *centrifugal* force acts in the direction away from the turn. This is most obviously apparent in a banking turn, in which the centripetal force is the increased lift on the wing. The centrifugal force results from the *inertia* of the aircraft and its occupants, or their tendency to continue in the same straight line. It acts perpendicularly to the wings, and downward relative to the aircraft and its occupants. Such a force may also be defined as a *radial acceleration* because its direction follows a radius from the centre of the turn. Since the force or acceleration increases with tightening the turn (shortening the radius), and also increases with the *square* of the velocity, accelerations many times the one G of normal gravity may develop in an aircraft in flight. It is well known to pilots that a sixty-degree bank imposes two G—twice the force of gravity—on the aircraft and its occupants, while six G is the permissible limit in civil aircraft certified for aerobatics. Military machines are designed to higher structural limits, and may exceed six G in pull-ups from dives, split Ss, or snap rolls. All these involve positive (head-to-foot) G forces; but negative (foot-to-head) forces may develop in high speed push-overs into dives, outside loops or inverted spins.

Taking the positive accelerations first, as these are more common during flight, the positive G forces act on the entire body, and also displace movable portions of it. At three G and above, a man is incapable of moving on his feet and the arms when lifted feel as if made of lead. Internally, the large organs of the chest and abdomen, heart, liver, spleen and intestines, flexibly attached to the skeleton, are dragged downward, the distance depending on the amount of the G force.[54] This does not cause any injury, however.

The blood, being a liquid, flows downward under the influence of G forces, collecting in the large vessels of the abdomen and in the legs. Blood pressure below the heart rises, but above the heart, and in the head particularly, it falls, with corresponding effects on the brain and retina. These organs are extremely sensitive to lack of oxygen, the retina particularly so. Thus, with decreased blood flow into the head, vision becomes dim at three to four G ('greyout'), and may shortly fail completely ('blackout') while the subject is still conscious, able to hear and move his limbs. Consciousness fails too, however, between three and five G. With reduction of G forces, consciousness returns first, followed by vision, and no permanent ill effects are experienced. It must be emphasized that high positive G forces must act for several seconds to displace the body's blood supply downward into the abdomen and legs; this explains why blackout and unconsciousness do not occur with brief application of high G forces, as in ejection-seat escape.

High negative G forces can be very unpleasant, though these are very rarely encountered even in military aircraft. Any negative G force tends to raise the blood pressure in the head, and this causes such pain and discomfort that humans cannot tolerate much more than minus 4·5 G because of intense pain in the eyeballs and severe headache. Experimental animals subjected to higher negative G forces suffer haemorrhages into the eyes and brain tissue, sometimes with fatal results.

Medical concern has been entirely with positive G forces in military air crew, 'blackout' being unknown in civil aviation other than aerobatics and air racing. Obviously a military pilot blacking out or suffering unconsciousness during combat manœuvres is ineffective and has little or no control over his aircraft. The problem of radial acceleration became urgent in the early 1930s with the development by the US Navy of the dive-bombing technique, in which the attacking aircraft plunged nearly vertically down on the target, releasing its bombs at low altitude and pulling up steeply to climb away. In these manœuvres, the pilots of F4B single-seater fighters and the F8C 'Helldiver' two-seater fighters experienced up to nine G, and suffered 'physiological embarrassment' including impairment of vision ('blackout') and sometimes loss of consciousness. Lieutenant Commander John R. Poppen (MC) undertook a study, the results of which were classified for several years, on the physiological origin of these phenomena. Carotid artery pressure was measured in large dogs, anaesthetized and strapped upright in the rear seats of dive bombers, during the pull-out, and a distinct fall in the arterial blood pressure to the brain was found. Later Poppen did further research with Dr Philip K. Drinker of the Harvard University School of Public Health, and established that 'blackout' resulted from anaemia of the brain as the blood, under the influence of high G forces, drained into the vessels of the abdomen and legs.

Experimentation on instrumented animals, not to mention humans, in the rear cockpit of dive bombers in flight was cumbersome and difficult, and other workers saw the possibility of developing large G forces in the laboratory by rotating their subjects in a centrifuge. With such a device, Armstrong and Heim were able to experiment on human and animal subjects as early as May 1935. The centrifuge was a light metal frame twenty feet in diameter and two and a half feet square, with an adjustable seat so arranged at one end that the subject, lying on his side, was subject to positive (head to foot) or negative (foot to head) acceleration; or, seated upright, he would experience transverse accelerations. The 'accelerotor', revolving in the horizontal plane at up to eighty rpm, produced up to twenty G.[55] With this apparatus, Armstrong demonstrated the drop in blood pressure in the carotid artery with six G of positive force. He emphasized the danger of high negative G forces, recording that humans found minus 4·5 G very unpleasant, while animals died with massive brain haemorrhages after exposure to minus 5 to 5·5 G. Transverse accelerations up to sixteen G were tolerated without significant symptoms.[56]

The *Luftwaffe* likewise took great interest in the problems of radial acceleration, having committed itself to the use of dive bombers in support of the German Army in land warfare. During 1934, Drs H. and B. von Diringshofen designed for the *Luftfahrtmedizinisches Forschungsinstitut* of Tempelhof a centrifuge thirty-eight feet in diameter and capable of developing twenty G. This was for years the envy of impecunious researchers in other countries. A larger centrifuge, 59·2 feet in diameter and driven by a 130 hp electric motor, was designed in 1937–39, but its construction was abandoned in 1943 due to air-raid damage. Other countries entered the centrifuge competition, the Japanese building in 1938 a huge and unwieldly affair forty-six feet in diameter.

Various procedures and devices were tried during this period to minimize the flow of blood from the brain into the lower part of the body under high G forces, without significant benefit. Crouching shortened the vertical distance over which the G force acted. Tensing the abdominal muscles limited to some extent the flow of blood into the abdominal vessels. Shouting during the pullout produced the same effect. As early as October 1933 Commander Poppen undertook development of an abdominal belt for the same purpose at the Naval Aircraft Factory in Philadelphia. This did little to minimize the tendency to black out, and in 1938, after two years of testing by Fleet and shore-based air activities, it was 'returned to a developmental status with a finding by the Commander Aircraft Battle Force that the advantages of this belt were not sufficient to offset its disadvantages.'[57] Armstrong advocated an inflatable belt, with a pressure of fifty to 100 mm of mercury, to cover the abdomen from the lower ribs to the pelvis, but there is no evidence that it was ever tested. Actually, the abdominal belt was not enough, and counterpressure over the legs was also necessary, as in the G suits evolved for fighter pilots during World War II.

The autopsy, a routine and indispensable feature of modern aircraft accident investigations, was a source of information as early as 1923. In the greatest air disaster up to that time, the French rigid airship *Dixmude,* a former Zeppelin surrendered as a war prize, disappeared with fifty persons aboard on the night of 20–21 December 1923 while returning to her base near Toulon after a three-day journey to In Salah in the Sahara Desert.[58] For days the French press carried fantastic accounts of the 743-foot craft drifting about the skies of Tunisia and Algeria. Then, on 30 December, came the shocking news that four days previously some fishermen of Sciacca, on the south coast of Sicily, had discovered in their nets the body of the airship's commander, the 31-year-old Lieutenant de Vaisseau Jean du Plessis de Grenedan. Witnesses were then found who had seen a big fire and explosion in the sky offshore about 2.15 am on 21 December, and small fragments of the airship's fabric outer cover and gas cells, as well as light metal debris, were picked up on land west of Sciacca. Dragging operations went on for weeks, but no large pieces of wreckage were located, and only one other body was ever recovered, four months after the disaster.

The corpse of her commander thus assumed unusual importance as evidence of what had happened to the *Dixmude,* and indeed, the autopsy provided mute indication of an explosion of extraordinary violence, which could only have been caused by ignition of two million cubic feet of hydrogen contaminated with air. Noting that du Plessis' watch had stopped at 2.27, Paris time, and that he was still wearing his fur-lined flight suit, the examiners further recorded:

No trace of fire was noted either on the body or on the clothing. The body exhibits multiple fractures, the face, the left arm and legs are shattered. The chest is crushed in on the left side, an injury which has ruptured the heart and the stomach. A wound, very deep and elongated, on the right side of the neck. Lacerations of the elbows and knees. The lungs are collapsed, which proves that death was not due to immersion. On the posterior aspect of the right thigh, a fragment of wood the size of a finger nail had been driven into the flesh, having pierced the clothing. The coveralls bore brownish stains identified by analysis as being stains of castor oil. The medical findings did not permit any conclusions as to the date of death.[59]

From the fact that the upper part of the body bore such extreme marks of injury on the left side, the investigators satisfied themselves that at the instant of the explosion, du Plessis was in the control car (his right hand was gloved), leaning half-way out of one of the open windows, when the blast, striking from his left rear, inflicted the severe injuries described above, slammed him against the window frame producing the lacerations of the neck, elbows and knees, and projected him out into space. Certainly the hypothesis explains why only du Plessis' body was recovered at the time of the crash.

The period between the wars saw the introduction on a large scale of the free-type, manually-operated parachute for the saving of life of air crew in an emergency, particularly in the military services. The successful design was created in the United States by Leslie Irvin, with the assistance of officers of the Engineering Division of the Air Service at McCook Field, Dayton, Ohio. Many foreign countries purchased these parachutes from the Irving[60] Parachute Company of Buffalo, New York, or manufactured them under license.

It will be recalled that the Germans, alone of all the wartime belligerents, succeeded in equipping their aircraft shortly before the Armistice with an attached-type parachute, and that numerous lives were saved thereby. The United States Army Air Service was unable to produce a suitable design for employment in France, but continued its research and development programme after the war. The parachute seemed a peculiarly irresistible challenge to inventors, and a large variety of models were made available to the Air Service for testing.

Most, like the German Heinicke, were of the 'attached' type. Some, now completely forgotten, were complicated to the point of impracticality:

Jahn parachute: This parachute, designed by Le Roy B. Jahn, Montevideo, Minnesota, depends for its recognition, principally, on its quick-opening device. This is accomplished by four steel springs sewn into the skirt, each spring being about 4 feet long when unfolded and about 1 foot when folded. This parachute has undergone numerous tests, which brought out that the springs may do more harm than good, and structural difficulties developed in the parachute itself. Its development has been dropped.[61]

The Irvin 'chute, a 'pack-on-the-back' design, initially had a rip cord attached to the aeroplane. This was modified so that the rip cord terminated in a D-ring attached to the parachute harness, to be pulled by the wearer when he desired to open the parachute. Pulling the rip cord opened the canvas parachute pack, permitting a small 'pilot 'chute,' constructed with steel ribs and springs, to eject itself into the airstream. This in turn simply drew the folded main parachute, twenty-eight feet in diameter, from the depths of the pack. Leslie Irvin made the first 'live' jump with his parachute at McCook Field on 28 April 1919 and its simple and positive action earned him a contract for three hundred more from the Army Air Service.

Though the Engineering Division favoured the free-type parachute, a final decision on its merits was not made until a tragedy at McCook Field in July 1919 demonstrated the fatal propensity of the 'attached' type parachute to foul the aircraft. The device in question, the 'Guardian Angel' developed by the E. C. Calthrop Co. of England, was criticized by McCook Field in the following terms:

The type which is packed between two aluminium discs is one of their development, and is considered entirely too bulky, although it opens positively and quickly. Both the parachute and its harness are considered too weak.[62]

None the less, Lieutenant R. R. Caldwell, RAF, was permitted to demonstrate the 'Guardian Angel' on behalf of its manufacturer. Incredibly, as he left the aircraft the life line fouled on a rocker arm of the engine, the harness failed under the shock, and Caldwell fell 600 feet to his death. The lesson was not lost on the spectators: the accident could not have occurred with the 'free' type parachute, and the Air Service standardized on the Irvin.

The standard version of the parachute, an improvement on Leslie Irvin's original model, was only twenty-four feet in diameter, with less weight and bulk, approximately the same rate of descent, and a faster opening time than the twenty-eight foot pioneer version. A twenty-four-sided polygon, made up of an equal number of triangular panels cut on the bias, the parachute was perfectly flat when laid on a level surface. Silk was the standard material, and only certain grades of Japanese-woven silk, cultivated on the Shanghai peninsula, were suitable:

The ability of this particular weight and weave of silk to withstand great impact of air pressure and the sudden 'hoop tension' that is applied upon the opening of the parachute under load at high speed, as well as its ability to resist the tendency to blow or tear out panels, is due extensively to its long 'time lag,' combined with the bias construction.

The 'time lag' on this silk was discovered in the Göttingen Tunnel in Germany during the last year of the war, and is 0·621 second for shocks applied at opening. The long 'staple' and method of weaving is mostly responsible for this 'time lag.'

The silks woven in this country have a much shorter 'time lag,' due mostly to the high tensions used in our looms.

The 7, 8 and 9 momme Japanese silk has a shorter 'time lag' than the 10 or 12 momme. However, the air friction per pore is too high in the 12 momme to let the effect of the open pores at the time of shock to be of maximum benefit; thus, under drop-testing, Shanghai 12-momme silk fails under an opening shock that 10-momme will withstand.[63]

The first life saved with the free back-pack parachute was that of a McCook Field test pilot, Lieutenant Harold R. Harris. On the afternoon of 20 October 1922 he was testing a Loening PW-2A monoplane fighter with experimental ailerons in a mock dogfight, when aerodynamic flutter (little understood at the time) caused the ailerons to disintegrate, and the wings to break up. Leaping just in time, Harris became the first member of the 'Caterpillar Club,' named in honour of the lowly silkworm whose product had saved him. Slowly other names were added—aviation was a small activity in the early 1920s. Only in 1922 was wearing of the parachute made compulsory in the Army Air Service. Some who saved their lives were test pilots, others were mail flyers. Charles Lindbergh jumped for his life four times before he flew to Paris, the last two occasions being when he was trapped aloft in fog in his DH 4 mail plane, with no hope of being able to land it safely.

As early as 12 June 1922 Captain Albert W. Stevens proved the efficacy of the parachute at high altitude by jumping from a Martin MB2 bomber at 24,200 feet over Dayton, Ohio. The bomber's Liberties were fitted with an early model of exhaust-driven supercharger, and gaseous oxygen flasks were carried in the forward and rear cockpits. Remarkably, Stevens wore strapped to his leg a seventy-cubic-inch oxygen flask, a 'bail-out bottle,' to maintain consciousness while falling from high altitude, anticipating by twenty years a development of World War II. Stevens breathed oxygen above 20,000 feet, and switched to the 'bail-out bottle' before diving over the side and pulling his rip cord. Actually he only 'took a few puffs from the tube,' feeling he did not need the gas as he rapidly descended to lower levels. The parachute opened with a 'violent jerk.' On the way down the 'chute oscillated 'like a wild thing trying to break free,' making Stevens airsick, and he broke some bones in his foot on landing.

During the twenty years between the two world wars, the aeroplane developed from the picturesque but low-performance fabric-covered biplane into a swift, powerful, long-range weight carrier linking the continents in peace and capable of determining their destinies in war. During the same period aviation medicine, formerly concerned only with physical standards for pilots, had accumulated through research a body of information concerning the special stresses to which flyers were exposed, and had pointed the way to the development of protective and safety equipment. Now, as World War II began, all this knowledge would be put to the test. Never before or since would so many men be exposed to the strains and the dangers of flight.

[1] Privileged to take several hours of dual recently in a Waco RNF dating from 1930, the author can testify to the exhilaration of communing with the elements, with the wind in his face, in an open cockpit on a pleasant summer's day. But for flying the family in chilly winter weather, he acknowledges the superiority of his heated and enclosed Cessna 170B.

[2] Harry Bruno, *Wings Over America* (New York: Halcyon House, 1944), p. 97.

[3] 'Aireview,' *The Fifty Years of Japanese Aviation 1910–1960* (Tokyo: The Kantosha Co. Ltd, 1961), book II, pp. 5–6.

[4] Andrew Boyle, *Trenchard* (New York: W. W. Norton & Co., 1962).

[5] C. H. Gibbs-Smith, *The Aeroplane: an Historical Survey* (London: HM Stationery Office, 1960), p. 96.

[6] Trenchard, an inarticulate prophet, apparently envisaged the strategic striking force as being composed of single-engined day bombers—improved versions of the Independent Force's DH 4s and DH 9s of 1918.

[7] Isaac Don Levine, *Mitchell: Pioneer of Air Power* (New York: Duell, Sloan & Pierce, 1943).

[8] Edward Arpee, *From Frigates to Flat-Tops* (published by the author, 1953).

[9] One of the thrills of the author's youth was to see *Saratoga's* 'Helldivers' playing themselves (with Wallace Beery) in a movie by that name in the early 1930s. Much later we learned that Japanese naval aviators were ordered to study its spectacular dive-bombing sequences when the movie came to Tokyo.

[10] Eugene Wilson, *Slipstream* (New York: McGraw-Hill, 1950), p. 72.

[11] Richard K. Smith, *The Airships Akron and Macon: Flying Aircraft Carriers of the United States Navy* (Annapolis: US Naval Institute, 1965).

[12] C. F. Andrews and W. G. Cox, *The Supermarine S.4-S.6B* (Leatherhead, Surrey: Profile Publications Ltd, 1965).

[13] Henry R. Palmer Jr, *The Story of the Schneider Trophy Race* (Seattle: Superior Publishing Co., 1962), p. 16.

[14] Merle C. Olmsted, 'Turbo-Supercharger Development,' *Journal of the American Aviation Historical Society,* vol. 12, no. 2, Summer 1967, p. 99.

[15] War Department: Air Service: Division of Military Aeronautics: *Air Service Medical* (Washington: Government Printing Office, 1919), p. 432.

[16] *ibid.*

[17] First Lieutenant John A. Macready, 'Exploring the Earth's Atmosphere,' *National Geographic Magazine,* vol. 50, no. 6, December 1926, p. 755.

[18] *ibid.* Yet the problem of cold at high altitude was never solved before the advent of the closed, heated cabin. As Armstrong admitted in 1939, 'in spite of a considerable amount of experimental study and research winter flying clothing remains . . . an admitted burden to personnel and quite ineffective for the low temperatures frequently encountered.' Small wonder that 'loss of morale, indifference or distaste for the mission' resulted. Harry G. Armstrong, *Principles and Practice of Aviation Medicine* (Baltimore: Williams & Wilkins Co., 1939), pp. 184–5.

[19] Macready, p. 773.

[20] His brother, Lieutenant Zeus Soucek, was also a naval aviator and set records in the PN-12 flying boat in 1928.

[21] Though one source claims he was breathing a mixture of eighty-seven per cent oxygen, 12·7 per cent carbon dioxide *(Journal of Aviation Medicine,* vol. 9, March–December 1938, p. 141).

[22] Armstrong, p. 320.

[23] Hy Steirman and Glenn D. Kittler, *Triumph* (New York: Harper & Brothers, 1961).

[24] Graham Wallace, *The Flight of Alcock and Brown* (London: Putnam & Co., Ltd, 1955).

[25] Charles A. Lindbergh, *The Spirit of St Louis* (New York: Charles Scribners Sons, 1954), p. 424.

[26] *ibid.,* p. 501.

[27] Between 29 June and 22 July 1928 John H. Mears and Charles D. Collyer circled the globe with a Fairchild cabin monoplane, but the aircraft crossed the Atlantic and Pacific oceans aboard ship.

[28] Richard Sanders Allen, *Revolution in the Sky* (Brattleboro, Vermont, The Stephen Greene Press, 1964), p. 80.

[29] Lieutenant Colonel Eldon W. Downs, 'Army and the Air Mail 1934,' *Air Power Historian,* vol. IX, no. 1, January 1962, p. 35.

[30] The Royal Air Force during this period engaged civilian physicians to care for the ordinary medical needs of their flyers on a contract basis.

[31] Mae Mills Link and Hubert A. Coleman, *Medical Support of the Army Air Forces in World War II* (Washington: Government Printing Office, 1955), p. 28.

[32] Armstrong, pp. 330–8.

[33] Wing Commander Robert Maycock, *Doctors in the Air* (London: George Allen & Unwin Ltd, 1957), p. 33.

[34] Major I. B. March (MC), 'Diary of Cold Weather Test Flight' *(Journal of Aviation Medicine,* vol. 6, no. 1, March–December 1935), p. 20.

[35] Robert J. Benford MD, *Doctors in the Sky: the Story of the Aero Medical Association* (Springfield, Illinois: Charles C. Thomas, 1955), p. 109.

[36] Armstrong, p. 304.

[37] Though photographs of Macready and other Army Air Corps high-altitude flyers show them wearing masks, these latter were mere leather shields to prevent frostbite, and the tube still led through them to the pipe-stem.

[38] W. M. Boothby and W. R. Lovelace, 'Oxygen in Aviation' *(Journal of Aviation*

Medicine, vol. 9, March–December 1938), p. 172.

[39] See pp. i–34, 35.

[40] Armstrong, p. 321.

[41] H. G. Armstrong, 'Medical Problems of Sealed High Altitude Aircraft Compartments' *(Journal of Aviation Medicine,* vol. 7, no. 1, March 1936), p. 2.

[42] Henry *(sic)* Seeler, 'Pressure Suits and Pressure Cabins in German Aviation,' *German Aviation Medicine in World War II,* prepared under the auspices of the Surgeon General, USAF (Washington: Government Printing Office, 1950), vol. I, p. 526.

[43] A. J. Jackson, *De Havilland Aircraft* (London: Putnam & Co., Ltd., 1962), p. 76.

[44] Macready, p. 768.

[45] Stanley B. Mohler, 'Wiley Post's Aerospace Achievements,' *The Air Power Historian,* vol. XI, no. 3, July 1964, p. 65.

[46] Henry *(sic)* Seeler, 'Pressure Suits and Pressure Cabins in German Aviation,' *German Aviation Medicine in World War II,* vol. I, p. 526.

[47] Isaac H. Jones, *Flying Vistas* (Philadelphia: J. B. Lippincott Co., 1937), p. 119.

[48] Charles L. Keller, 'Automatic Pilot, 1913 version,' *Sperry Engineering Review,* October 1960, p. 20.

[49] Even today the turn indicator is the one gyro instrument indispensable for instrument flying, in conjunction with the bank indicator, airspeed meter, altimeter and magnetic compass.

[50] The first version of this instrument was produced by Sperry as early as 1919, with a miniature biplane superimposed on the artificial horizon. Robert J. Scheppler, 'Aviation Instruments, Part I' *(Journal of the American Aviation Historical Society,* vol. 6, no. 3, Autumn 1961), p. 169.

[51] Charles H. Gorman, 'CO Poisoning' *(Journal of Aviation Medicine,* vol. 8, March–December 1937), p. 42.

[52] *ibid.*

[53] Armstrong, p. 340.

[54] For what it is worth, the author's personal belief is that displacement of abdominal organs by G forces is the immediate cause of airsickness, a subject on which there is a great deal of controversy. Sixty-degree banks at one time were sure to make the author nauseated, until he practised them deliberately and succeeded in desensitizing himself.

[55] William H. White, *A History of the Centrifuge in Aerospace Medicine* (Santa Monica, California: Douglas Aircraft Co., 1964), chapter II.

[56] H. G. Armstrong, 'Effects of Acceleration' *(Journal of Aviation Medicine,* vol. 9, March–December 1938), p. 199.

[57] Van Wyen and Pearson, *United States Naval Aviation 1910–60* (Washington: Government Printing Office, 1961), p. 75.

[58] Douglas H. Robinson, 'The Mystery of the "Dixmude",' *Journal of the American Aviation Historical Society,* vol. 9, no. 2, Summer 1964, p. 96. One of the missing was Médecin Iere Classe Léopold Pelissier, attached to the Cuers airship base—the only medical man to lose his life in an airship accident.

[59] Jean du Plessis de Grenedan, *Les Grands Dirigeables,* vol. I: *Leur Passe, Leur Avenir, l'Experience du 'Dixmude'* (Paris: Plon-Nourrit et Cie, 1925), p. 268.

[60] The company was so titled, even though the inventor spelled his name otherwise.

[61] Bureau of Aeronautics, US Navy, *Rigid Airship Manual 1927* (Washington; Government Printing Office, 1928), pp. vii–2.

[62] *ibid.,* pp. vii–3.

[63] *ibid.,* pp. vii–6.

5

Aviation Medicine Comes of Age: World War II, 1939–45

During the six-year struggle between the United Nations and the Axis Powers, the air weapon, growing beyond all expectations, played a major role as a third arm and as a strategic offensive force. Thousands of planes, hundreds of thousands of men, ranged the skies of Europe, Asia and Africa on combat missions, carrying the youth of the belligerent nations to altitudes and distances attained only by experimental aircraft a few years previously. Anoxia, aero-embolism, airsickness, fatigue, threatened the efficiency of the air forces on which victory depended. The knowledge of the aeromedical researcher in the laboratory, and of the flight surgeon in the field, were vital to the accomplishment of the Air Force mission.

What the mission should be was a matter of debate throughout the war. Generals and admirals saw the aeroplane as an auxiliary to land and sea forces, serving the foot soldier as airborne artillery, and the battleship as a scouting aid. More and more as the struggle progressed the aeroplane assumed an independent strategic role. This was predominantly the case in the British Royal Air Force and the United States Army Air Force, which, from the teachings of Marshal of the RAF Lord Trenchard and Brigadier General William Mitchell, had evolved a common doctrine holding that the aeroplane, acting independently of the ground forces, could achieve decisive results through strategic bombing attacks on the enemy's industry and population.[1] For the Japanese and the United States Navies the aeroplane, through the development of the fast carrier striking force, superseded the battleship and became the primary offensive weapon of sea power.

Traditional domination of the German military establishment by the Army prevented the German Air Force from achieving a strategic role. The newest of the aerial contestants of 1939–45, founded in 1933 after Hitler's seizure of power, the *Luftwaffe* might have been expected to develop and implement air power theory untrammelled by the conservative military traditions prevailing in the democracies. Instead, it was fated to be, first, a propaganda weapon to terrify European neighbours into submitting to the will of the *Führer,* and secondly, to

149

serve as the striking arm of the mobile armoured spearheads of the new German Army. The vacillating leadership of the vainglorious hero of *Karinhall, Reichsmarschall* Hermann Goering, denied the *Luftwaffe* the opportunity to develop an independent strategy, and a trained and qualified staff.

The new German Air Force, unveiled with great éclat on 1 March 1935, was revealed as a training organization with very limited offensive capability. Open-cockpit biplane fighters, and the corrugated-metal Junkers Ju 52 transport converted into a makeshift bomber, comprised its combat strength. These were the aircraft which went to Spain with the Condor Legion in 1936 to fight in the Spanish Civil War. Their successes were meagre, but in the next year better results were obtained with the first of the *Luftwaffe's* mass-produced advanced combat types, most of which were still in service when World War II broke out two years later.

With the emphasis on Army co-operation, short-range bombers received most attention. In particular, Ernst Udet, Goering's old flying buddy and head of the *Luftwaffe* technical department, had brought back from America the dive-bomber concept, and one of the aircraft produced in quantity was the Junkers Ju 87 *Sturzkampfflugzeug,* or 'Stuka,' an ugly, angular two-seater monoplane with inverted gull wing and fixed landing gear. Screaming down in sixty-degree dives, a big bomb swinging down on a fork to clear the propeller, and pulling out with the aid of an automatic device even if the high G forces caused the pilot to black out, the *Stuka* was a terrifying weapon against armies overwhelmed by the *Blitzkrieg,* and unprotected by their own air forces. A number of clean twin-engine bombers were also coming along—the Heinkel He 111, the Dornier Do 17 'flying pencil,' and the Junkers Ju 88, a versatile aircraft which, with modifications, served through the war as a bomber, a high-altitude reconnaissance aircraft, a heavy anti-bomber weapon and a night fighter. Excellent by the standards of their day, these were all-metal monoplanes with engines of approximately 1000 hp, the Heinkel having a particularly pleasing geometry with its gracefully streamlined body and elliptical wings and tail. All had self-sealing fuel tanks, to minimize the risk of fire, but no armour. They shared also the common defect of inadequate defensive armament—single hand-operated rifle-calibre machine guns, difficult to aim through the slipstream.

For the offensive-minded *Luftwaffe,* sharing the Master Race's disdain for its opponents, the defensive fighter was something of an afterthought. In particular, it was considered that the new bombers, by virtue of their speed, could outrun enemy fighters and hence needed no protection. In the pre-war period, however, the most famous German fighter aircraft of World War II, the Messerschmitt Me 109, was designed and produced, making its first flight in September 1935. A low-wing monoplane with retractible landing gear, it carried 20 mm. cannon even before 1939. Initially it was handicapped by an inadequate range, but like its famous contemporary, the Spitfire, the Me 109 proved adaptable, and with increasingly powerful engines and modifications to the airframe and armament, it remained the mainstay of the German fighter force to the end.

The *Luftwaffe's* experience in Spain, fighting against the disorganized hodge-podge of French, Russian and US aircraft which comprised the Loyalist Air Force, encouraged the Nazi planners to believe that air superiority could be easily gained, after which their fast bombers and screaming *Stukas* could batter at will the armies and transport of the enemy. The four-week lightning campaign in Poland in the autumn of 1939 seemed to confirm the *Luftwaffe's* feeling of superiority, with the Polish air force bombed out of existence on its airfields in the first two days, and the *Stukas* and the bombers then racing ahead to clear the way to Warsaw for the tanks and motorized infantry. Undoubtedly the *Luftwaffe's* finest hour was the conquest of the *Armée de l'Air* and the overwhelming of much of the ground opposition in the defeat of France in the spring of 1940.

Fighter Command of the British Royal Air Force was no push-over, however, and in the three-month Battle of Britain in the summer of 1940, the German Air Force failed to win the control of the air that was a necessary preliminary to invasion. Where Air Chief Marshal Dowding showed great moral courage and tenacity of purpose in husbanding reserves and refusing to squander the fighters on which Britain's future depended, his amateurish opponent, *Reichsmarschall* Goering, changed his objectives, abandoned attacks on Fighter Command's airfields when success seemed within his grasp, and switched to militarily meaningless terror raids on London, finally turning to night bombing. Inadequately armed and armoured German bombers fell in large numbers to the eight-gun Hurricanes and Spitfires, particularly the slow and clumsy *Stukas,* while the Me 109s were too few in number, and too short-legged, to protect their heavier aircraft. Above all, and unsuspected by the Germans, who were only developing such equipment, the British had created in the nick of time a workable early warning system based on radar installations around the coast, which enabled ground controllers to vector their few and overworked fighters against the German formations before they reached their targets.

In frustration, the *Führer* drew back from England and turned on the hereditary foe in the East, where the *Luftwaffe* played its traditional ground-support role in the advance that led in the summer of 1941 to within sight of Moscow, and in the grim attacks and counter-attacks of the next three years.

In other theatres it was all downhill thereafter. Gradually the *Luftwaffe* was forced back on the defensive. With increasingly heavy bomber assaults on the cities of the *Reich* after the Casablanca directive of January, 1943, instituting the Combined Bomber Offensive by the RAF by night, and the USAAF by day, the Germans had to build up fighter strength at the expense of bomber production. To stop the American B-17s in daylight seemed more feasible than to find and shoot down the RAF's four-engined bombers by might. For attacks on the heavily-armed and armoured Flying Fortresses, the Me 109G carried two 13 mm machine guns and two electrically-driven 20 mm MG 151 cannon firing at the incredible rate of 750 rounds per minute. And the Focke Wulf firm had produced in the FW-190 a compact fighter built around a 14-cylinder radial engine of 1800 hp. Armoured with plating up to eight mm thick, the Focke-Wulf carried two machine guns on the cowl, two MG 151 cannon in the wing roots, and a pair of Oerlikon 20 mm cannon in the wings outside the propeller arc, firing at the rate of 280 rounds per minute. In the early 8th Air Force attacks deep into Germany the enemy's single-seaters were joined by twin-engine fighters such as the Me 110 and the Ju 88 carrying as many as six 20 mm cannon and 21 cm (8 in.) rockets. The German defensive day fighters succeeded in inflicting such unacceptable losses on the American daylight bombers that fighter escort had to be provided. In the last year of the war, with swarms of P-51 Mustangs accompanying the 'Forts' over Germany, the *Luftwaffe* often lay low during the daylight hours, only to vent its wrath on the lumbering, underarmed Lancasters and Halifaxes of RAF Bomber Command by night. Radar-equipped, vectored towards the bomber streams making their way across Germany under cover of darkness, the black-painted night fighters achieved such successes as the destruction of ninety-five out of 795 Lancasters and Halifaxes sent against Nürnberg on the night of 30–31 March 1944 and remained a threat right to the end. It was in fact the success of the Allied bombing attack on oil-producing facilities and transportation which brought about the final defeat of the *Luftwaffe* in 1945.

Britain's Royal Air Force, the world's first independent air arm, upheld as doctrine the Trenchard belief in the decisive role of strategic bombing of the enemy's industry and civilian population, yet failed to create a bomber force able to execute this mission. Partly this originated in the short-sighted economy policies of successive governments, both Tory and Labour, who starved the fighting services

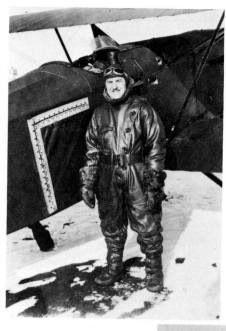

23. Winter flying clothing of the U.S. Army Air Service, 1924. (Air Force Museum)

24. Wiley Post in his 1934 pressure suit; 'Winnie Mae' in background. (Air Force Museum)

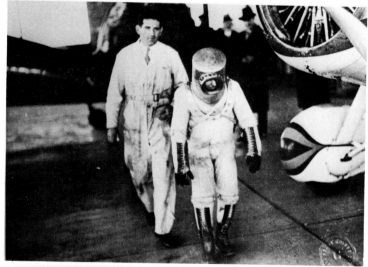

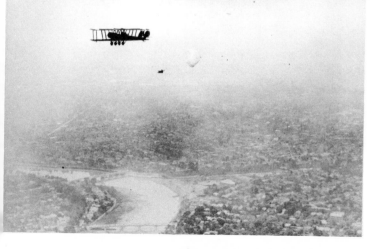

25. Parachute test at Dayton 1919: 'pull-off from a Martin MB-I bomber. (Air Force Museum)

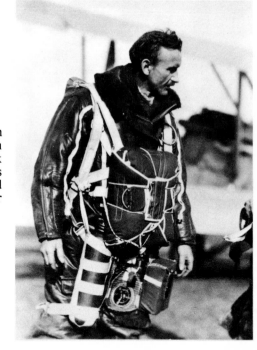

26. Captain A.W. Stevens dressed for high altitude parachute jump from a Martin Bomber on 12 June 1922. Note chest pack parachute, white tapes running down his arms which are electric leads for heated gloves, and oxygen bottle with regulator strapped to his leg. (Air Force Museum)

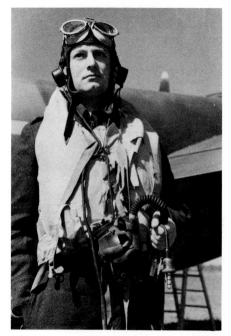

27. Mosquito pilot, wearing Mae West life jacket and holding tubing of his oxygen mask with quick-disconnect fitting, and plug-in for electrically heated flight suit (1944). (Imperial War Museum)

28. Focke-Wulf Ta. 152 H-I. German fighter with pressurized cockpit under development at the end of the war (1945). (Imperial War Museum)

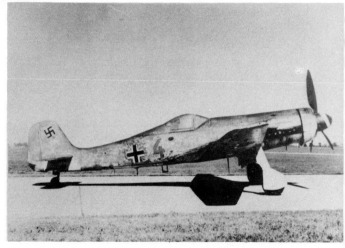

while publicly advocating collective security and universal disarmament. Partly this was due to the minuscule Air Force, treated by the senior services as a temporary inconvenience, finding its chief justification in controlling troublesome tribesmen in Iraq and on the North-West Frontier of India—hardly training for modern warfare. At home, up until 1938, the fateful year of the Munich surrender, the equipment of the RAF bomber squadrons was little improved over the Handley-Page 0/400 of World War I, and inferior in range and load-carrying ability to the four-engined Handley-Page V/1500 of 1918. In 1934, however, the Baldwin Government decided to build up the bomber force, and furthermore, with larger, heavier and faster all-metal monoplanes of greater range and speed than the existing biplanes. In a far-sighted decision, power-operated gun turrets were specified, the Nash and Thompson versions most commonly fitted in nose and tail carrying two or four ·303 calibre machine guns. The Hampden, the Armstrong-Whitworth Whitley, and the Vickers Wellington formed the backbone of Bomber Command during the first three years of the war. Their successors, large aircraft worthy of the strategic bombing concept, were ordered as early as 1936. These included the four-engined Short Stirling and Handley-Page Halifax, and the twin-engined Avro Manchester, which, reworked as the Lancaster with four Rolls-Royce Merlin engines, became the RAF's most famous and effective bomber.

The test of war demonstrated that Bomber Command of the Royal Air Force was neither equipped nor trained for its role of crushing the enemy through strategic bombing. Early daylight attacks on warships off the German coast proved that even the 235 mph Wellington with four machine guns in power-operated turrets was no match for defending Messerschmitt Me 109 and 110 fighters. Perforce, Bomber Command switched to night operations, but during the months of the 'phoney war' their aircraft were dropping propaganda leaflets ('nickelling'), not bombs, over the *Reich*. The night bombing offensive again German industry commenced only after the invasion of France, in the spring of 1940. Only gradually did it dawn on Bomber Command, and on the leaders of the British Government, that these early attacks were completely ineffective: when photographic equipment was installed in the night-bombing aircraft, the flash photographs showed that only one-third of the attackers had placed their bombs within five miles of the target. Navigation was largely to blame: dead reckoning and star sights, as used in World War I, were quite unequal to the precise location of a target, even a city, at night. The British Air Staff might have learned this lesson from reading their own history[2] describing the ineffectiveness of the Zeppelin raids on

England in World War I, but evidently they did not do so.

Under the inspired leadership of Air Chief Marshal Sir Arthur Harris, who became Commander-in-Chief of Bomber Command on 22 February 1942, the heavy bomber grew to be the means of destruction of the enemy's war-making potential that Trenchard and Mitchell insisted it could be. The first 'thousand-plane raid' on Cologne on the night of 30–31 May 1942 was a tremendous stimulant to morale of the Command and of the people of Britain. At the same time, with the knowledge of responsible government leaders, the policy of bombing German industry and communications was quietly shelved, as such targets could not be pin-pointed at night, and replaced by incendiary area-bombing of German cities designed to disrupt the economy by killing or rendering homeless the German working population. Radio navigational aids—'Oboe' and 'Gee' directing the aircraft from England, and 'H$_2$s,' an airborne radar clearly indicating at night built-up areas and bodies of water, led the attackers to the designated targets. Ground or airborne flares, dropped by especially skilled crews of the Pathfinder Force (many flying the phenomenal 400 mph twin-engined De Havilland Mosquito) enabled the crews of the Halifaxes and Lancasters to salvo their bombs within 1000 yards of the aiming point. And the bomb loads became progressively heavier—up to seven tons of assorted incendiaries and explosives in the Lancaster, some of which might weigh 4000, 8000 or 12,000 pounds each—even a monster 22,000 pound explosive bomb, the 'Grand Slam,' which protruded partly from the bomb bay. Raids on German cities in the last two years of the war became as complex as a five-ring circus, with a constant radio commentary from a 'master bomber' cruising above the target, and an infinite repertoire of acts—'Corona' and 'Cigar,' designed to confuse enemy night-fighter directors, 'Musical Parramatta,' 'Musical Newhaven,' and 'Musical Wanganui,' describing the various means of flare-marking the target for the bombers which might number many hundreds. The results were fatal for thousands of the spectators, with unprecedented destruction caused by the 'fire-storms' that raged for days in the catastrophic blows against Wuppertal, Hamburg, Kassel and ultimately on the night of 13 February 1945, against Dresden, where 135,000 persons died—more than in the atomic bomb attacks on Hiroshima and Nagasaki together. But the men in the air paid a price also. Incapable of ascending much above 20,000 feet, cruising at about 200 mph, pitting rifle-calibre machine guns against multiple cannon, emitting constant radar transmissions on which the German night fighters could home with their 'Naxos' equipment, all too many of the big four-engined bombers flamed, exploded, and went down in pieces over Germany with their seven-man crews. Unlike the American 8th Air Force, RAF's Bomber Command never found a direct counter to the German defences, and had to resort to evasive routing and deception measures. Only with the collapse of the ground-control organization after the Allied invasion of the Continent did the German night fighters lose their effectiveness. But they, more than any other weapon, were responsible for Bomber Command's 47,268 dead in combat operations.[3]

In contrast to the re-worked variations of the World War I Handley Page which had equipped the bomber squadrons during the lean years of 'collective security,' British fighter designers had led the world. The Hawker Fury, first fighter anywhere to exceed 200 mph, was the fastest in the world when it entered squadron service in 1931. But the defensive fighter arm was overshadowed by the Air Staff's emphasis on the strategic offensive, and further down-graded by the pessimistic view of Britain's leaders confronting the nightmare of air attack on their sprawling capital. Against the opposition of the Air Ministry, Fighter Command was born in 1936 and nurtured by the incumbent Secretary of State for Air, Viscount Swinton, who realized that London and its citizens could not be left naked to the growing threat of the Nazi *Luftwaffe*. That Fighter Command succeeded when put to the test in the Battle of Britain was due to two miracles unforeseen in 1933 when Prime Minister Stanley Baldwin predicted that 'the bomber will always get through': the low-wing monoplane fighter, and the invention of radar, which gave advance warning of attack to ground controllers who could then vector the fighters against enemy bombers at a distance.

As is well known, two fighters representing a revolutionary advance over the traditional biplane were developed in the short years of expansion before 1939—the Hawker Hurricane and the Supermarine Spitfire. Its reputation overshadowed by that of the Spitfire, the Hurricane was the first in squadron service in December 1937 and comprised the bulk of the fighters available at the beginning of the war. The Spitfire, which entered service in June 1938, was a more sophisticated aircraft which owed something to the Supermarine S 5, S 6 and S 6B Schneider Cup racers of the early thirties. Of aeromedical interest is the fact that both aircraft had bullet-proof glass windshields and armour plate in front of and behind the pilot. On the other hand, many surviving air crew were badly burned before self-sealing fuel tanks were fitted in September 1940 and even then the upper fuselage tank ahead of the pilot in the Spitfire could not be so modified. (German fighters were constructed with self-sealing tanks, but only after the battle commenced did they carry improvised cockpit armour).

After some tentative sparring with *Luftwaffe* units during the 'phoney war,' and after a sharp encounter with German bombers at Dunkirk, the untried British fighter squadrons were put to the test in defence of their homeland during the Battle of Britain. Three Air Fleets of the *Luftwaffe* in Norway, Belgium and France set out to win air superiority by destroying the Royal Air Force in the skies and on the ground, using their bombers to draw British fighters into the air. In opposing them, the slower Hurricanes, inferior in performance to the Messerschmitt Me 109s, went for the poorly armed and armoured bombers. The *Stukas* were slaughtered in droves and withdrawn before the end of the battle, and the twin-engined Dorniers, Heinkels and Junkers suffered unacceptable losses. For lack of drop-tanks, the Me 109s could not give their bombers cover beyond London, denying the *Luftwaffe* true strategic capability. Combats took place from 25,000 feet down, contrary to earlier expectations, with the bombers coming over at 16,000 feet or lower, and the Me 109s at 20,000 feet or higher. In dogfights at high altitude with the crack German *Jagdgeschwader,* the Spitfire showed itself as fast as the Me 109 and more manœuvrable.

The acute danger of defeat in the air and invasion passed in September 1940 but night attacks continued over the length and breadth of England until June 1941 when the assault on Russia called away the *Luftwaffe,* never to return in strength. The 'night blitz' is symbolized by the shattering attack on Coventry on 14 November 1940 but there were also heavy raids on London, that on 29–30 December being particularly destructive. The answer to the night bombers lay in radar, and early versions of the night fighter carrying airborne radar were barely operational by the winter of 1940–41. Large aircraft with good endurance and weight-lifting capacity were required, carrying a crew of two—the pilot, especially skilled in instrument flying, and the radar operator who, led by the ground controller, hopefully might pick up the 'blip' of the enemy aircraft with his 'black box,' and guide his pilot to the close vicinity of the quarry. At the last minute—ideally—exhaust flames would come in sight, and a belch of 20 mm cannon shell would obliterate an enemy who never knew what had hit him. The secret of airborne radar was carefully guarded, and the night-fighter successes explained by a cover story to the effect that the pilots were being crammed with vitamin A to produce hyperacute night vision. For a period, credulous flight surgeons in the United States forced butter and carrots in great quantities on their unwilling flight crews! Converted twin-engined Blenheim bombers won the first night-fighting successes, but the aircraft which ultimately became the scourge of the *Luftwaffe* in the night skies over Britain was the Bristol Beaufighter. Its armament of four 20 mm cannon in the nose and six ·303 calibre machine guns in the wings could saw a bomber into fragments in seconds.

Unlike the Royal Air Force, which had faith without works, the United States Army Air Force battled unceasingly to realize the strategic vision of its martyred leader, Brigadier General Billy Mitchell. Yet the institution of the long-range bomber force could not be called into being before a suitable instrument had been created. In August 1935 the first of the immortal Boeing B-17s was delivered for testing to the Material Division at Wright Field, Dayton, Ohio. Though the first was destroyed in a tragic takeoff crash, thirteen YB-17s were ordered and delivered during 1937. With these aircraft, strategic bombing became possible. Almost from the beginning, the B-17 was planned to be a high-altitude bomber, and General Electric turbo-superchargers on the YB-17A gave it a ceiling of more than 30,000 feet. The thirteen originals, together with the experimental XB-15, were the only four-engined bombers in the Army Air Corps when World War II broke out. Minor improvements were made between then and Pearl Harbor, and twenty B-17Cs were supplied to the Royal Air Force. These, flying in small numbers to extreme altitudes up to 39,200 feet, made a number of daylight raids on German naval bases in the summer of 1941. Losses were heavy, and the resulting redesign produced in the B-17E, entering service at the time of Pearl Harbor, a craft featuring a heavy defensive armament of twelve ·50 calibre machine guns (including two in the tail and four in twin power-operated turrets), self-sealing fuel tanks, and heavier armour. Other bombers were also ready when Japan threw down the gauntlet, notably the B-17's less publicized but ultimately more numerous rival, the four-engined Convair B-24, with its efficient Davis laminar-flow wing and great range.

The years before World War II found American fighter (or 'pursuit') strength woefully deficient, and its role in the Army Air Corps mission under a cloud. No less a person than the Asistant Chief of the Air Corps, Brigadier General Oscar Westover, had asserted that 'bombardment aviation has defensive firepower of such quantity and effectiveness as to warrant the belief that with its modern speeds it may be capable of effectively accomplishing its assigned mission without support.'[4] Thus, pursuit aviation saw itself rejected in its traditional role of bomber escort. At the same time, interceptors were not required as the Atlantic and Pacific Oceans guarded America against enemy bombers. None the less, three superb fighters were under development at the time of Pearl Harbor.

The Lockheed P-38 Lightning, with two supercharged 1150 hp Allison engines turning contra-rotating propellers, carried its pilot in a nacelle between the engines, and the armament of one 20 mm cannon and four ·50 calibre machine guns was concentrated in the nose. The Lightning had superb high-altitude performance and range, but although it was used initially for bomber escort over Europe, it proved too big and heavy to dogfight with Messerschmitts. Many were sent to the Pacific, where the top-scoring American ace of World War II, Major Richard Bong, ran up his score of forty kills in a P-38. The greatest day of the twin-boom fighter came on 18 April 1943 when sixteen Guadalcanal-based Lightnings flew 435 miles to Kahili airfield on Bougainville and shot down two Japanese 'Betty' bombers, one carrying the redoubtable Commander-in-Chief of the Japanese Combined Fleet, Admiral Isoroku Yamamoto.

Powered by a 2000 hp Pratt & Whitney eighteen cylinder radial engine, the massive Republic P-47 Thunderbolt, with supercharger in the rear fuselage, was originally designed as a high-altitude fighter. Later in the war the 'Jug,' as it was affectionately known, gained a tremendous reputation as a fighter-bomber, showing astonishing strength and ability to fly home after sustaining very severe damage. A long-range variation produced for the Pacific war, the P-47N, escorted Superfortresses in attacks on Japan. Eight ·50 calibre machine guns were mounted in the wings, plus bombs and rockets up to 2500 pounds in the fighter-bomber role.

Remembered by many pilots as the greatest fighter of World War II, comparable only to the Spitfire in gracefulness of form and dazzling performance in a dogfight, the North American P-51 Mustang was designed before Pearl Harbor for the British Purchasing Mission, and came only belatedly to the USAAF. Much of the secret of its high-speed performance lay in its laminar-flow wing, but with the Allison engine, both the USAAF and the RAF could only see the Mustang in a minor ground-attack role. Its greatness came from its marriage to the British Rolls-Royce Merlin with two-stage supercharger. Following the severe defeats of the unescorted 8th Air Force heavy bombers over Germany in the autumn of 1943, the P-51 appeared in the nick of time as an escort fighter with both long range and unsurpassed combat performance. Beginning in March 1944 the P-51B with two seventy-five gallon drop tanks was able to escort to a point 650 miles from base, and with two 108 gallon tanks had a range of 850 miles, sufficient to reach Berlin and beyond. Without the P-51 escort fighter, the daylight strategic bombing campaign against Germany could well have been defeated with unacceptable losses in 1944.

Quite rightly, the strategic bombing campaign against Germany commands major attention in this study, if only because 77·6 per cent of all Air Force overseas casualties were sustained in the European and Mediteranean theatres of operations. In the face of scepticism by the British, who had earlier suffered disaster in sending heavy bombers over Europe by day, the United States 8th Air Force began in 1942 to demonstrate its conviction that close defensive formations of heavily armed B-17s, bombing precisely from high altitude, could do more damage than the night bombers in area raids on German cities. Early attacks by small formations against targets in the occupied countries involved slight losses, partly because RAF Spitfires could escort the bombers all the way to these near-by objectives. Flying at altitudes of 22,000 to 26,000 feet, the air crews, particularly the waist gunners at open windows amidships, first experienced frostbite and anoxia. That the effort could not be more rapidly expanded was due to the 8th's reinforcements being siphoned off to the fighting in North Africa. When longer-range missions were laid on in the following year, losses to the determined German fighter defences rose alarmingly as the 'Forts' ventured beyond the reach of Spitfires, P-38s and later P-47s. Armed with only one ·30 calibre hand-held gun in the nose, the earlier B-17s were very vulnerable to head-on attacks initiated at this time by cannon-firing Focke-Wulf 190s and Messerschmitt Me 109Gs. In a long double mission on 17 August 1943, with one group bombing the Messerschmitt factory at Regensburg and then continuing to North African bases, and the other striking the ball-bearing factories at Schweinfurt and returning to England, the *Luftwaffe* threw in everything it had—single- and twin-engined fighters, armed with machine guns, cannon, rockets and mortars, many aircraft making more than one attack. Three hundred and seventy-six B-17s were dispatched—the largest number sent out in any 8th Air Force raid to date—and 315 attacked, dropping 724 tons of bombs. Thirty-six aircraft were destroyed from the Regensburg Force, twenty-four from that sent to Schweinfurt, representing an unacceptable sixteen per cent of the bombers dispatched, and nineteen per cent of those which attacked. On 14 October 1943 followed 'second Schweinfurt,' a disaster with far-reaching consequences. Of the 291 B-17s dispatched, a badly-mauled force of 228 reached and bombed the target. Losses totalling sixty bombers amounted to over twenty per cent of the force that left England.[5] 'The fact was that the Eighth Air Force had for the time being lost air superiority over Germany.'[6]

Without air superiority the invasion of Europe—already in everyone's mind—would be impossible. Therefore the German Air Force, now in the ascendant, would have to be beaten down. Long-range fighter escort was part of the answer: on 13 December 1943 a force of 710 bombers was sent against Bremen and Kiel, with escort all the way by P-38s, P-47s and P-51s. Heavy bomber losses dropped gratifyingly to acceptable levels. Then, in February 1944, came the

'Big Week,' during which the 8th's heavy bombers concentrated on German fighter aircraft production. Over 3300 B-17s and B-24s were dispatched from England during the six raiding days, and only 137 were lost, thanks to long-range escort, despite heavy German fighter opposition. German losses were in fact severe, and henceforth, their efforts against the American day bombers declined. In March the heavy bombers were sent all the way to Berlin with P-51 escort, before turning to attack German flying bomb sites in northern France, and the French railway network behind the invasion coast. When the heavies came back in the fall to attack oil refineries and installations and the German transportation system, the *Luftwaffe* was a shadow of its former self, though its morale remained unbroken to the end. Such was the eventual success of the 'oil plan' that in the last days of the Thousand-Year *Reich,* new, fully-equipped Focke-Wulfs and Messerschmitts remained on the ground for lack of fuel while the enormous American bomber formations roamed unopposed except for the anti-aircraft fire, the 'flak,' which was always a menace.

The Mediterranean Allied Air Forces, their heavy bombers comprising mostly B-24 Liberators, lent their weight to the strategic air campaign by bombing the so-called 'soft underbelly of the Axis.' One mission from North African bases, the attack on the vital oil refineries at Ploesti in Rumania on 1 August 1943, has gone down in Air Force tradition, along with Regensburg and First and Second Schweinfurt, as an epic of courage, discipline and self-sacrifice.[7] A hundred and seventy-seven B-24s set off in formation soon after dawn from bases around Benghazi to fly the unprecedented distance of 1200 miles to the city which supplied a third of Germany's oil requirements. By late afternoon the Liberators—their number reduced to 165—were swooping down on the tall smoke-stacks and cracking towers of the ugly refineries with the lyrical names—Concordia Vega, Astra Romana, Colombia Aquila, and the others. Literally on the deck, in the face of intense flak and German and Roumanian fighters, they planted their delayed-action bombs in the refineries. For the Liberators of the Ninth Air Force, Operation TIDAL WAVE was the end, as fifty-three planes failed to return to base—most of them victims of light anti-aircraft fire around the heavily defended town. Three hundred and ten American airmen died—one out of every five who reached the target—but they left behind them a legend and a memory that will outlast that of the Charge of the Light Brigade.

Following the Italian surrender, the Fifteenth Air Force, composed of B-17s and B-24s based around Foggia, was called into being on 1 November 1943. From then until V-E Day its bombers, alternating with those of the 8th in England, whipsawed the tottering *Reich* and its dependencies in southern and eastern Europe.

In the Pacific, the USAAF story was one of light and medium bombers, ground support, and long-range fighter strikes and escort missions against an enemy who at first seemed superior everywhere. Distances were enormous, long flights over water the rule, but altitudes were moderate and oxygen frequently was not necessary.

The real drama in this theatre derived from the strategic attacks by the XX Air Force that played a decisive role in the downfall of the Japanese Empire. Considering the vast distances in the Pacific, the B-17 and B-24 (dubbed by comparison 'medium bombers') would not do, and the chosen instrument was the first of the VHBs (Very Heavy Bomber), the Boeing B-29 Superfortress. Development of this craft started in 1940 with a requirement for a bomber to carry 2000 pounds of bombs for 5333 miles at 400 mph. A miracle in itself, the giant bomber—141 feet in span, 99 feet long, and grossing 62 tons at takeoff—was made possible only by a succession of smaller miracles. The new Wright R-3350 radial engines of 2200 hp were themselves a step in the dark, and initially, all too many caught fire on takeoffs, with disastrous results. The crew of ten were housed in compartments forward and aft, pressurized to a differential of 6·55 pounds per square inch, and connected by a tunnel. The armament—eight ·50 calibre machine guns in four power turrets (plus two ·50 calibre and one 20 mm cannon in the tail) were remotely controlled by gunners handling computer gun sights in blisters amidships. The first B-29 flew on 21 September 1942 and in the early summer of 1944 the first VHBs struck at Japan from primitive bases in the heart of China. At the end of a long and difficult supply line—everything, even bombs and gasoline, had to be flown over the Himalayas from India—the Chinese fields were abandoned in favour of new installations on the captured islands of Guam, Saipan and Tinian in the Western Pacific. The campaign from the Marianas got under way on 24 November 1944 with 111 B-29s being sent against Tokyo. Flying at 27,000 to 33,000 feet, the big bombers were more handicapped by 120-knot winds than by defending Japanese fighters. The high-altitude bombing campaign—retarded by bad weather and mechanical malfunctions—limped along until spring. Missions were few and far between, damage to the Empire was insignificant in proportion to the effort, and morale dropped. Noteworthy was the unexpected prevalence of very high winds of up to 200 knots at bombing altitudes above 30,000 feet. It was the USAAF's first encounter with the jet stream.

Forced to concede that high-altitude day bombing was not producing results, Major General Curtis E. LeMay, heading the XXI Bomber Command, threw away the USAAF's cherished doctrine and switched to low-altitude night attacks. The effect was immediate and devastating: with the Japanese years behind in radar, their defences were crippled, and the huge bombers, able to dispense with guns and armour and to operate at comfortable altitudes under 10,000 feet, were freighted with massive loads of incendiaries, up to 16,000 per plane. It was immediately apparent that the end of the Pacific war was in sight when on the night of 9 March 1945 a force of 334 B-29s burned twelve square miles of flimsy Japanese buildings in the heart of Tokyo. Over 80,000 died. In grim succession LeMay's bombers put the torch to the major Japanese cities—Nagoya, Osaka, Kobe, Yokohama. On 6 August 1945 the B-29 'Enola Gay,' flying at 31,600 feet, dropped the first atomic bomb on Hiroshima in a daylight attack. Three days later 'Bock's Car' dropped the second on Nagasaki. The B-29s had helped to force the Japanese surrender without the need for a costly invasion.

To a large extent, the war in the Pacific was the Navy's war, and Navy air spearheaded the drive from Pearl Harbor to Tokyo. On 'The Day that will Live in Infamy' the battleship was still queen, the United States Navy had only seven carriers in commission, and their air groups had barely entered the monoplane era. It was the three flat-tops *Yorktown, Enterprise* and *Hornet* which, almost alone against the Japanese Combined Fleet, sank all four first-line enemy carriers and won the decisive Battle of Midway on 4 June 1942. The vain sacrifice of thirty-eight out of forty-two Douglas TBD Devastator torpedo bombers of the three carrier air groups drew down the enemy's 'Zeke' fighters to sea level and enabled the Douglas SBD dive bombers, plunging down from 19,000 feet, to plant their 1000-pound bombs in the vitals of *Akagi, Kaga* and *Soryu*. Later in the day a scratch team of dive bombers set fatal fires in *Hiryu*.

As the war continued, new planes were brought forward, and the carriers went from strength to strength. Perhaps the real measure of naval air power was the destruction of the *Yamato*, the greatest battleship the world has ever seen, armed with 18·1 inch guns and displacing 72,000 tons full load, on 7 April 1945. Where Britain's Royal Navy four years earlier had taken four days to cripple and sink the 42,500 ton *Bismarck*, the Japanese giantess was put down in two hours by 280 Hellcats, Corsairs, Helldivers and Avengers from the carriers *Hornet, Wasp, Bennington, Belleau Wood, San Jacinto, Essex, Bunker Hill, Cabot*, and *Bataan*—about half the carrier force covering the fighting on Okinawa. Dive bombers put five medium bombs into her, but it was the ten torpedo hits from the ninety-eight torpedo bombers participating that sent the Japanese superdreadnought to the bottom. The Americans lost ten planes.

The strike at Pearl Harbor—a tactical masterpiece, though politico-strategically, a blunder of the first magnitude—destroyed for ever the myth that the Japanese were a nation of myopic copyists. While their Army aviation was designed to play a subordinate role in a land war against Russia, it is no exaggeration to state that their naval air arm ruled the Pacific in the first six months of the war, and in numbers, training, and quality of *material,* out-classed United States naval aviation. Japanese designers showed themselves to be as bold and imaginative as their pilots were aggressive and self-sacrificing. Fortunately for us, these high qualities were not enough in the absence of a powerful industrial base for aircraft production, and of an adequate flight training organization geared to the needs of a long war.

Three hundred and fifty-three planes, from six large, fast carriers, made the attack on Pearl Harbor. Seventy-nine of these were fast, low-wing fighter monoplanes with retractible landing gear, absolutely unknown to American intelligence agencies, though they had made their military debut in the war in China in August 1940—the Mitsubishi A6M-2 Zero (nicknamed 'Zeke' in the Allied identification system). For months it out-climbed and out-turned heavier American Curtiss P-40 Tomahawks and Grumman F4F Wildcats, and not until the attack on Dutch Harbor, on 3 June 1942, was an example of this Japanese fighter captured and put in flying condition. One hundred and forty-three high-level bombers and torpedo bombers did most of the execution in the Pearl Harbor raid, while one hundred and thirty-one dive bombers participated. There was also a remarkable twin-engined land based bomber, sleek of form, with a maximum speed of 264 mph and a range of 2500 miles—the Mitsubishi G4M-1 ('Betty'). In a convincing demonstration of their capabilities, a squadron of these craft torpedoed and sank the British battleships *Prince of Wales* and *Repulse* off Malaya on 10 December 1941. Yet all these aircraft bought manœuvrability and range at the price of defence. As a Japanese authority quaintly puts it, the early engagements 'proved that the Navy's principle of placing priority to attack at the cost of defence—fighter without armour plate, torpedo bomber with no bullet-proof tanks—was a mistake after all.'[8]

Japan's aeronautical engineers never gave up. Lacking the earth-moving equipment which enabled the Americans to turn a coral island into an airstrip in a week, the Japanese Navy relied heavily on seaplanes and flying boats operating from tenders in the lee of captured islands. There was the Kawanishi N1K1 'Kyofu' ('Rex'), a powerful float-plane fighter with four 20 mm cannon and a top speed of 300 mph. Converted to a land plane ('George'), it fought on even terms with the Hellcat in the last days of the war. There was the barrel-shaped Mitsubishi J2M-1 fighter, 'Raiden' ('Jack'), heavily armoured, armed with four 20 mm cannon, and able to reach 380 mph. No dogfighter, 'Jack' scored many of the successes against attacking B-29s. There was a four-engined bomber, the Nakajima G8N-1 'Renzan' ('Rita'), intended to attain 375 mph at 29,500 feet. Four only were completed before V-J Day. At the end the Japanese, in desperation, turned to *kamikaze* tactics—the suicide crash—grisly but effective against the 'small boys' of the US Fleet off Okinawa. Not only were obsolete 'Zekes' and other aircraft flown by the half-trained suicide pilots—there was even a manned, rocket-propelled flying bomb, the 'Ohka' ('Cherry Blossom,' code named 'Baka' or 'fool' by the Allies), with 1760 pounds of explosive in its nose, which, with rockets lighted off, dived into its target at more than 400 mph.

World War II proved beyond doubt the special qualifications, the strong sense of professional dedication, and the contribution to military effectiveness of the flight surgeon. All too often a mere 'hail fellow well met'[9] in the early days of sketchy training and indoctrination, he had become by 1945 a skilled specialist, the trusted confidant of his subordinates, and an indispensable adviser to his commanding officer. Many flew with their men to give them confidence and also to experience the stresses of combat at first hand, and some went down to their deaths along with the flight crews.

The Germans initially did not assign flight surgeons to combat units, as did the USAAF. Medical care in peacetime was provided by station personnel attached to the air base. This proved inadequate under wartime conditions, particularly with units frequently changing their location, and early in 1940 flight surgeons were added to the strength of flying units—one to each squadron *(Gruppe),* or in reconnaissance units, to each flight *(Staffel).* So well did they do their work that the outstanding leader of the German fighter arm, Major General Adolf Galland, 'once ascribed a large part of the aggressiveness and fitness of the flying units to the activity of the flight surgeons.'[10] In the desperate days of 1944 and 1945, when German fighter and bomber units were being decimated by the overwhelming might of the Allied air offensive, they came to occupy a unique morale-building position:

In most cases, the flight surgeon was not only the senior in years and experience in his unit, but also the officer with the longest service within the unit: he knew the flying and military careers of all the men. He often had enough flying experience himself to be able to judge things from this viewpoint. The importance of his position often became obvious, when group commanders were killed one after the other and the flight surgeon—better than many a young officer—was able to inform the new commander of the human aspects of his unit.[11]

Many of these medical men indeed were qualified to pilot military aircraft, and there are records of the German flight surgeons conducting examinations in an aircraft in flight to determine a man's actual fitness to return to full flying duty after amputations.

In wartime the squadron medical officers of the Royal Air Force were expected to give attention to the morale of air crew and their psychological problems:

A squadron medical officer's duties included completely identifying himself with the air crew by being present at briefing, visiting them while they were waiting at their dispersals before take-off, being on the spot at take-off and return and by being on instant call during the interim period in case aircraft returned early or damaged. At interrogation, by wandering quietly among the crews he learned what experiences they had met and their reactions to them.[12]

In addition, numerous medical officers flew constantly as part of their routine duties. Particularly was this true of the Flying Personnel Medical Officers appointed in 1939 to co-ordinate the work of medical researchers in the laboratory with the requirements of the air crew flying the new high-performance equipment being issued to the expanding RAF. Taking part in operational sorties over Germany, the Flying Personnel Medical Officers in Bomber Command investigated such matters as turret comfort and habitability (taking the place of the gunner themselves); visibility of radar displays and training in reading them; and unsatisfactory air-crew performance in identifying, marking and bombing their targets. In Fighter Command there were investigations of oxygen equipment at high altitude; blackout in sharp turns; and fatigue caused by repeated exposure to radial accelerations, often by medical officers themselves qualified to pilot the Spitfire and Hurricane fighters. Some of these physicians even flew with the squadrons into combat—covered by their squadron mates, as they were legally non-combatants—and one, Group Captain H. Corner, Deputy to the Principal Medical Officer of Fighter Command, went missing and presumed dead when his damaged Spitfire went down in the Channel short of fuel while returning from a sweep over France. So valuable was this type of work with the squadrons that a number of RAF medical officers went through the full pilot training course, ending up flying Spitfires in aerobatics, formation flying, and air gunnery training.[13]

The USAAF had no comparable programme. Before the war, American flight surgeons had received flight instruction to the point where they were qualified to operate training and utility aircraft, but this practice was discontinued during the war years. The accelerated programme at the School of Aviation Medicine, at Randolph Field, Texas, included ten hours of dual flying for those who desired the experience, the medical student pilot occupying the front cockpit of the BT-13 Vultee Valiant basic trainer. Overseas, commanding officers of bomber formations showed an ambivalent attitude towards the medical officer participating in combat operations. Some physicians threatened to become too absorbed with air fighting to the neglect of their professional functions. The surgeon of the 15th Air Force 'established the definite policy that participation in a few such missions should be encouraged, but that no flight surgeon should go on more than 10 such missions.'[14] The Ninth Air Force surgeon in October 1944 forbade flight surgeons to go on combat missions, asserting 'personally I feel that no medical officer as such serves any good purpose on combat missions and we therefore risk a critical item—the medical officer—for a very questionable gain.'[15] On three of the first five missions of the B-29s from China, a flight surgeon went along as an observer. In the United States Navy, flight surgeons served afloat in aircraft carriers, either as ship's company or attached to air groups. In the 'Essex' class carriers which spearheaded the drive across the Pacific, there was a senior medical officer and three junior medical officers, operating a well-equipped sick bay on the third deck, with thirty beds, doctors' offices, two dental chairs and an operating room.

The work of the flight surgeon with air crew in combat was backed by a tremendous research organization in the Zone of the Interior in the three leading air-power nations. In Germany it was the *Erprobungsstelle* at Rechlin, the *Institut für Flugmedizin* of the *Deutsche Versuchsanstalt für Luftfahrt* (DVL) at Berlin-Adlershof, and the *Institut für Luftfahrtmedizin* in Munich. In England it was the RAF Physiological Laboratory at Farnborough. In the United States the most significant advances were made by the Aero Medical Laboratory at Wright Field, Ohio, the Army Air Force's School of Aviation Medicine at Randolph Field, Texas, and the Navy's School of Aviation Medicine at Pensacola, Florida. Many research projects were farmed out to universities, medical schools, and medical centres, notably the Mayo Clinic at Rochester, Minnesota. All these institutions made their contribution to the efforts of their respective air forces to fly higher and faster, with less risk of death or injury.

This was not the case with Japanese aeromedical research, hamstrung by bitter interservice rivalries and by the vagaries of the Japanese temperament. An American medical officer who investigated Japanese aviation medicine and research immediately after V-J Day characterized it as a 'mixture of the feudal and the modern,' and 'deeply steeped in folklore, while at the same time interspersed with careful and detailed fundamental research.'[16] While 'in actual practice, flyers available were so definitely short, and their life expectancy equally short, that not much actual preventive work was done,' the Army laboratory at Tachikawa, and the Navy facility at Yokosuka, diverted themselves with detailed and irrelevant research projects on air sickness and special diets. The Navy claimed to have developed a shark and ox pituitary extract which so improved night vision that 'if there were a quarter moon it was as if there were a full moon.' Remarkable specificity was claimed for 'Pleasant Feeling Drugs' (barbiturates and hypnotics), 'Strength drugs' (carbohydrates, liver and vitamin preparations), and 'Fighter, Attack and Bomber Power Flying Pills' (vitamin and liver combinations).

In the realm of oxygen equipment, the Germans, with their large-scale research into aeromedical problems commencing with the Nazi assumption of power in 1933, were well ahead of the United Nations. As early as 1937, *Luftwaffe* medical officers, acting both as pilots and observers, were making high-altitude investigations aboard Heinkel He 111 and Dornier Do 17 bombers, and formulating rules for the use of oxygen on all flights above 13,100 feet, and above 8200 feet on long journeys. They demonstrated also that oxygen equipment then available provided adequate protection up to 26,200 feet, and that pressure cabins were not necessary for operations below this altitude. On the other hand, actual symptoms of dysbarism were investigated at altitudes above 26,200 feet, one of the observers, a Dr Hornberger, being particularly susceptible to 'the bends.'[17]

All of the early oxygen systems were of the *constant flow* type, that is, they delivered a constant flow of oxygen through a regulator manually adjusted by the user to increase the amount with altitude, either to a pipe-stem or a mask. Even when the flyer was exhaling, the flow continued, thus wasting a large proportion of the gas and shortening the time that the aircraft could remain at altitude with a given quantity of oxygen on board. In 1936, however, the *Auergesellschaft* of Berlin developed the first demand regulator to be manufactured and used in quantity by any air force. The Auer A-824 conserved oxygen in two ways: it shut off the flow of oxygen when the flyer was exhaling, and opened to pass oxygen only when his inspiration created a slight vacuum. Furthermore, it saved oxygen by diluting it with air at lower altitudes where one hundred per cent oxygen was not physiologically necessary. There were four diluter settings, 0 delivering forty per cent oxygen, 4 about sixty per cent oxygen, 6 about eighty per cent oxygen, and 8 about one hundred per cent oxygen. Since the settings were manually controlled, flyers tended to make long flights on position 8, even when flying at relatively low altitude, thereby wasting the gas. Therefore the next demand regulator, the 10-38, manufactured after 1937 by the *Auergesellschaft* and the *Drägerwerke* of Lübeck, had an aneroid control which gradually closed the air intake as the aircraft ascended, until at 26,200 feet the regulator delivered one hundred per cent oxygen.

The ordinary demand regulator, operating by negative pressure during the flyer's inhalation phase, carried with it the danger that at high altitude any leakage of air into the mask might cause anoxia. Indeed, with the blood oxygenation falling off beyond 33,000 feet even with one hundred per cent oxygen, the only safe procedure above this height was to deliver one hundred per cent oxygen under pressure, whereby air could be prevented from leaking in around the mask. As early as March 1939 the *Erprobungsstelle* at Rechlin had developed the 10-137 demand regulator which, at altitudes above 26,200 feet, delivered oxygen under pressure. Whereas other air forces required the flyer to change controls manually to obtain oxygen under pressure, 'in Germany, after careful consideration, the use of manual adjustment from negative pressure to positive pressure was rejected, since an oxygen regulator is, above all, safety equipment.'[18] The 10-137 demand regulator was in general use by the *Luftwaffe* from early 1941 until the end of the war, and permitted adequate (eighty-seven per cent) oxygenation of the blood up to 39,400 feet.

In the design of oxygen masks, the Germans again led the way, with a fundamental development, the quick-disconnect, being introduced by the *Drägerwerke* as early as 1934. This was a fitting which enabled the flyer easily to couple or uncouple his mask hose to the oxygen supply with a force of between 15·5 and 18·7 pounds. A set of springs could be tightened or loosened to maintain this force; if the disconnect force was too small, the flyer might inadvertently uncouple from his oxygen supply with disastrous results at high altitude. German researchers early experienced difficulty with the moisture of the exhaled breath condensing and freezing in the mask or hose, sometimes blocking the inflow of oxygen, and sometimes sticking open the expiratory valve so that the flyer at high altitude breathed air. Pre-heated oxygen was found excessively drying to the respiratory passages; an electrically-heated mask was tried; but in 1939, the mask HM 51 (10-67) was developed in which the warmth of the exhaled air prevented freezing within the mask. Towards the end of the war the *Luftwaffe* was about to adopt a copy of the American A-10-A oxygen mask, as the latter's design prevented its tearing off the face during bail-out from aircraft; but due to the general military collapse, the German 44 mask did not go into production.

The *Luftwaffe* likewise devoted much attention to the supply of

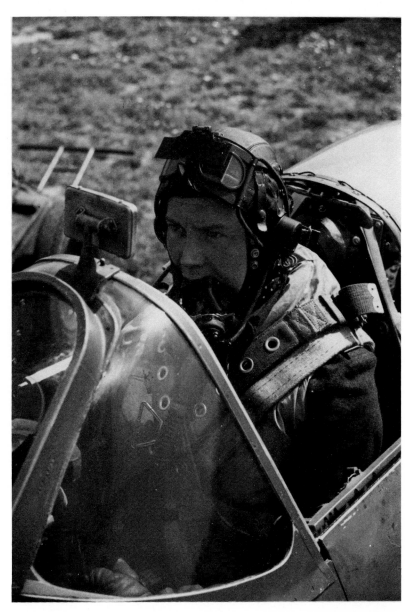

29. Battle of Britain Spitfire pilot in cockpit with protective equipment: helmet with ear phones, goggles, sun shades, oxygen mask with microphone, Sutton harness with shoulder straps crossing over his chest, worn over parachute harness. (Imperial War Museum)

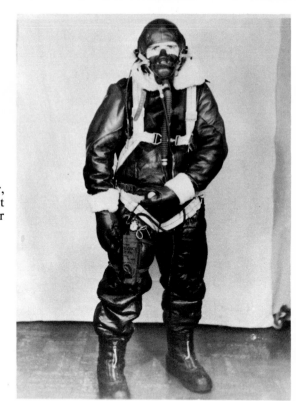

30. U.S. Army Air Forces flight gear, showing oxygen mask and bail-out bottle strapped to right leg (1944). (Air Force Museum)

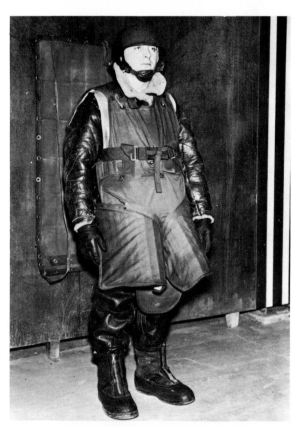

31. Armoured 'flak suit' as worn by US Army Air Forces bomber personnel. Armoured 'flak curtain' hangs behind subject (1944). (Air Force Museum)

oxygen in aircraft. Much time and effort was expended by the *IG Farben Gesellschaft* of Bitterfeld on an apparatus for producing oxygen chemically in an aircraft. Cartridges containing manganese dioxide were heated in an autoclave and gave off oxygen free of contaminants at a pressure of eighty-five psi, which could be stored in bottles in the aircraft. Unfortunately the cartridges had a tendency to explode spontaneously for reasons the manufacturer was unable to determine, and after a Ju 52 aircraft was badly damaged in 1937 by such an explosion at 19,700 feet, development of the chemical system was discontinued. Some of the earliest efforts at carrying oxygen in aircraft involved the liquefied gas, but certain problems of using liquid oxygen—the impossibility of measuring the amount left in the double-walled containers as the liquid slowly vaporized, problems of storage and availability, were never solved before the war. Hence, compressed gaseous oxygen was used by the *Luftwaffe* throughout World War II. Though they were vulnerable to gunfire, the Germans employed high-pressure cylinders with a two-litre volume and a working pressure of 2133 psi, providing 290 litres of oxygen at normal pressure. One cylinder was installed for each man-hour of high altitude flight, with two cylinders per man in fighters and four to five per man in bombers.

By contrast, the Royal Air Force in 1939 was not really equipped to fight at high altitude. Bombing and fighter exercises had been carried out for years at comfortable levels below 15,000 feet, and as late as the Munich Crisis in 1938, none of Fighter Command's twenty-nine squadrons (five equipped with Hurricanes and the rest with obsolete biplanes—five with Gladiators, three with Furies, nine with Gauntlets, and seven with Demons) could operate above 15,000 feet as their guns were not heated.[19] The official medical history admits that in Bomber Command in 1939–40:

There existed a lack of appreciation of oxygen among flying personnel, either due to the fact that the majority of pilots in the war of 1914–18 had little experience of its use and little appreciation of the disastrous effects of oxygen lack or because the inter-war generation had little or no experience with such matters, for the reason that the older type of bomber aircraft could not operate at heights where the use of oxygen was essential.[20]

Crews had not been indoctrinated, equipment was inadequate, and Bomber Command, in the long 'nickelling' flights over Germany in the first winter of the war, were using a wasteful continuous-flow type of mask. Promptly it appeared that the amount of oxygen carried was inadequate for the endurance of the aircraft, even with the oxygen not being used below 15,000 feet. In the Hampden, with a crew of four and an endurance of ten hours, the oxygen sufficed for only four hours sixteen minutes at 15,000 feet. In some aircraft the number of high-pressure bottles, each containing 750 litres at atmospheric pressure,[21] had to be increased. Thus, in the Blenheim, which, with a three-man crew and three bottles, had an oxygen 'duration' at 20,000 feet of 3 hours 20 minutes, the number of bottles was increased to four. The RAF never employed the diluter-demand regulator during World War II,[22] but in 1942 the 'economizer' was introduced—essentially a rebreather bag which held the oxygen during the expiration phase, instead of wasting it. Since Bomber Command aircraft rarely exceeded 20,000 feet, this supply system was retained until the end of the war. The early high-altitude daylight raids with American Boeing Fortress Is (B-17Cs) at altitudes of 30,000 feet or more, exposed their British crews to extreme low temperatures, and masks froze up. In 1942 the 'G' type mask was developed, which remained standard for the rest of the war, but a shroud to enclose the expiratory valve, and electric heating for the microphone, had to be evolved to prevent freezing above 23,000 feet in winter. Oxygen accidents occurred most commonly in the early years of the war, due in large part to inadequate indoctrination. A typical experience of euphoria with anoxia befell a crew member of a four-engined Halifax on the night of 28 April 1942:

The rear gunner stated that while over the target area he began to feel queer, the feeling gradually increasing until he started to gasp and wondered if he could have been wounded without being aware of it. He then realized that his oxygen might have failed and informed the captain of this possibility. The flight engineer was then dispatched to the rear gunner with a portable oxygen bottle. The gunner did not, however, trouble to use this as the aircraft was then over the target area and he had to keep a sharp look-out. He remembered getting angry with the engineer and after leaving the target area at 20,000 feet the gunner was heard talking to himself on the intercommunication system in a 'thick' voice and saying in no uncertain terms that he 'was not worrying about night fighters'. . . . This particular failure was traced to a leak in the indicator at the point beside the flare chute. The oxygen failure was therefore due to a defect in the oxygen pipeline and not to mask or economizer.[23]

In one month, November 1943, forty-two sorties out of 5727 flown in Bomber Command were abandoned due to oxygen failures. Thereafter the ratio improved, thanks in no small measure to strict training of all personnel in portable low-pressure chambers.

For the American 8th Air Force, bombing by day from altitudes of 25,000 to 30,000 feet, the oxygen supply and delivery problem was much more serious. In the first and hardest year of operations in England, there were many accidents, and numerous deaths from anoxia, reflecting both faulty equipment and inadequate indoctrination.

The apparatus was primitive in relation to the demands of the high-altitude mission: the early B-17Es had a high-pressure oxygen system with flasks charged to 1800 psi, even though actual firing tests had shown these shattered when hit by bullets. This delivered oxygen through the A-8A constant flow regulator to the A-8 mask, which essentially was the old B-L-B with rebreather bag. With this, it will be remembered, the oxygen-rich air in the upper respiratory passages was blown into the bag, and when this was filled, the last of the expired air, with a high carbon dioxide content, was exhausted into the atmosphere through the ports filled with sponge rubber. Since the amount of oxygen required increased with altitude, the rate of flow had to be set manually by the user to a number on the regulator corresponding with the flight altitude. With a relatively small amount of oxygen being delivered at low altitude, the quantity in the rebreather bag would be exhausted during inhalation, and for the remainder of the inspiration, air would enter through the sponge-rubber ports—a primitive kind of diluter system. In practice, the B-L-B mask and A-8A regulator demanded more attention than busy crew members, fighting for their lives in the skies over Germany, were able to give them. The pilot had to call out over the intercom the changes in altitude so that crew members could re-set their regulators; but they might not hear him, or might set them incorrectly. Above all, in the bitter cold at high altitude, condensed moisture in the breath froze and blocked the sponge-rubber ports or filled the rebreather bag with ice. Accidents and fatalities occurred at all the altitudes at which missions were flown during 1943: eight deaths at 30,000 feet or higher; eleven between 25,000 and 30,000 feet; and three below 25,000 feet. The surgeon of the VIII Bomber Command felt obliged to recommend that no bombing missions be flown above 25,000 feet, and that each crew member be given an extra A-8 mask in case the original one froze and became useless. Eventually the continuous-flow equipment was downgraded for use by passengers in transport aircraft, with the directive that it should not be used above 25,000 feet!

There were many reasons for switching from continuous-flow to diluter-demand equipment. During the Battle of Britain, Captain Otis Benson Jr (MC) had obtained from the British some Auer demand regulators found in shot-down German aircraft, and had delivered them to the Aero Medical Laboratory at Wright Field on 20 June 1941. These served as the basis for the design of an American diluter-demand regulator, the A-12, which was generally issued early in 1944. Operating in the usual way, set on 'normal' or 'automix,' the aneroid control delivered a varying mixture of air and oxygen, from plain air at sea level to one hundred per cent oxygen above 34,000 feet. When set on '100 per cent oxygen,' this was delivered with each inspiration, this setting being used, for instance, to breathe pure oxygen on the ground before takeoff to wash out blood nitrogen and mimimize the incidence of 'the bends.' An 'emergency' setting provided one hundred per cent oxygen by the constant-flow system, useful to revive an unconscious crew member, or to maintain normal arterial oxygen saturation with heavy exercise at high altitude. This was very wasteful and rapidly depleted the oxygen supply.[24]

With the A-12 regulator came a low-pressure system utilizing shatterproof cylinders charged to a pressure of 450 psi. Several types of masks were used with this system—the A-9, the A-10 (which the Germans thought enough of to copy, and which had the reputation of being proof against freezing), and the A-14, which, after proving successful in fighters, caused some accidents by freezing in the much colder interior of the bombers. The next development was a pressure-breathing diluter demand regulator, the A-14, introduced in the autumn of 1944. The object, as in the German regulator, was to raise the combat ceiling of the aviator above 40,000 feet. Unlike the German 10-137 regulator, which automatically delivered oxygen under pressure above 26,200 feet, the American apparatus required the flyer to turn a switch on the dial of the A-14 to obtain one hundred per cent oxygen under pressure. Up to 30,000 feet the A-14 functioned as a normal demand apparatus. On the 'safety' setting it delivered the gas under 2 mm of mercury pressure, ensuring full oxygenation up to 40,000 feet in spite of possible leaks around the mask. To ensure adequate blood oxygenation at higher altitudes, the '41 M' setting offered a pressure of 8 mm of mercury; '43 M' equalled 11 mm, '45 M,' 15 mm, and 'above 45 M', 23 mm of mercury pressure. At the higher pressure settings, the lungs inflated without effort, but increasing force had to be used to exhale, making pressure breathing over any length of time a fatiguing exercise.[25] Still, at 45,000 feet pressure breathing would maintain useful consciousness, and permit normal activity, for half an hour.[26] Masks sealed to the face, to retain oxygen under pressure, had to be developed for use with pressure breathing, the A-13 and later the A-17 masks being standard.

Even with newer equipment, anoxic accidents still occurred. One 8th Air Force mishap in a combat mission in February 1944, in which four of the ten crew members of a B-17 lost consciousness, was unusual in the number of men involved, but not in the sources of difficulty. At 1010, while en route to the target at 27,000 feet, the ball-turret gunner felt he was not receiving sufficient oxygen.[27] He discovered that the quick-disconnect fitting on his hose had pulled out. Becoming more and more panicky, he was unable to re-connect the coupling to his oxygen supply, and lost consciousness. At 1015, when the navigator called all stations on the intercom for an oxygen check, he received no reply from the ball-turret gunner and ordered the left-waist gunner to check on his condition. The left-waist gunner disconnected his hose from the main line and plugged into a portable walk-around bottle, which should have contained a thirty-minute supply of oxygen at 450 psi. On reaching the ball turret, however, the left-waist gunner felt he was not getting enough oxygen and returned to his station, where he plugged into the main line. The radio man then tossed another walk-around bottle to the right-waist gunner, who plugged into it, went to the ball turret, disconnected his own hose and tried to plug the ball-turret gunner's hose into the bottle, but failed because of the faulty connection. The right-waist gunner, breathing air too long, then lost consciousness. The radio man, connected to the main oxygen line by a long hose, tried to walk aft to aid his unconscious comrades, but shut off his oxygen supply by stretching the hose, and lost consciousness. The bombardier then started aft carrying two A-4 walk-around bottles, but while changing his own hose to one of the bottles in the bomb bay, the bomb bay doors began to open during the run-up to the target; he dropped both bottles and ran to the radio room where he lost consciousness. The pilot released the bombs and in view of the emergency, dived the B-17 from 25,000 to 5000 feet. The co-pilot went aft and during the twenty-minute descent, gave artificial respiration and emergency oxygen to the ball-turret gunner; the other three revived spontaneously in the denser air at low altitude. The ball-turret gunner had been unconscious for one hour and ten minutes, of which forty to forty-five minutes had been at 28,000 feet. The right-waist gunner was unconscious for twenty minutes at 28,000 feet. The left-waist gunner did not lose consciousness, but was hypoxic for fifteen minutes at 28,000 feet. The radio operator was unconscious for fifteen minutes, and the bombardier for ten minutes, at 28,000 feet. Investigation showed that the main oxygen line from which the A-4 walk-around bottles were charged was probably leaking.[28]

Not all anoxic accidents ended so happily. In the early days of the daylight bomber offensive over Europe, most fatalities were caused by freezing of the oxygen masks. When this problem was overcome, the quick-disconnect fitting became the chief culprit. In a B-24 training mission, the aircraft flew for four hours at 14,000 feet, then began a climb to 30,000 feet. When the waist gunner failed to answer an oxygen check at 29,000 feet, the tail gunner was ordered to leave his station and investigate. At 30,000 feet the pilot tried again to raise the waist gunner; being unsuccessful, he sent the top-turret gunner aft to the waist and started to descend. The waist gunner and tail gunner were both found unconscious. Their oxygen supply was restored and artificial respiration given, but both men were pronounced dead on landing, only fifteen minutes after the descent commenced. Both men's quick-disconnect fittings were found to pull out of the regulator with a force of one and two pounds respectively, instead of the stipulated twelve pounds.[29]

Towards the end of the war, the proportion of anoxia incidents decreased. A major reason was thorough indoctrination and training of all 8th Air Force personnel in simulated flights to high altitude in three pressure chambers. During 1943 alone, 1004 air crew members received this training, with the result that anoxia due to faulty discipline 'practically disappeared.'

Special problems of high-altitude physiology were the routine lot of the photographic reconnaissance units of all the major air forces. Operating alone over enemy territory, the PRU squadrons, flying unarmed camera-equipped aircraft, could find safety from enemy fighters only in extreme speed and altitude. Early in the war the British used the Spitfire IV for such flights at 32,000 to 33,000 feet; later the Mark X and XI made photographic reconnaissance at 38,000 to 42,000 feet. With the standard oxygen equipment, symptoms of anoxia could and did develop, as when an experienced pilot became confused and photographed Dresden by mistake for Berlin. In 1943 the RAF photo reconnaissance squadrons received several sets of pressure-breathing equipment with inflatable jackets which provided counterpressure over the chest by means of oxygen-inflated bladders, which also served as rebreather bags. With this equipment, Spitfire XI aircraft were able to fly to 42,000 feet or higher, one pilot spending four hours above this altitude—two of them at 44,000 feet. The pressurized waistcoat, or corset, had the disadvantage of forcing venous blood and body fluids into the extremities, but it showed the way to the post-war pressure suits. It was not used by American photo-reconnaissance flyers, whose favourite mounts were the F-5 (modified Lockheed P-38) and F-6 (modified North American P-51). In these aircraft the A-14 pressure demand regulator was fitted. The comprehensive answer to the high-flying photographic pilot's problems was of course the pressure cabin.

From the medical point of view this was the ideal solution, maintaining at moderate altitudes a pressure of air such that oxygen masks need not be used, or at higher altitudes, permitting survival with oxygen where life otherwise would be impossible. From the engineering point of view there were disadvantages, in terms of added weight involved in fabricating a pressure-resistant enclosure; and added equipment such as the compressors to force air into the cabin, exhaust valves, etc.

Aiming to produce a bomber that could fly above the flak and fighters, the British Air Ministry in 1939 had drawn up a specification for a pressurized machine. This led to the Vickers Wellington V, extensively modified with a cigar-shaped pressure cabin, which in August 1940 attained 30,000 feet, and with its wing span extended twelve feet, 40,000 feet. Sixty-four similar Mark VIs were built with Merlin engines, and saw some service in 1941 with 'Oboe,' a line-of-sight blind bombing aid whose range over Germany was extended by flying at the highest possible altitude.

For a period before the war the Germans had considered pressurized cabins for their second-generation bombers, but had decided otherwise after their medical personnel in 1937 had proven that contemporary oxygen equipment afforded full protection up to 26,200 feet. Still later the *Luftwaffe* ruled that personnel could ascend to 39,400 feet with pressure-demand oxygen equipment, and perhaps higher with 'acclimatization' through daily ascents to 16,400 feet in a portable pressure chamber. This would not suffice at the great heights at which the long-range photo-reconnaissance aircraft were forced to fly, and as early as 1941 the Germans brought out the Ju 86P, a drastic modification of one of the *Luftwaffe* bombers of the early expansion period, with supercharged engines and a full-view pressurized cockpit which accommodated two men. Flying at 43,000 to 54,000 feet, the Ju 86P astonished the British by making reconnaissance flights over Britain and the Nile delta, beyond the reach of contemporary Spitfires. The RAF was forced to reply, and brought out the pressurized Spitfire VI, of which a hundred were built. With a two-stage supercharger on the 1415 hp Merlin engine, and a wing span increased by four feet to 40 feet 2 inches, the ceiling approximated 45,000 feet, particularly if the armament of four ·303 calibre machine guns and two 20 mm cannon were reduced. The pilot had to breathe oxygen at this altitude, as the pressure differential between the inside and the outside of the cockpit was not more than three psi.

Other pressurized aircraft were built in small numbers by both sides. A hundred and forty Spitfire VII fighters were produced, commencing in 1942. Pressurized Spitfires were also used by the high-flying photo-reconnaissance units, beginning with sixteen of the unarmed Mark Xs in 1942. Curiously, pilots did not like them as the power taken from the engine by the cabin compressor decreased their speed; in addition, their canopies fogged up, a defect which the Germans had avoided in the Junkers with double hermetically-sealed panes, and with calcium chloride pellets inserted to absorb moisture. An early pressurized Mosquito, the Mark XVI appearing in 1943, was the target of similar complaints. In the last year of the war, more powerful pressurized aircraft—the Spitfire XIX with 2050 hp Griffon engine, and the Mosquito 34—performed more acceptably to the exacting standards of the photo reconnaissance units. These last had a ceiling of 43,000 feet. The Germans also pressurized a few of their Messerschmitt Me 109Gs, and the Focke-Wulf Ta 152H, under development at war's end, had a pressurized cockpit with double panes of glass in the canopy.

As already mentioned, the American Very Heavy Bomber, the Boeing B-29 Superfortress, was the first pressurized aircraft ever produced in quantity. With a pressure differential of 6·55 psi, these aircraft maintained an equivalent altitude of 8000 feet up to 30,000 feet. Inasmuch as the United States Army Air Forces had had no previous operational experience with pressurized aircraft, the B-29 was something of an unknown quantity, and the dangers of 'explosive decompression' with sudden loss of cabin pressure were considerably exaggerated. In fact, pressure-chamber experiments showed that no danger resulted from sudden expansion of air in lungs, intestines or middle ears. Before the first B-29 wing entered service, all its flight surgeons and many of its officers were 'exploded' from 8000 to 30,000 feet in 0·075 seconds in the pressure chamber at Wright Field. While this rate corresponded to what might occur if a hole twelve feet in diameter were blown in the pressure cabin while flying fully pressurized, in actual firing tests on the XB-29 with ·50 calibre and 20 mm ammunition, the largest opening made was when the sighting blisters, thirty inches in diameter, were shattered. In fact, all instances of explosive decompression with the B-29 during the war involved the sighting blisters.

An actual incident occurred on 30 September 1943 when a side gunner's blister of a B-29 blew out at 30,000 feet with the pressure differential at 6·55 psi. The crew of nine had been well briefed in advance for this emergency, with the pilot and one crew member in the rear compartment actually wearing their oxygen masks at all times above 15,000 feet. The remainder, having their helmets on and oxygen masks attached and connected to regulators, were able to fasten their masks over their faces before losing consciousness. In fact, it soon appeared that the greatest risk connected with explosive decompression was that of being sucked out of the opening. During a raid on Nagoya on 3 January 1945 gunfire caused a sighting blister to blow out at 29,000 feet aboard the B-29 *American Maid,* and the gunner, Sergeant James Krantz, together with his gunsight, was blown out of the opening. His life would have been lost had he not been wearing a restraining harness of his own design; but such was the force of the slipstream that the sergeant could not pull himself back in and after three minutes he lost consciousness. The central fire-control gunner and right-blister gunner together were unable to pull him in, and ultimately it required the added strength of the radar operator and co-pilot to rescue him. Though suffering from severe frostbite, the doughty sergeant opened his eyes when given oxygen, and within twenty minutes he began to recover from his harrowing experience.[30]

Dysbarism, or 'the bends,' proved less of a problem than anticipated in combat flying in World War II. This condition obtains when gases dissolved in the blood and tissues come out of solution in the form of bubbles, just as the bottle of soda fizzes with bubbles when the cap is removed and the pressure decreased. 'The bends' were initially identified as a hazard in deep-sea diving, where the nitrogen dissolved in the blood at pressures obtaining below 32 feet, at which depth the pressure is two atmospheres. For the flyer, the atmospheric pressure has to fall to less than half before symptoms appear. These have been observed at altitudes as low as 23,000 feet when the subject is doing heavy physical work, and the risk of dysbarism is always present in unpressurized flying above 30,000 feet. The effects can be serious and even crippling, depending on the location where the bubbles lodge in the circulation. Should they block the smaller blood vessels supplying the brain, disturbance of vision, headache and sometimes temporary paralysis of one or more extremities may occur. Bubbles of nitrogen in the smaller vessels of the lungs lead to a sense of pressure in the chest, burning pain, fits of coughing and a sense of difficulty in breathing (the 'chokes'). Sometimes bubbles under the skin cause itching and crawling sensations. Most common is gritty, aching pain in the joints ('the bends'), caused by bubble formation in the joint fluids. Occasional fatal cases have occurred in pressure-chamber 'flights,' invariably with symptoms of severe brain damage.

In actual flight operations in World War II, even with rates of ascent exceeding three thousand feet per minute in propeller-driven fighters such as the P-38 Lightning, the P-51 Mustang, and the Griffon-engined Spitfire, actual symptoms were rare. This was largely due to the common practice of washing out the nitrogen in the blood and body fluids by breathing one hundred per cent oxygen on the ground before takeoff. Half the nitrogen dissolved in the body can be eliminated in thirty minutes by this method. More commonly, 'the bends' were observed in personnel doing heavy work, such as bomber crew men handling flexible machine guns at high altitude. Dysbarism was most commonly noted in pressure chamber 'flights.' In a three-hour 'flight' by 177 cadets at 38,000 feet, with 'ascent' at two thousand feet per minute, thirty had to be brought down due to 'the bends.' One author reported fatal collapse after seventy-two minutes at 38,000 feet in the chamber; neurological abnormalities were also noted, such as transient hemiplegia and homonomous visual-field defects. Fifteen minutes of oxygen inhalation at sea level reduced by fifty-five per cent the incidence of 'the bends' in 1800 cadets exposed to 38,000 foot altitude for two hours. In these pressure-chamber studies, it was found that exercise could bring on symptoms as low as 22,000 feet.[31]

In this day and age of shirt-sleeve comfort in pressurized jet aircraft flying up to 60,000 feet, it is hard to conceive of the hardships which flight crews suffered in World War II at high altitude; but now, as then, the temperature at 20,000 feet often falls to sixty-seven to seventy-six degrees below zero F. The fighter pilot, snug in his enclosed cockpit behind a big engine, was well protected, but the bomber crewman, particularly the powered-turret gunners, and in the B-17s and B-24s, the waist gunners standing at open windows amidships, all too often became victims of frostbite.

The British encountered the problem in night raids over Germany even before our 8th Air Force reached Europe (here it must be mentioned that British bombers with liquid-cooled engines—the incomparable Rolls-Royce Merlin in the Whitley, certain marks of the Wellington, the Halifax and Lancaster—were more effectively heated by the engine coolant than the American bombers with air-cooled power plants, which used small gasoline stoves located in the fuselage). The British early discovered that the face, fingers, hands, toes and feet were most commonly affected, and that anoxia was a contributing factor, deficient blood oxygenation rendering tissue particularly susceptible. To prevent facial frostbite, many crew members did not shave for six hours before a flight, to leave the natural protective oils on the skin. Lanolin or other greases were applied for several years, but any water content increased the liability of frostbite of the face, and the use of grease was discouraged by Air Ministry order after October 1944. Heavy flying clothing and Balaclava helmets were issued and, after January 1942, electrically heated gloves, socks and underwear were available. Frostbite casualties still occurred, however, from failure of the electrical clothing, from inadequate or improper clothing, and above all, from boarding the plane with flight clothing moist with rain or perspiration. Carelessness was recognized to be such a large contributing factor that in one Group of Bomber Command, frostbite injuries were held due to own misconduct if proven to be caused by carelessness, and disciplinary action was taken. 'Air-crew cloakrooms' were also established to ensure that flight clothing was properly dried out between missions.

Severe frostbite casualties were part of the aeromedical nightmare that featured the 8th Air Force's first year of operation over Europe. Lack of experience, faulty indoctrination, defective or inadequate equipment were the culprits, as gunners removed their gloves and froze their fingers to clear jammed guns, or to exchange a frozen B-L-B mask for a spare one. Bare flesh froze instantly on contact with cold metal at seventy-six degrees below zero F. Waist gunners froze their faces at open windows. During eight-hour missions ball-turret gunners were forced to urinate in their clothing because no relief tubes were fitted; severe and crippling frostbite of buttocks and thighs followed, with sloughing of muscle tissue. 'This a real emergency ... many men seen in the hospital will not return to duty for months—if ever.'[32] Grimly, the 8th Air Force medical author recommended the Russian proverb, 'the only way to treat frostbite is to wait for everything to drop off that is going to drop off and then see what you can do with what is left.'[33] Electrically-heated clothing was at first undependable; electrical systems were overloaded, and early suits might burn the groins and popliteal spaces, while the back, hands and feet of the unfortunate flyer froze. Electrical elements of the suit were at first connected in series instead of in parallel, so when one part failed, others went out of action too. 'How did I freeze my right hand? My goddam left boot burned out!'[34] Strict discipline was enforced, 'private' flight clothing seized and issued from a common pool, and enlisted men trained to dry and maintain the clothing. Efficient heated suits, gloves and boots, together with muffs (five per heavy bomber) and electrically-heated casualty bags or blankets were developed and issued. Frozen faces still occurred in waist gunners until two officers of the 8th Air Force (who won the Legion of Merit for their efforts) devised a plexiglas waist window which still permitted free movement of the ·50 calibre Brownings. With this last refinement, installed early in 1944, frostbite in high altitude bomber crews became almost a thing of the past.

Aero-otitis media was the cause of much sick time in the European Theatre. Curiously, it was not the fighter pilot, making rapid dives from high altitude, but the bomber crewman who suffered most from this condition. Apparently duration at altitude was the most significant factor, the highest incidence being in the 8th Air Force bombing missions over Germany, while the 15th Air Force, flying lower-level missions in the Mediterranean, had only one-fourth the incidence of aero-otitis media. The existence of an incipient upper respiratory infection before flight certainly predisposed to the development of aero-otitis media. Many men were hospitalized during the 8th Air Force's first year overseas:

The usual story is that a mission is flown, followed by subsequent grounding for several days or weeks because of aerotitis, and then the cycle is repeated. In the end, these men take up a lot of time of the Unit Surgeons, occupy hospital beds, and are not available for combat duty a third of the time.[35]

Beginning in October 1944 three specially-trained nose and throat specialists were sent to England to treat cases of aero-otitis media with radium therapy. This procedure shrank the chronically hypertrophied lymphoid tissue blocking the Eustachian tubes to the ears, and was reported by one medical facility as 'contributing immeasurably to the prevention of recurrent aero-otitis.'[36]

A variety of combat injuries were seen that did not occur in peacetime flying, the treatment of which taxed the resourcefulness of surgeons, physicians and psychiatrists. Despite armour plate in the aircraft, men were killed or maimed over the skies of Europe by penetrating missiles. For those struck directly by the plane-smashing weapons of defending *Luftwaffe* fighters there was no hope, the quarter-pound explosive shell of the Mauser MG-151 20 mm cannon, with a muzzle velocity of 2590 feet per second, having an incredibly disruptive effect on human flesh and bone that meant instantaneous death. But as early as October 1942 analysis of combat wounds in 8th Air Force bomber crews showed that seventy per cent were caused by low-velocity missiles—flak splinters or fragments of exploding cannon shell. This inspired Brigadier General Malcolm C. Grow (MC), then surgeon of the 8th Air Force, to promote development of body armour that might stop such fragments.[37] The Wilkinson Sword Co. of London produced a vest of overlapping 1 mm thick manganese steel plates which stopped ·45 calibre bullets at thirty paces and, by March 1943, a hundred and twenty suits, sufficient for twelve B-17 crews, were being tested in combat. In four cases where men were struck in areas protected by body armour during the test period (one man being a tail gunner hit by a machine-gun bullet from an attacking Focke-Wulf 190) no injury occurred. Quantity production was undertaken in the USA and by 1 January 1944 some 13,500 'flak suits' had been sent to England. Statistics proved their effectiveness, many men being struck in the chest and abdomen sustaining no injuries whatever. A later study of 116 men struck in the thoracic or abdominal region while wearing body armour showed that 74·15 per cent suffered no injury whatever, 18·12 per cent were slightly wounded, and 7·5 per cent were killed. Eighty of these men were struck by flak fragments, twenty by 20 mm cannon shell splinters, and four by machine-gun bullets. Compared to the injuries of unarmoured personnel, the fatility rate for thoracic wounds was reduced from thirty-six to eight per cent, and for abdominal wounds from thirty-nine to seven per cent.

It is curious to note that 8th Air Force flight surgeons had much trouble squelching a superstition among combat crews that the flak suit provided more protection when laid flat on the floor of the plane than when worn on the person. This seems to have originated from the erroneous belief that most flak fragments entered from below through the floor of the aircraft. As late as April 1945 it was recommended that 'a strong directive be issued from Headquarters, Army Air Forces, forbidding the improper use of the flak suit as a floor mat. [38]

A steel helmet completed the twentieth-century suit of mail worn by many World War II flight crew members. During the Tunisian campaign and the invasion of Sicily and Italy, Colonel Otis C. Benson, Surgeon of the 12th Bomber Command (later the 15th Air Force) had publicized the saving of lives from wearing the standard M-1 infantry helmet, which sometimes had to be spread with a jack screw to accommodate earphones. An improved version designed by General Grow, the M-4, made of numerous manganese steel plates and able to turn a ·45 calibre bullet fired from six feet, was widely manufactured and used by the 8th Air Force. Sixty-four and four-tenths per cent of the men wearing it when struck in the head were uninjured; 15·2 per cent were severely wounded, and 17·4 per cent were killed.[39]

Due to the lack of self-sealing tanks in RAF Spitfires and Hurricanes, the Battle of Britain produced a considerable literature on the treatment of burns. With flaming gasoline gushing back at them from ruptured fuselage tanks, flyers suffered most on the unprotected areas of the body—the face, head and hands. Only in combat did men learn that helmets, goggles and heavy gloves might well prevent severe disfigurement and disability. Surprising to many victims was the lack of pain experienced as the aircraft went down with flame-filled cockpits, and the months in hospital that followed. Equally surprising to medical personnel was the alertness, cheerfulness and animation of men brought in with recent flash burns over considerable areas of the body, who slipped into coma and died a few hours later of irreversible shock. When I was a medical student in 1939, tannic acid was the latest miracle and the standard treatment for severe burns: infection, severe scarring and contractions caused RAF surgeons promptly to discard it, and to substitute soothing vaseline gauze. Deservedly renowned was the work of the plastic surgeon, Sir Archibald McIndoe, in rehabilitating many of the badly burned and disfigured Battle of Britain pilots. A great humanitarian, McIndoe's question as he worked with dermatome and scalpel was, 'when their bodies are whole again can we also rebuild something of their lives?'[40] His memory lives on in the 'Guinea-Pig Club,' an association of those men whose very selves, as well as their faces and hands, were restored by his exertions, and in the writings of many of his patients, among them Richard Hillary, the author of one of the literary milestones of the war, *The Last Enemy*.

Richard Hillary's death thirty months after the Battle of Britain was not without significance for aviation medicine. Haunted by survivor's guilt ('why have I been saved?'), closer to his lost squadron mates than to the living around him, he was driven to apply for flying duty, and succeeded in being posted to night-fighter training although he clearly was not fit, either physically or psychologically.[41] His close friends sensed that his immeasurable loneliness could be assuaged only by joining his former comrades in death. The current night fighter in the autumn of 1942 was the twin-engined Bristol Blenheim I. Because of his scarred hands with the fragile grafts covering the stiffened fingers, Hillary started on the Bisley, an underpowered Blenheim variant:

> The Bisleys have a switch to shut the gills—the Blenheim a wheel somewhere behind the pilot that needs about 50 turns. The Bisleys have a simple lever up and down to raise and lower the undercarriage—the Blenheims have a catch out from the handle which must be pushed in with the thumb before the undercarriage can be pulled up.[42]

On the night of 7 January 1943 Richard Hillary's Blenheim crashed and burned on a training flight. Icing might appear to have been the immediate cause of the accident, but it is easy to conclude that his handicap prevented him from operating the controls properly. Thus 'the last of the long-haired boys' found the death which he had sought. Granted that he may have had the right to risk his own life when he should have been grounded—how could he take with him his radar observer, Walter Fison?

Other men broke in mind rather than in body. These were the victims of the neuroses of war—but in a fighting service, this designation rapidly became an epithet. The euphemisms were legion, the occurrence universal. In the *Luftwaffe* 'the diagnosis of *hysteria* or *neurosis* was forbidden for political reasons and therefore either ignored by physicians or camouflaged as organic disease. . . . Concepts like *inner conflict reactions* or *abnormal reactions to stress* were used instead.'[43] In the Royal Air Force 'the term "Flying Stress" was generally applied in the instance of air-crew personnel who broke down and became unfit for duty on medical grounds under the strain of flying.'[44] In the American forces, where one American general had dealt with the problem of the skyrocketing neuropsychiatric casualty rate during the North African campaign by administrative order:

'There will be no further psychoneuroses in this command,'[45] the euphemisms were 'combat fatigue' and 'operational fatigue.' In all cases of emotional breakdown under combat stress (excluding the examples of 'lack of moral fibre' or 'fear of flying' where there had been no significant combat exposure) a conflict existed between the man's conscious motivation to serve, to uphold the reputation of the unit, and above all, to be worthy of his fellow crew members or squadron mates; and the unconscious fear of death or mutilation, originating in repeated exposures to traumatic combat situations, or sometimes, to a single overwhelming event. In the end the ego was overpowered and characteristic symptoms developed such as irritability, anxiety, insomnia, terrifying combat nightmares, weight loss, nausea, excessive drinking and—if the victim felt guilty over the death of a comrade—depression. Some men turned themselves in to sick bay; some, from an excess of zeal or fear of being considered cowards, were turned in by their fellows as their symptoms created danger for others; some were taken off duty by the flight surgeon. The latter, if he was interested in his work and possessed the confidence of his men, could do much to prevent a serious breakdown by taking air crew off flying duty temporarily and sending them to a rest home for a week or so, where freedom from military discipline, rest, recreation, liberty in near-by towns and contact with the opposite sex[46] worked wonders, and enabled many a hard-pressed man to finish out his tour of duty. A definite number of missions to be flown, known to personnel in advance, helped combat flyers to hold out till the end was in sight. Good leadership, superior aircraft and success of the unit in combat helped to hold down the N-P casualty rate; heavy losses raised it, Major Douglas D. Bond, Director of Psychiatry in the Central Medical Establishment of the 8th Air Force, noting a sharp rise in cases of war neurosis when the rate of aircraft losses first exceeded eight per cent at the time of the Schweinfurt and Regensburg raid in August 1943.[47] As for the men who had to be admitted to the sick list with 'operational fatigue' or 'combat fatigue,' Bond believed that simple removal from the actual danger of combat flying was more effective than any active psychotherapeutic measures. There was much disagreement on this point, the average civilian psychiatrist-in-uniform, with a background of State Hospital work or psychoanalytic training, being more impressed by the disturbed flyer than by the disturbing situation he was reacting to, and tending to feel that severe symptoms, as in civil life, made for a bad prognosis. These medical men failed to realize that even the strongest ego has its breaking point, but the ego capable of withstanding much combat stress before temporarily collapsing has strong recuperative powers. Most 'combat fatigue' victims made a good recovery with minimal treatment, though the technique of 'narcosynthesis'—helping a man to talk out a recent terrifying experience with the help of intravenous drugs such as sodium amytal or sodium pentothal—accelerated the recovery of many from the effects of gross psychic trauma.

What was it like—that moment of truth, after too many high-altitude missions over Germany, too many 'Forts' going down in flames with no 'chutes opening in their wakes, too many empty bunks in the barracks on the night after a big raid, too many mutilated, bloody corpses hauled out of shattered turrets and cockpits back on the hardstands, when a man realized he had 'had it,' that he could take no more? For one B-17 bombardier it came during the attack on Kiel on 13 June 1943 when twenty-two out of sixty attacking bombers were shot down by German fighters—'a sobering defeat,' according to the official air historian:[48]

The Kiel raid was his worst. His gun was frozen and he sat helplessly watching repeated fighter attack and heavy flak. The plane in which there was a General was on his wing and he saw it crippled and spin down through the clouds over the target. No one got out that he saw. In rather quick succession on his plane the tail gunner passed out from anoxia, all but 2 guns froze, the No. 2 engine was hit, and caught fire and the plane on the other wing was hit, went out of control and side-slipped directly underneath them so close that the pilot of his plane had to pull up sharply to avoid a crash. This plane then crashed into the B-17 on their opposite side; they had to do evasive action to to miss pieces of B-17s that were flying in the air. He saw the ball turret knocked off and go down 'like an apple' with the gunner still inside. He saw another man jump with a burning parachute and fall 'like a hunk of lead.' Shortly after another neighbouring ship did a loop and spun in. He saw another lose its wings and the fuselage go down end over end, no parachutes being seen. He saw another snap-roll and one wing came off. His own plane was badly damaged and had to be salvaged after this raid. On coming in to land after this raid, the plane ground looped in landing. This raid was a disastrous one for his group. Ten out of nineteen planes failed to return, the remainder were well shot up, and several including his own were wrecked on landing, the General was missing, and everyone was stunned by what had happened. The patient felt pent-up and restless during the interrogation, and after it began crying and weeping. That night in the barracks he broke down again while the clothes of his missing room-mates were being packed up. He tried drinking to relieve his anxiety but it didn't help much. That night he had his first battle dreams, couldn't sleep because of vivid nightmares of crashing and falling and one time woke up sweating profusely and was told that he had been screaming and yelling in his sleep. This raid marked the onset of a severe nervous state and by now throughout the day and night he was tense, anxious, tired, depressed, things seemed unreal, and he had difficulty concentrating.[49]

Ninety-six hours of narcosis therapy and a week at a rest home failed to help him, and he was discharged with the diagnosis of 'operational fatigue, not recovered.'

Most poignant of all was the problem of 'survivor's guilt' in the flyer—often a bomber crew member—whose comrades had died, while he had lived:

The dead appear in dreams at night, happy dreams of former good times, which are now a mockery, or fearful dreams of dying, which are exact reproductions of what happened, or fantastic elaborations of it. In the dream, the agony is the helplessness and suffering of the dead and the anguish of not having helped or not being able to help them. The dead also appear in waking reveries and in associations of places and people. The identification is too strong to be dissolved by the physical fact of death, and, since the dead live within the living just as they did before they died, they cannot be expected to remain in their watery or fiery graves.[50]

Where 'combat fatigue' labelled the men who broke emotionally in the face of the *Luftwaffe's* fanatic onslaught against the strategic bombing of Germany, 'operational fatigue' was frequently the diagnosis used for men in less active theatres who were worn down by the strain of dangerous missions, and unwholesome and isolated living conditions, in the absence of severe enemy action. Two excellent papers appeared on this subject during the war, one describing fatigue in P-38 Lightning pilots flying long missions from Adak, Shemya and Amchitka in the Aleutians, the other being a general survey of fighter pilots in the south-west Pacific area flying P-38s, P-47s, and the three-place Northrop P-61 Black Widow night fighter.[51] In both theatres pilots could agree that 'a good fight is always a morale builder for the survivor.' Pilots had confidence in their aircraft, and there was no serious morale problem. But in the long-range twin-engined P-38 squadrons, thirteen pilots during two months' time flew seventy patrols and combat sorties of more than six hours' duration, as well as numerous shorter missions. One pilot made seven such missions, one six, three made five each, three made four each, two made three each. During the two-month period there were only four enemy contacts. On the long missions, it was considered that a pilot could remain fully alert for the first thirty to forty-five minutes, and partially alert for the next three to four hours, but eventually would become so fatigued that he could not properly search the sky even though he knew his life depended on seeing the enemy before he was attacked. The threat of bad weather caused tension and anxiety, five pilots being killed by the Aleutian weather in three months. To get under the deep, low-hanging clouds, much of the flying was done just above the icy water. Here at least there was no trouble with anoxia and little with cold. The docile P-38 did not require constant attention, and could be trimmed to fly hands-off. Cockpits, however became very uncomfortable on six-hour missions. There was no room to stretch the legs and body, and tall flyers bumped their heads on the transparent canopy. Sitting in one position for long periods caused soreness of the buttocks ('parachute ass'), severe in eight cases, and subsequently, some could not sit through a meal. Seven men had trouble urinating in flight, and one would not use the relief tube at all. The plegmatic type of pilot suffered less, while the more emotional ones fatigued rapidly. Fear of flying, palpitations, dry mouth, inability to relax after flight and insomnia were listed as symptoms of operational fatigue. 'A sense of loneliness, helplessness and futility, greatly exaggerated on single plane flights, was noted by all.' Living conditions at the base were held to contribute, particularly in the hot, muggy jungle climate of the south-west Pacific. Here men lived in tents amidst dust or mud, ate monotonous canned rations, lost weight because the diet lacked appeal and were nagged by their superiors with 'take your atabrine,' 'dry out your clothes,' 'stay away from native villages,' etc. Men returning from seven-day leaves in Australia brought back whisky; 'an occasional indulgence benefits the individual by allowing relief of pent-up energy and emotions.'

Flying fatigue was not only a problem overseas; it was a threat in the training commands at home. A study of 172 student aviators training at Pensacola, Florida, showed that excessive fatigue was undermining physical and psychological fitness, emotional stability, desire to fly and general offensive spirit, and was a factor in some crashes. The authors labelled as 'overfatigue' a condition not relieved by a night's rest, or only briefly relieved. 'Fatigue syndrome' described the extreme degree continuing for days. Physical illness was a predisposing cause, but also gave some students a chance to rest. Fatigue was not related to the number of hours flown per week, but night flying after day flying the same day was a potent cause. Instructors exaggerated the problem when they habitually spoke indistinctly, handled the controls roughly, kept silent, shouted, used profanity, lacked interest or criticized incessantly.[52]

That overfatigue contributed to flying accidents was precisely demonstrated during the war by the so-called 'Cambridge Cockpit Studies' in England. One hundred and forty test subjects 'flew' blind for two hours in a simulated Spitfire cockpit which was never steady due to a 'rough air' device which required constant attention to the instruments and controls to maintain a straight and level course. Deviations in terms of side-slip, air speed, attitude and compass heading, were plotted and scored. Side-slip and air-speed scores deteriorated by fifty per cent by the end of the two-hour period.

Attitude-holding and compass course-holding improved initially with practice, then deteriorated. Some subjects later 'flew' the cockpit until exhausted, some lasting six or seven hours, and showed progressive deterioration of ability despite high interest and motivation. Specifically, the scores revealed: (1) 'Timing was suffering more and more as fatigue developed,' (2) as fatigue increased, the subjects 'became increasingly willing to accept lower standards of accuracy and performance,' (3) with increasing fatigue, they tended to concentrate on one or two instruments at a time, and 'at the end of the experiment 60 per cent were paying no attention to their side instruments,' (4) with awareness of the approaching end of the experimental run, four out of seven showed a sudden increase in errors. 'Apparently a tired airman has an almost irresistible tendency to relax when the crisis is past and home is in sight.' This correlates with the known high proportion of accidents occurring during landing after a long flight.[53]

To enable tired flight crews to complete vital wartime missions, benzedrine sometimes was used as a stimulant on order of the unit commander and under medical supervision. Five milligrammes (one tablet) every three hours was laid down as the dose for mental alertness, and ten milligrammes every six hours for maintaining physical efficiency. Not more than six tablets were to be taken each week.[54] The peacetime Air Force prefers to limit the demand on its flyers, rather than push them with stimulants.

Airsickness, practically unknown in the peace-time Air Force where standards could be kept high and those subject to motion sickness eliminated, suddenly became a problem in wartime, when huge numbers of men were being processed through the training centres. The condition is not essentially different from the malady affecting travellers aboard ship, or even in automobiles, and is considered by medical men to be merely one form of motion sickness. It is generally known that the symptoms of feeling unwell, followed by nausea, vertigo, vomiting and even prostration, occur when the victim is subjected to motion; that the symptoms rapidly disappear once the sufferer is on solid ground; and that nobody ever died of the condition, though many in the acute throes of motion sickness may have wished they would. Certain individuals are more susceptible than others, and the initially susceptible frequently adapt, so that after repeated experiences they can easily tolerate motion which previously would have made them violently ill.

A small handful of fearful and suggestible persons can develop symptoms of motion sickness in the absence of motion, simply from thinking about it, as in the case of the person who becomes ill in a ship alongside a dock. In such individuals a predominantly emotional cause is operating. In the great majority, the condition has nothing to do with fear, but represents a physical susceptibility to motion. There is continuing debate concerning which systems are involved. Stimulating the vestibular apparatus of the inner ear through the accelerations produced by motion plays a large part, and conversely, individuals who have had their vestibular organs destroyed by disease never have motion sickness. Vision plays a part, with individuals who can fix their eyes on the earth or horizon outside the aircraft, and thus maintain a sense of reference to the ground, being less susceptible to airsickness than those whose eyes are inside the cabin. On the other hand, persons seated on a stationary chair inside a 'witch house' structure that rotates around them become violently ill, even though the vestibular apparatus is not stimulated at all. Respectable researchers testify that internal motion of the intestines and other large organs in the abdomen produces nausea and other symptoms of motion sickness. A lot of interesting observations have received credence: that one is less susceptible lying down than sitting up; that overindulgence in food and alcohol are predisposing factors; that warmth, odours and stagnation of the air in the compartment aggravate the problem; and that pilots handling the controls never become airsick,[55] while they may fall victims to the ailment when dead-heading in the cabin with the passengers. Because the disease is self-limiting and never serious, it never received the study it deserved until World War II, when it was found to be a serious military handicap both for flight crews and paratroopers.

Some investigators insisted on seeing the problem as a purely emotional one and a result of neurotic tendencies, one medical author (who evidently did not experience it himself) alleging that the motion of the aircraft caused unacknowledged anxiety, and that writers on the subject who had been airsick themselves feared to admit this fear, and rationalized the entire problem in terms of motion susceptibility instead.[56] In a paper marked by careful observation and strict objectivity, McDonough and Bond divided the airsick into two groups—those who were responding to anxiety, and those who had a physical susceptibility to motion, which decreased with exposure to flying. The former type, comprising ten per cent of cases seen, was a cause for elimination from flight training, and included men who had nausea in anticipation of flying, or ten to fifteen minutes after takeoff on a smooth day; the nausea being severe, not relieved by vomiting, and continuing throughout flight. These men were hypersensitive to odours, heat and poor ventilation, and their symptoms, particularly nausea and headache, continued for up to seventy-two hours after a flight. By contrast, the ninety per cent majority were airsick only in very rough weather or violent aerobatics, felt comfortable between vomiting episodes, and did not experience headache, dizziness or difficulty in thinking. Their symptoms disappeared on landing, and with continued flying they adapted, with less frequent airsickness, and generally completed flight training successfully.[57]

No new antidotes to motion sickness came out of the extensive World War II studies, the traditional seasickness remedy, hyoscine, still being the most successful preparation. The superior antihistamine-derived preventatives today in use, under the trade-names of Bonamine and Marezine, were evolved only in the period following World War II.

Earlier studies on radial acceleration had indicated that 'blacking out' in sharp turns and pull-outs was caused by a relative anaemia of the brain, resulting in turn from blood pooling in the legs and abdominal vessels under the influence of high G forces. It followed that mechanical pressure applied externally to the lower portion of the body would force the blood upwards towards the heart and mitigate the cerebral anaemia. A large number of schemes were tried before a 'G suit' was devised that was simple and effective enough to be issued to the combat air forces. The Franks water suit, a non-stretch garment enclosing fluid-filled reservoirs covering the lower body, exerted counterpressure automatically under G load by simple hydrostatic force, and elevated the blackout threshold by at least 1·5 G in centrifuge tests. Pilots objected to the water suit on grounds of weight, bulk and restriction of movement. Research then switched to air-filled suits, but because it was believed at first that the ankles, calves, thighs and abdomen should be pressurized at different levels, the early 'gradient pressure suits,' with seventeen bladders and three-way air valves, were unduly heavy and complicated. The G-2 suit, with five bladders all inflated at the same pressure, was much simpler, the weight being reduced from ten to four and a half pounds. Eventually the G-3A suit was manufactured and issued in quantity. Weighing altogether three and a quarter pounds, it had a single-piece bladder system exerting pressure on the abdomen, thighs and calves, the bladders being encased in a close-fitting outer garment of oxford-weave nylon. When acceleration during manœuvres reached two G, a valve admitted air from the engine intake to the bladders in the suit, the pressure rising approximately 1 psi per G. Thus protected, the pilot's tolerance for blackout was raised by 1 to 1·5 G. The necessary air valves were installed in all first-line USAAF fighters, the P-38, P-47 and P-51, but not in the P-61 night fighter nor in the second-rate P-39, P-59 and P-63.

Available only in the last year of the war, and generally used only in Europe, the G suit was praised in one paper by a flight surgeon with a P-51 fighter group of the 8th Air Force. One hundred and forty-two pilots flying escort on the big bombers had their G suits inflated on an average of 3·4 times during an average escort mission, with much higher frequency if combat occurred with German fighters. Depending on the ammunition load and the amount of fuel in fuselage and wing tanks, the P-51 Mustang could tolerate 6·3 to 7·1 G without structural damage. With the G suit functioning, the pilot could, however, tolerate eight G without blacking out, meaning that he could remain conscious and in control of his aircraft in manœuvres which might damage it, and which would cause his opponent to black out. Of 118 P-51 pilots, eighty-two per cent had experienced over five G, and fifty-seven per cent had exceeded six G. Thirty-one per cent had at some time performed manœuvres which had exceeded the structural limitations of the aircraft. In a group of 173 pilots flying without the G suit, seventy-three per cent had experienced grey-out, and twenty-four per cent had blacked out. Among forty-eight pilots using the G suit, grey-out had occurred in thirty per cent, and blackout in only ten per cent. Not only did the G suit minimize fatigue, but it paid off in combat, permitting tight manœuvres which would have been impossible without it. A table headed 'Relationship Between Use of G Suit and Enemy Aircraft Shot Down' showed:[58]

	No. of A/C shot down	No. sorties	No. operational hours	No. A/C shot down per 1000 sorties	No. A/C shot down per 1000 operational hours
Wearing G suit	87	3048	13,059	29	67
Not wearing G suit	58	3911	17,362	16	33

During World War II, for the first time, aircraft crashes were extensively investigated on a scientific basis. This involved an examination of the physical effects of linear deceleration and impact on the human organism. Deceleration refers to the application of force to slow or halt the movement of a body or object. The amount of force needed is proportional to the square of the speed of the object, and a corresponding amount of energy is absorbed by the object. Very abrupt deceleration may cause the forces to build up to a level which has a disruptive effect on structure, including the organs, tissues and skeletal framework of the human body. Here again the magnitude of forces involved is expressed in multiples of gravitational force. Normal braking in an automobile involves a decelerative force of less than two G; in aircraft crashes survival is possible with abrupt deceleration of as much as fifty G. In any aircraft mishap involving contact with the ground, efforts will be made to cause the deceleration forces to be applied as gradually as possible—the 'controlled crash.' Yet the fact remains that most deaths in flying are caused by violent impact with the ground at high speed, involving abrupt deceleration with the human body required to absorb an intensity of G forces beyond its structural limitations. Medically, the resulting diagnosis is 'injuries, multiple, extreme.'

Survival for air crew in an uncontrolled crash depends both on design and protective equipment. The former, whose importance was not appreciated until about 1940, is the province of the engineer; the latter is that of the medical man. Obviously, air crew will be seriously or fatally injured in a crash if the structure of the cockpit collapses and crushes them, or if they are thrown against interior surfaces. Many deaths, it must be remembered, are caused by heads being smashed against instrument panels. It is also the engineer's concern that the seat attachments do not fail under G forces in a crash. The protective equipment involves restraining straps and belts, designed to prevent the air crew from being thrown against the structure.

The Germans, at least, attempted fundamental research on the effect of deceleration at high G forces on the human body. At the *Institut für Flugmedizin der DVL* at Berlin-Adlershof they began before the war the construction of a 'catapult' in which a light-weight instrumented cabin for the test subject ran on rails extending for 410 feet, the whole enclosed in a long shed. The pull of a descending weight—actually a tank able to contain seventy-five tons of water—accelerated the cabin over the first 262 feet to a maximum velocity of 163 mph. During the last eighty-two feet of the track, brakes decelerated the cabin gradually or abruptly.[59] Allied bombing destroyed the 'catapult' before it could be put to use, but it pointed the way to the far more powerful rocket-sled deceleration test equipment in the post-war years.

During World War II, US Army Air Force Regulation 62-14 required Accident Investigation Committees to be set up by commanding officers to investigate all accidents in which personnel were killed or severely injured, or an aircraft extensively damaged. Each committee consisted of three experienced pilots, an intelligence officer, and a medical officer, the latter reporting on AAF Form 205 which was forwarded to the Air Surgeon for evaluation.

These soon led to some systematic studies of crash injuries. A series of papers by Captain George M. Hass (MC) of the School of Aviation Medicine drew attention to the high proportion of head injuries in crashes (in eighty to ninety per cent of aircraft accidents) and the frequent occurrence of severe internal injuries in individuals who showed few symptoms immediately after a crash.[60] Head injuries were almost invariably caused by the body jack-knifing forward at the moment of impact, with the face or forehead striking the instrument panel, or what the medical researchers labelled the 'cowling-instrument panel-cockpit assembly.' At least, this produced brief unconsciousness and an amnesia for the few minutes antedating the crash; at worst, skull fracture with severe brain injury, massive haemorrhage and death. Not all severe injuries resulted from impact of the body on the interior of the cockpit: some individuals, properly strapped to their seats, lost consciousness and died of unsuspected internal haemorrhage. The inertia of the blood-filled internal organs might cause them to tear loose from their skeletal attachments, or rupture the organs themselves. The heart might burst, the heart valves be torn, or the aorta, the large blood vessel leading from the heart, be ripped across. The spleen and liver, massive organs enclosed in a flimsy epithelium, might rupture and lacerate. Tears of the intestines were common in severe crashes, and surgeons were advised to suspect them in surviving air crew. Haemorrhage into injured lungs might cause delayed shock and death. With crashes at the high speeds of which World War II aircraft were capable, not only might the cockpit longerons and structure collapse, crushing the occupant, but the heavy organs of the body might be torn entirely free and burst out of the thorax or abdominal cavity.

What could be done to minimize the staggering number of deaths in aircraft crashes, particularly in the training commands? To supplement the traditional lap belt, a shoulder harness was developed that greatly reduced the incidence of severe head injuries so prevalent even in minor crashes. A pair of one and three-quarter inch webbing straps, when properly secured, held the pilot firmly against the back of the seat. The so-called inertia reel automatically locked the harness tight in a crash whenever the load on the harness rose to two to three G. In a study of 234 belly landings of fighter aircraft between 1 January and 30 June 1944 it was found that with the harness in use, 175 survived uninjured, forty were injured and three were killed (the seats failing in all cases). Without the shoulder harness none escaped unscathed; fifteen were injured and one killed. The fear that a man's neck might be snapped if his shoulders were restrained was not borne out: in a study of all fighter-type crashes within the United States after 1 September 1943 only nine vertebral fractures were found. Two were fractures of the neck vertebrae, but in both cases the shoulder harness was not used.

Flight surgeons found much that was dangerous to the flyer in the design of the aircraft, and began a collaboration with engineers and designers that removed or mitigated many unnecessary hazards. Carbon monoxide poisoning was shown to be related to design, in that it was commonest in the pilots of single-engined fighters with radial engines. In the P-47, with its complicated exhaust collection system, leaks were common in the packing of the exhaust collector rings, and eighteen pilots in a squadron flying this aircraft at low altitude without oxygen were found to have a blood carbon monoxide level of 11·1 per cent.[61] A study of visibility from fighter cockpits showed, as might have been expected, that the 'Jug,' the P-47 Thunderbolt, with its big eighteen-cylinder R-2800 radial engine blocking the view over and around the nose, had the highest proportion of taxiing accidents. The P-51, with its slim in-line Rolls-Royce Merlin in the nose, had a favourable ratio, and the P-38, with excellent view forward and downward from its nacelle between the two engines, had the lowest rate of all. Designers were criticized for using curved glass or plexiglas in cockpit panels, to improve streamlining, which at the same time severely distorted vision. In the early B-17G the nose gunner saw two targets through the curved forward panels. The deviation error in plexiglas turret panels was the largest cause of foresighting errors. Curved plastic panels in the pilot's compartment of the B-29 had to be replaced with flat plexiglas because of distortion.[62] The cockpit itself was not safe: controls were too close together, or difficult to differentiate, so that (in the C-54 transport, for instance) it was possible to raise the landing gear instead of the flaps, or to hit the feathering button for the wrong propeller by accident. In the B-24 bomber, the top turret was insecurely supported and could fall on personnel in a crash. In training planes, instrument panels were moved forward, sharp edges and projections were eliminated, and crash bars or roll-over bars were fitted over the top of the cockpit to protect the pilot's head if the aircraft nosed over. In future designs, the cockpit structure was reinforced, and seat attachments strengthened.

Flight surgeons made their contributions to the success of night fighting through research in night vision as early as the Battle of Britain. It was of course known that an entirely separate eye mechanism—the rods—was responsible for night vision, with the cones functioning by day, and before the war tests of night visual acuity with red vision had been devised. While it was known that vitamin A played an important part in night vision, early studies showed that with a normal diet, excessive vitamin A did not improve visual performance at night. On the other hand, the rods were excessively sensitive to anoxia, with night blindness being nearly complete at 12,000 feet without oxygen. Therefore, oxygen was ordered from the ground up for night-fighter air crew. Further, as it was known that strong light bleached the rods of their functioning porphyrin pigments for periods of thirty minutes or more, night-fighter pilots, to maintain 'dark adaptation,' had to wear dark goggles in ready rooms before boarding their planes. Later, as it became known that red light did not affect the rods, it was possible for pilots wearing red goggles to see adequately by artificial light, without destroying their dark adaptation.

The US Navy, which did more night flying in formation than the Army Air Forces, became interested in the phenomenon labelled the *autokinetic illusion*. A pilot in formation at night tended to develop an almost hypnotic fixation on his leader's dim tail light, to the exclusion of his instruments, and not only might believe the light was moving when it was not, but could even react to the *apparent* movement ('because the lead pilot weaves about so much') with manœuvres dangerous to himself or others.[63] Hypnosis and self-deception could progress to the point where the victims accused the lead pilot of attempting a wing-over in night formation! and if they dived away to evade, they might strike the water before realizing the true situation. It is possible that one of the Navy's greatest fighter pilots, Lieutenant Commander Edward H. ('Butch') O'Hare, Medal of Honor winner and victor in twelve combats, died because of this phenomenon. On 26 November 1943, in the first attempt at night fighter interception from a carrier, O'Hare, flying an F-6F Hellcat, mysteriously went down while closing the formation leader, a radar-equipped TBF Avenger. All personnel were warned of the danger of the autokinetic illusion in night formation flying, while Captain Graybiel, using a North American SNJ Texan trainer and a twin-engined Beech SNB Kansan assigned to him at Pensacola, discovered that the phenomenon was much less severe if the lead plane carried two or more lights to divide the attention of the following pilots.

Parachutes were worn generally by all air crew in World War II, except in transport aircraft. The Germans, as usual, were ahead of the Allies in development, experimenting with ribbon-canopy parachutes for high-speed bail-out, and an aneroid controlled automatic parachute release which pulled the rip cord at 13,100 feet. They also introduced the explosive ejection seat, which was responsible for saving approximately fifty pilots in emergency bail-outs from Me 109, FW 190, and jet-propelled Me 262 aircraft in the last few months of the war.

In the American service the B-8 twenty-four-foot diameter parachute was standard, with webbing harness and manual release, little changed during the past twenty years except that nylon had been substituted for silk. Pilots of fighters and trainers wore this as a seat pack. Others, particularly bomber crew members, wore the detachable chest pack. Wearing the harness alone, they could comfortably move about and perform their duties, and in an emergency, quickly attach the parachute pack by snap hooks and D rings. Of course there was always the risk that the parachute might not be within reach when bail-out was ordered, or could not be attached in time.

All too often the parachute failed in its function of saving life. Noting that there were four emergency jumps from Army Air Forces aircraft daily within the continental limits of the United States, the author of a 1944 paper reported that twenty-five per cent of the jumps from fighter and single-engined trainer aircraft led to fatal results, while the rate was less than five per cent in bail-out from twin-engined trainers. Four hundred escape attempts resulted in fifty fatalities, three-quarters of which originated from three causes: jumping at too low an altitude (forty-eight per cent), jumper's body striking part of the aircraft structure (twenty per cent), and parachute fouling the aircraft (ten per cent). Medical officers were advised to instruct flight personnel: (1) don't wait too long to bail out. (2) dive out head first to clear plane. (3) look around before opening the 'chute and be sure you are clear of the plane. (4) straighten legs and keep feet together before pulling the rip cord, in order to avoid tangling yourself in your gear. Surprisingly, the author did not enter the debate prevailing among single-engine pilots as to whether it was better to dive out of the cockpit towards the outside or the inside of a spin. It would appear that by choosing the inside, there was less chance of being struck by the tail.[64]

With increasing speed and radial acceleration forces, the point was reached where men in spinning aircraft were unable to escape unaided. This fact, not generally known even to the flying fraternity, undoubtedly took many men to their deaths in crippled bombers over Germany and Japan who otherwise could have saved themselves. Too often it was assumed that the crew of the falling aircraft, 'rooted to the spot' by fear, were too panic-stricken to move. A few survivors' accounts circulated to flight surgeons in 1944 indicated that they were paralysed by G forces.

The pilot of a B-24D aircraft attempted to bail out while the aircraft was in a flat spin. From the flight deck he attempted to jump through the open doors of the right forward bomb bay: .

Instead of falling out of the right forward bomb bay, I landed in the left forward bomb bay, the door of which had not opened. It felt as if some invisible force was pressing me against that door, and I found it very difficult to move my arms or legs. Only by tremendous exertion was I able to grasp the edge of the catwalk. I tried in vain to pull myself over this catwalk. The ship gave a sudden lurch and I was catapulted out of the bomb bay. My parachute opened immediately, and as my body was swinging to a position directly beneath it I hit the ground. It's my opinion that the effect of the centrifugal force was not strong enough to hinder my escape until the ship had made one complete turn. After that, except for reaching out with my hand, it was impossible to move.[65]

A gunner, pinned to the floor and unable to drag himself to a hatch, shoved his parachute out the hatch, pulled the rip cord, and was forcibly hauled out by the opening parachute, suffering numerous lacerations and abrasions. The need for an ejection escape system was apparent, but this vital survival apparatus did not come for American airmen until after the war.

With the increasing high-altitude capability of the newer aircraft, American flight surgeons were worrying even before Pearl Harbor about anoxia in high-altitude bail-out. With an open parachute, a man would certainly die during the ten minutes he would require to descend from 35,000 to 20,000 feet. With free fall and closed parachute, the 15,000-foot drop could be made in one minute. In 1940 an experiment was run in a pressure chamber at the Mayo Clinic to determine if a man at 35,000 feet could remain conscious long enough without oxygen to bail out (thirty seconds) and then to free fall to 20,000 feet and open his parachute (one minute). The results were alarming. The subject, Lockheed Aircraft's experienced test pilot Milo Burcham, turned cyanotic and began to lose consciousness after thirty seconds of simulated struggle to escape from the cockpit. He forgot to open the valve of the emergency oxygen cylinder and had to be persuaded to do so by the observer. After five seconds more Burcham was unconscious, the emergency oxygen apparatus fell from his mouth, and he moved convulsively. Revived by the observer, Burcham did not realize he had been senseless and was 'surprised when the observer said he had given him an exciting experience.'[66] 'If delayed parachute opening descent were the only alternative open to aeroplane crews in dire emergency there might well develop among aviators a distaste for high-altitude missions and a lowering of morale throughout flying commands.'[67] The authors accordingly proposed that a small cylinder containing a ten minutes' supply of oxygen at 1800 psi be carried in a leg pocket of the flying suit, to supply oxygen during bail-out via the regular B-L-B mask.

Colonel Lovelace, in the best tradition of the flight surgeon, chose himself to demonstrate that with the 'bail-out bottle' he could survive a fall from 40,000 feet with open parachute. On 23 June 1943 he went out of the open bomb bay of a B-17 at 40,200 feet. Attached to the aircraft by a static line, his parachute deployed immediately. The opening shock was unexpectedly violent: brought up against his harness with terrific impact, Lovelace instantly lost consciousness. Fortunately his oxygen mask stayed in place and he recovered while floating down at 30,000 feet, to discover that the gloves had been torn off his hands when the parachute snapped open. A thin nylon liner glove protected his right hand, but the bare left hand was frostbitten.

Lovelace's self-sacrificing experiment was actually the highest parachute opening on record up to that time. No research had been done previously on the subject, and it had simply been assumed that with decreasing air density with increased altitude, the parachute opening shock would diminish in proportion. The totally unexpected violence of Colonel Lovelace's experience indicated that the opening shock at high altitude might well involve forces greater than the human frame could withstand. A research project was put in hand, using 200 and 145 pound hard rubber dummies, and eventually a 145-pound St Bernard dog, dropped from the bomb bay of a B-17 Flying Fortress. The standard 24-inch nylon B-8 'chute was employed, opened by a 25-foot static line, with the dummies instrumented to measure the G forces. Tests at a constant speed—232 mph—showed that with the 200-pound dummy, the force of the opening shock increased with altitude as follows:

Altitude, feet	No. of openings	Mean forces in lb.	at final peak in G
3,000	6	2400	12·0
7,000	13	2300	11·5
15,000	9	3300	16·5
20,000	5	5300	26·5
26,000	10	5300	26·5
33,000	3	5800	29·0
40,000	9	6600	33·0

Another series of tests showed that with increased launching speed, the opening force at final peak increased, particularly at higher altitude. At 175 mph true air speed—terminal velocity of a falling body at 26,000 feet—the G force was 14·0, but at 232 mph at the same altitude it was 26·0 G. Small wonder that parachute harnesses failed in the higher-altitude launchings, and men were injured. Here was another reason for free fall to lower altitudes before opening the parachute.[68]

The reasons for the paradoxical increase in opening shock with less-dense air have been worked out on theoretical grounds. Terminal velocity, the speed at which the acceleration of a falling body is balanced by air resistance, is a factor. Opening shock increases with terminal velocity, which itself increases, because of lesser air density, from 127 mph at 10,000 feet to 200 mph at 40,000 feet. At the latter altitude, the falling body has nearly three times as much kinetic energy as at the 10,000-foot level, thereby tripling the force which the man–parachute assembly have to withstand in high-altitude bail-out. At high altitude also, the canopy opens at a faster rate because the less-dense air does not resist its expansion as much as near sea level. This rapid deployment abruptly decelerates the man–parachute assembly producing higher peak loads. Lastly, the opening parachute during deployment sets in motion a large volume of air which it scoops in, the mass of which decelerates the man wearing it. The mass of less-dense air at high altitude is less than that at lower levels, resulting in less deceleration before full deployment of the 'chute, and a higher peak force of the opening shock.

Thus the flight surgeons of the major air powers played their part in World War II. But even before V-E Day in Europe, they were faced with a new challenge—the fantastic speed and altitude performance of the new jet-powered aircraft, and the stresses they imposed on their human operators.

[1] The myth persists that the Italian general, Guilio Douhet, through his 1921 book, *The Command of the Air,* first conceived and promulgated the doctrine of strategic air power. It was in fact jointly evolved by Trenchard and Mitchell from their World War I experiences in Europe (where Trenchard had commanded the so-called Independent Force, and Mitchell the Air Services of First Army Group, AEF). Not until about 1933 did Mitchell's American supporters (among them the future wartime Commander-in-Chief of the United States Army Air Forces, General H. H. Arnold) 'discover' Douhet and add his writings to their arguments.

[2] Sir Walter Raleigh and H. A. Jones, *The War in the Air* (Oxford: at the Clarendon Press, 1922-35), 6 vols.

[3] Sir Charles Webster and Noble Frankland, *The Strategic Air Offensive Against Germany* (London: HMSO, 1961), vol. III, p. 287.

[4] Wesley Frank Craven and James Lea Cate, *The Army Air Forces in World War II* (Chicago: The University of Chicago Press, 1948), vol. I, p. 65.

[5] See Martin Caidin, *Black Thursday* (New York: E. P. Dutton & Co., Inc., 1960).

[6] Craven and Cate, vol. II, p. 705.

[7] See James Dugan and Carroll Stewart, *Ploesti* (Random House, New York, 1962).

[8] The Staff of 'Aireview,' *General View of Japanese Military Aircraft in the Pacific War* (English text) (Tokyo: Kanto-Sha Co. Ltd, 1956), p. 57.

[9] Mae Mills Link and Hubert A. Coleman, *Medical Support of the Army Air Forces in World War II,* Office of the Surgeon General, USAF (Washington: Government Printing Office, 1955), p. 548.

[10] Hubertus Strughold, 'Development of Aviation Medicine in Germany,' *German Aviation Medicine in World War II,* prepared under the auspices of the Surgeon General, USAF (Washington: Government Printing Office, 1950), vol. I, p. 43.

[11] *ibid.,* p. 43.

[12] Squadron Leader S. C. Rexford-Welch, *The Royal Air Force Medical Services* (London: HMSO, 1955), vol. II, p. 71.

[13] See Wing Commander Robert Maycock, *Doctors in the Air* (London: George Allen & Unwin Ltd, 1957). Maycock himself went through the fighter pilot training course.

[14] Link and Coleman, p. 452.

[15] *ibid.*, p. 666.

[16] Major Norman Malamut, AC, 'Notes on Japanese Aviation Medicine and Research,' *Journal of Aviation Medicine,* vol. 18, February–December 1947, p. 64.

[17] Theodore Benzinger, 'High Altitude Flight Breathing Oxygen,' *German Aviation Medicine,* vol. I, p. 429.

[18] Henry *(sic)* Seeler, 'German Altitude Equipment (Ground Servicing and Aircraft Equipment) from 1939 to 1945,' *German Aviation Medicine,* vol. I, p. 466.

[19] Robin D. S. Higham, *The Armed Forces in Peace Time* (Henley-on-Thames: G. T. Foulis, 1962), p. 186.

[20] Rexford-Welch, vol. II, p. 17.

[21] These were proof against ·303 calibre bullets, but by the end of 1940 they had to be replaced with wire-wound bottles designed to resist cannon fire.

[22] Letter, RC London, Mechanical Engineering Department, Royal Air Force Establishment, Farnborough, England, 12 August 1965.

[23] Rexford-Welch, vol. II, p. 99.

[24] Captain L. D. Carlson, 'Concise Description of the Demand Oxygen System,' *Air Surgeon's Bulletin,* vol. I, no. 1, January 1944.

[25] In a pressure chamber 'flight' to 43,000 feet, we were told to inhale passively, count to five, then exhale forcibly. I noted that I had to exhale quite sharply or the lungs would fill up and there would be no tidal air exchange. The amount of force required when exhaling against 11 mm pressure was quite uncomfortable.

[26] Lieutenant Colonel A. P. Gagge and Captain S. C. Allen, 'Pressure Breathing,' *Air Surgeon's Bulletin* vol. I, no. 9, September 1944.

[27] From the context, it is clear that the diluter-demand system was installed in this aircraft.

[28] Captain Gordon W. Wormley MC, 'An Anoxia Accident in the 8th Air Force,' *Air Surgeon's Bulletin,* vol. I, no. 9, September 1944.

[29] *Air Surgeon's Bulletin,* vol. I, no. 3, March 1944.

[30] Kenn C. Rust, 'Bomber Markings of the 20th Air Force,' *Journal of the American Aviation Historical Society,* vol. 7, no. 3, Autumn 1962, p. 169.

[31] *Air Surgeon's Bulletin,* vol. I, no. 11, November 1944.

[32] Captain Wm. F. Sheeley MC, 'Frostbite in the 8th Air Force,' *Air Surgeon's Bulletin,* vol. 2, no. 1, January 1945.

[33] *ibid.*

[34] *ibid.*

[35] Quoted in Link and Coleman, p. 656.

[36] Quoted in Link and Coleman, p. 657.

[37] Brigadier General Malcolm C. Grow MC and Lieutenant Colonel Robert C. Lyons, 'Body Armour, a Brief Study of its Development,' *Air Surgeon's Bulletin,* vol. 2, no. 1, January 1945.

[38] Link and Coleman, p. 628.

[39] *ibid.*, p. 635.

[40] Edward Bishop, *The Guinea Pig Club* (London: Transworld Publishers, 1963), p. 56.

[41] Since writing the above, I find Marshal of the Royal Air Force Lord Douglas of Kirtleside blaming himself for Richard Hillary's return to flying duty and subsequent death, in that he allowed Hillary to extract from him a promise to assign him if the

doctors passed him as fit. 'I said that because I felt quite certain that the doctors would never pass him as fit for any sort of operational flying'. *Years of Command* (London: Collins, 1966), p. 156.

[42] Lovat Dickson, *Richard Hillary* (London: Macmillan & Co., 1951), p. 186.

[43] Immo von Hattingberg, 'Medical Care for Flying Personnel,' *German Aviation Medicine,* vol. II, p. 1063.

[44] Rexford-Welch, vol. II, p. 122.

[45] The late Edward A. Strecker MD, personal communication.

[46] However, 'for a month at Ifrane (in Morocco), when the personnel was almost exclusively officer, a venereal disease rate of 1400 per 1000 per annum was attained'! (Link and Coleman, p. 498).

[47] Douglas D. Bond, *The Love and Fear of Flying* (New York: International Universities Press, Inc., 1952), Appendix I, p. 181.

[48] Craven and Cate, vol. II, p. 670.

[49] Major Donald W. Hastings MC, Captain David G. Wright MC and Captain Bernard C. Glueck MC, AAF, *Psychiatric Experiences of the 8th Air Force, First Year of Combat (July 4, 1942–July 4, 1943)* (New York: Josiah Macy Jr Foundation, August 1944), p. 291.

[50] Lieutenant Colonel Roy R. Grinker MC and Major John P. Spiegel MC, AAF, *Men Under Stress* (Philadelphia: Blakiston, 1945), p. 114.

[51] (1) Major Mavis P. Kelsey MC, 11th AF, 'Flying Fatigue in Pilots Flying Long-Range Single-Seater Fighter Missions,' *Air Surgeon's Bulletin,* vol. 1, no. 6, June 1944. (2) Lieutenant Colonel James B. Hall MC and Major Frank K. Borse MC, 5th AF, 'Fighter Pilot Survey in the South-West Pacific,' *Air Surgeon's Bulletin,* vol. 2, no. 6, June 1945.

[52] Graybiel, Horwitz and Gates, 'Problems of Fatigue Among Student Pilots at the Naval Air Training Center, Pensacola, Florida,' *Journal of Aviation Medicine,* vol. 15, February–December 1944, p. 9.

[53] Ross A. MacFarland, *Human Factors in Air Transportation* (New York: McGraw-Hill Book Co., Inc., 1963), pp. 348–9.

[54] *Air Surgeon's Bulletin,* vol. 1, no. 2, February 1944.

[55] I confess that in my early student days I once developed nausea of near-critical proportions while flying my PA-11 in rough air with my instructor as passenger. The pilot is definitely less susceptible than the passenger, however, not only by virtue of his past experience, but because he can better anticipate the motion of the aircraft, and indeed, creates this himself to an extent with the controls, unconsciously avoiding such a degree of motion as will cause him discomfort.

[56] Captain D. M. Green MC, 'Air Sickness in Bomber Crews,' *Journal of Aviation Medicine,* vol. 14, February–December 1943, p. 366.

[57] Major Francis E. McDonough and Captain Douglas Bond MC, 'Management of the Airsick Aviator,' *Air Surgeon's Bulletin,* vol. 1, no. 3, March 1944.

[58] Captain Milton Mayer MC, 8th AF, 'The G Suit in Combat: Relationship between Use of G Suit and Enemy Aircraft Shot Down,' *Air Surgeon's Bulletin,* vol. 2, no. 8, August 1945.

[59] Siegfried Ruff, 'Brief Deceleration: Less than One Second,' *German Aviation Medicine,* vol. I, p. 586.

[60] Captain George M. Hass MC, 'Internal Injuries of Personnel Involved in Aircraft Accidents,' *Air Surgeon's Bulletin,* vol. 1, no. 1, January 1944.

[61] *Air Surgeon's Bulletin,* vol. 1, no. 7, July 1944.

[62] Major E. A. Rumson and Captain A. Chapanis, 'Visual Factors in Design of Military Aircraft,' *Journal of Aviation Medicine,* vol. 17, February–December 1946,

p. 115.

[63] Graybiel, A. and Clark, B., 'The Autokinetic Illusion and its Significance in Night Flying,' *Journal of Aviation Medicine*, vol. 16, March–December 1945, p. 111.

[64] 'Injuries Associated with Parachute Escapes,' *Air Surgeon's Bulletin*, vol. 1, no. 5, May 1944.

[65] Captain George W. Hass MC, 'Unsuccessful Use of Parachutes, and Cases Resulting from Forces Generated in Aircraft Spins,' *Air Surgeon's Bulletin*, vol. 1, no. 10, October 1944.

[66] Boothby, Lovelace and Burchell, 'Necessity of Emergency Oxygen Unit for Use in Parachute Escapes at High Altitude,' *Journal of Aviation Medicine*, vol. 12, March–December 1941, p. 126.

[67] Boothby, Lovelace and Benson, 'Emergency Oxygen Unit for Use in Parachute Escape or in Case of Failure of Regular Oxygen Supply at High Altitude,' *Journal of Aviation Medicine*, vol. 11, March–December 1940, p. 59.

[68] Captain G. A. Hallenbeck MC, Lieutenant K. E. Penrod AC and Major Ross MacCandle AC, 'Magnitude and Duration of Parachute Opening Shock,' *Air Surgeon's Bulletin*, vol. 2, no. 3, February 1945.

6

The Jet Age

The great revolution in aircraft propulsion has taken place in my lifetime. Forty-three years ago it was the mosquito hum of fifty 450 hp Pratt & Whitney 'Wasp' radials as a corresponding number of Army Air Corps P-12B biplanes from Selfridge Field, Michigan, passed overhead in a long straggling formation en route to a concentration at Mitchell Field, Long Island. Today the heavens are filled with the distant thunder of jet engines from aircraft passing over so high, so far ahead of their own sound, that I rarely see them unless they are pointed out by their own contrails pencilled across the sky.

Of course, we heard in those days of jet power—the possibility of discarding the whirling propeller and driving the aeroplane by a blast of heated and expanded air. At the 166 mph top speed of the Boeing P-12B—the stubby open-cockpit fighter which every red-blooded youngster dreamed of flying when he grew up—the jet engine would be grossly inefficient in terms of fuel consumption. At 500 mph, with the speed of the jet blast more nearly approaching that of the aircraft, efficiency would improve. But like the theoretical atomic power plant which could drive the *Mauretania* across the Atlantic on the nuclear energy in a glass of water, the jet engine would never be built. The world's speed record had been set at 357·7 mph in 1929 by a British propeller-driven seaplane, the Supermarine S-6, built for the Schneider Trophy contest. Five hundred miles per hour was an unattainable dream.

In the summer of 1940 the aeronautical magazines heralded the 'first' jet aircraft—the Caproni-Campini 'flying barrel.' Shaped like an oversize oil drum with wings, with its two-man crew riding in a nacelle on top, it had a compressor inside the barrel turned by a 900 hp piston engine, and flew for ten minutes on its first flight on 27 August 1940 at a disappointing 200 mph. Those funny Italians, we thought. They would never beat the jewel-like Rolls-Royces, Daimler-Benzes and Hispano-Suizas which powered the world's premier fighter planes.

But the turbo-compressor jet was no laughing matter, and in fact, had flown in secret exactly a year earlier near Rostock, Germany. Even while piston-engine design and development were daily setting new records, some men were fascinated by the theoretical advantages of the turbine jet engine. Fewer moving parts, less friction, and greater reliability: instead of a thrashing mass of reciprocating pistons, connecting rods and cranks, only a smoothly spinning turbine and compressor. Greater efficiency: where the four-cycle piston engine made three idling strokes for every power stroke, the one-cycle jet produced power through what might be called a continuous explosion. Elimination of the propeller: at speeds above 450 miles per hour, with its whirling tips reaching supersonic velocity, the propeller's efficiency fell sharply, while the jet was just coming into its own and its actual horsepower output increased with speed. Two obstacles stood in the way of producing this revolutionary power plant: the inability of contemporary metals to stand up to the stresses on the turbine blades revolving at 16,000 rpm at temperatures up to 1600 degrees F, and the large amount of engineering effort needed to develop the theory into a practical prime mover.

The first problem was solved by the metallurgist, and the modern jet turbine became feasible only through the creation of exotic non-ferrous alloys such as stellite,[1] retaining their hardness and stiffness even when incandescent. The second problem was gradually overcome by the persistence and vision of a few pioneers who believed in the jet principle, coupled after the commencement of World War II to the resources of industry in Germany, Great Britain and the United States.

Actually the first jet aircraft had flown on 27 August 1939 representing the fruits of three years of effort by a young physicist, Hans von Ohain, with the private backing of the prominent German aircraft manufacturer, Ernst Heinkel. The Heinkel He 178 tested that morning was powered by von Ohain's centrifugal-flow He S3B turbojet engine, with a maximum thrust of a modest 1102 pounds. Yet it was a beginning, and the Heinkel was faster than all but a few piston-engine fighters.[2]

The Heinkel first jet flight was a secret kept until after V-E Day. Knowing nothing of the German effort, a British Royal Air Force officer, Frank Whittle, had been working on his own plans for a centrifugal-flow turbine engine since 1935. The Air Ministry, at first disinterested, permitted Whittle's early patents to be published—thereby giving encouragement and guidance to his German rivals. By 1939 officialdom was more encouraging, and on 15 May 1941 Whittle's W 1 centrifugal-flow jet, with a thrust of 850 pounds, made its first flight in a Gloster E 28/39 built as a test bed for the engine. General Henry H. Arnold, the Chief of the US Army Air Forces, immediately realized the value to the United States of this innovation, and succeeded in having a Whittle engine, and British technicians, brought to America shortly before Pearl Harbor.

Despite the great amount of time and effort devoted to jets during World War II, the propeller-driven, piston-engined aircraft remained predominant right to the end. Low thrust output, short engine life, excessive fuel consumption and aerodynamic unsuitability of the airframe for speeds near that of sound, diminished the jet's theoretical advantage. Germany, which had the longest lead, failed to exploit it, though it used jet aircraft in combat during the last months of the war. No Heinkel aircraft entered service, but the Messerschmitt Me 262 flew with some success as a fighter, after a characteristic inspiration by the *Führer* had wasted time trying to modify this 515-mph speedster to serve as an anti-invasion bomber. Its two Jumo 004 engines, with a thrust of 1984 pounds each, had a useful life of less than twenty-five hours. Appearing at last in small numbers in attacks on the massed bomber formations of the 8th Air Force, the 'Schwalbe' (Swallow), as the Germans called it, caused much anxiety to the USAAF command. Fuel shortages, insufficient training of personnel, and the impending general collapse of the Thousand-Year *Reich* prevented the Me 262 from achieving decisive results, and it was mastered by the P-51 Mustang and other piston-engined fighters, though by numbers and tactics rather than by superior speed. The Germans also had a remarkable rocket-powered interceptor, the Messerschmitt Me 163 'Komet.' Tailless, with a swept-back wing, it could attain a speed of 621 mph. Its rocket motor, with a thrust of 3750 pounds, was fuelled with hydrogen peroxide as an oxidizer and a mixture of hydrazine hydrate thirty per cent in methyl alcohol, a treacherous combination which caused the deaths of many of its pilots. Even if the fuels did not explode in a bad landing they could cause serious burns if sprayed over personnel.[3]

Like the Germans, the British installed two jet engines in their first combat aircraft because of the inadequate thrust of the early Whittle units. The Gloster Meteor prototype first flew on 5 March 1943 but it was not until July 1944 that production aircraft, fitted with engines of 1700 pounds thrust, first entered squadron service. With a maximum speed of only 410 mph at 30,000 feet, these aircraft were slightly slower than the premier contemporary propeller-driven RAF fighter, the Hawker Tempest. They had some success against the V 1 flying bombs. In April 1945 just before the German collapse, Meteors went to the Continent, but no combat with German jets ensued.

Despite intensive effort, and direct British assistance, the United States did not succeed in getting jet aircraft into action before the end of World War II. The Whittle W 1 engine was copied by the General Electric Company, already experienced in turbine and supercharger design, and two of these were installed in the first American jet, the Bell P-59 Airacomet. With a top speed of only 413 mph at 30,000 feet, the Airacomet was a disappointment in comparison with contemporary piston-engined fighters, and the sixty-six built were used for training. The first jet accepted for operational service was the Lockheed P-80, a thoroughbred alongside the clumsy two-jet Bell, with a powerful 4000-pound thrust General Electric J-33 jet buried deep in its sleekly streamlined body and thunderously exhausting out of the tail-pipe at the rear. The speed was 558 mph at sea level, and six ·50 calibre machine guns were grouped in the nose. First delivery of the Shooting Star production model was in October 1944 and two of them reached Italy just before V-E day but were not flown in combat.

In the post-World War II period, piston-engined aircraft, left over from the vast stocks accumulated for global combat, equipped the bulk of the operational units. But with increasingly powerful turbine engines being developed, the superiority of performance of jet aircraft was obvious, and the organization of the United States Air Force—the third military arm—on 18 September 1947 accelerated the trend. Through the years, a succession of jet aircraft have taken their places in the three Air Force combat commands.

Tactical Air Command, charged with air operations in support of the ground forces, and equipped with fighter-bombers and light bombers, carried the brunt of the air fighting in the Korean War between 1950 and 1953, and is generally deployed in overseas bases in the Far East and in Europe. The original jet fighter, the Lockheed F-80 Shooting Star, scored the first victory in jet versus jet combat over the Russian-built Mig 15 in Korea on 8 November 1950 but proving too slow to combat the swept-wing Migs, it was relegated to ground-strafing and fighter-bomber roles. The swept-wing North American F-86 Sabre, with a General Electric J-47 engine of 5200 pounds thrust, out-fought the faster Migs by virtue of superior training and manœuvrability, and established a kill ratio of fourteen to one.

In the period immediately after World War II, the Air Defence Command, charged with protecting the continental United States, was neglected in view of the American nuclear monopoly. Following Russia's development of her own atomic bomb in 1949, there was a rush to equip the command with jet fighters superior in speed to Russian propeller-driven long-range bombers. The first major version was the Lockheed F-94 Starfire, a modification of the tried and proven F-80. The original fighter had been lengthened to produce a two-seater jet trainer, the T-33; this in turn was modified to create a two-seater interceptor. 'All-weather capability' was the requirement for the defensive fighter, and the second seat was for the radar operator whose ahead-searching equipment would lead the pilot to the target through cloud and darkness. Early models carried four ·50 calibre machine guns in the nose, but later ones set a new style in armament, carrying rockets only. The Starfire's successor was the Northrop F-89 Scorpion. Fifty-two of the 2·75 in. rockets were carried in out-size pods on each wing tip, aimed in the final F-89J model by a computer fire-control system.

Of the three major commands, it was the Strategic Air Command which was charged with implementing the American policy of 'massive retaliation' with airborne nuclear weapons. It was the wartime Boeing B-29 Superfortress which had dropped the first atomic bombs on Japan, and up until about 1950, a diminishing number of the big piston-engined planes operated in bomb groups of the Command. A modified version, the B-50 with more powerful engines, entered service in 1947. In order to give the 5000-mile bomber intercontinental capabilities, the Air Force developed in-flight refuelling, using at first modified B-29 tankers, and later the KC-97 tanker, a transport version of the Superfortress. To prove the long-range capability of the B-50 with air-to-air refuelling, SAC sent the 'Lucky Lady II' around the world non-stop in ninety-four hours in February 1949 refuelling over the Azores, Arabia, the Philippines and Hawaii. True intercontinental capability came with the Convair B-36 in 1947. The biggest, though not the heaviest aircraft ever flown by the US Air Force, the B-36 had been conceived in the dark days after the fall of France in 1940, when it appeared that America might have to fight alone without allies against a Germany controlling both the British Isles and the European Continent. The B-36 was therefore required to carry a 10,000-pound bomb load 5000 miles and return, in order to be able to bomb targets in Europe from US bases. Development was slow during the war years, but in the first reaction to the Communist declaration of 'cold war,' the B-36 was ordered in considerable numbers because of its ability to reach Russian targets from American bases. The tubular fuselage, 162 feet long, bore twelve 20 mm cannon in six twin turrets, remotely controlled. The pressurized crew compartments fore and aft were connected by an eighty-foot tunnel along which ran a wheeled cart, and the flight deck was so far forward of the six pusher-mounted Pratt & Whitney 3500 hp piston engines that the pilots could barely hear them in flight.

With the jet engine a reality, the B-36, for all its size, was merely a stop-gap weapon in the race for air superiority, and a pure jet bomber was eagerly awaited. This aircraft, the gracefully swept-wing Boeing B-47 Stratojet, had been under development since the autumn of 1943. First flown on 17 December 1947, the B-47 attracted national attention when on 8 February 1949 it flew from Moses Lake, Washington, to Andrews Air Force Base, Maryland, at an average speed of 607 mph. In many ways the B-47 represented a complete break with tradition, and set styles and fashions in American design of large jet aircraft that could be traced for years, even in the products of rival manufacturers. Despite its dimensions of 109 feet in length, 116 feet in wing span, and a gross weight which finally attained over a hundred tons, the Stratojet was handled by a crew of three—pilot and co-pilot under a fighter-type canopy atop the nose, and bombardier/navigator seated below them. Because there was no room for a retractable landing gear in the thin, laminar-flow wing, the main gear—a pair of 'bicycle wheels' mounted in tandem—retracted into the body. The flexible wing drooped under its own weight on the ground, but bent upwards at a dihedral angle in flight. The tall fin and the stabilizers were swept back like the wings. The six jet engines were carried beneath the wing in 'pods'—in pairs inboard, singly under the tips—easily accessible, and not likely to injure vital wing structure in the event of a turbine failure. While its speed of over 600 mph was impressive, the Stratojet was less than intercontinental, with a range of only 4000 miles even in the later models. This problem was overcome by basing the B-47 wings in foreign countries—a solution with political drawbacks—and by in-flight refuelling. The jet B-47 was badly mismated to the 375 mph propeller-driven KC-97 tanker, however, having to drop down from its 40,000-foot ceiling to the 20,000 foot level of the slow tanker, where the jet's fuel consumption increased mightily. In 1957, with 1800 B-47s in service, the type reached the peak of its employment in SAC. As the Russian defences improved, the B-47 bit by bit lost its superiority. In an attempt to keep the big bomber at a distance from the heaviest defences, the 'toss-bombing' technique was developed, whereby the B-47, during a climb, released its bomb to soar upward in a great arc into its target city miles away, while the plane, continuing upward, half-looped and then rolled upright, to speed away in the opposite direction. Beginning in 1964 the B-47 was phased out as obsolete.

The intercontinental jet bomber, the Boeing B-52, entered service in the year 1954. Similar in design and appearance to the B-47, and only slightly faster, the much bigger Stratofortress, with an all-up weight of 488,000 pounds, achieved a range of over 10,000 miles without refuelling. Eight jet engines were paired in pods under the wings. The crew was increased to six, with two pilots, a bombardier, a radar navigator, an electronic countermeasures operator and a tail gunner, who handles his remotely controlled ·50 calibre machine guns or 20-mm 'Gatling gun' in the tail from a position amidships. And with a suitable tanker mate, the four-jet Boeing KC-135, the prototype of all the famous Boeing jet transports, the Stratofortress could and did reach out to all parts of the world from bases within the continental United States. In recent years the thermonuclear 'Hound Dog' and 'Skybolt' air-to-surface missiles have enabled the B-52 to strike its lethal blow from beyond the circle of close-in target defences. With 600 in service, the B-52 is still the backbone of Strategic Air Command, and with 'iron' (conventional) bombs has played a major role in the Vietnam conflict.

The Navy initially viewed the advent of jet aircraft with mixed feelings. Having developed the fast aircraft carrier with its air group of fighters, scout bombers and torpedo bombers into the weapon that played a decisive role in winning the Pacific war against Japan, the Navy could not accept the early, underpowered jets, with their slow acceleration and takeoff runs exceeding the length of a carrier's flight deck. For several years the Navy aimed to have the best of both worlds by combining the jet with the piston engine. The first of these hybrids, the Ryan FR-1 Fireball, was being groomed in the summer of 1945 to go into action against the Japanese Kamikazes. With a nine-cylinder Wright Cyclone engine of 1350 hp in its nose driving a three-bladed propeller, and a Whittle-type General Electric J-31 jet with 1600 pounds thrust in its tail, the Fireball was intended to take off and cruise with the economical piston engine, and turn on the fuel-hungry jet for additional thrust in combat. Both power plants together gave it a maximum speed of 419 mph. Some testing was done with the Fireball after V-J Day, but in June 1947 it was withdrawn from Fleet service.[4]

As early as 21 July 1946 a pure jet fighter succeeded in taking off and landing aboard a Navy carrier, the big *Franklin D. Roosevelt*. The aircraft was the McDonnell FH-1 Phantom, a war-conceived design which, like the other early jets, had two power units because of their low thrust. Perhaps the greatest significance of the event was that the Westinghouse J-30 turbojet engines of 1600 pounds thrust each were an entirely American axial-flow design, destined for much greater development than the Whittle centrifugal-flow type. Yet the Navy's carrier force had to be revamped out of all recognition in the eventual conversion to jet power—new giants of the 'Forrestal' class over a thousand feet in length, while older vessels which had led in the destruction of Japanese sea power spent months, even years, in Navy yards being fitted with canted flight decks, steam catapults, and mirror landing systems. Fighters quickly became all-jet, with Grumman maintaining its lead as during the war period, with the straight-wing F9F-5 Panther being replaced by the swept-wing F9F-8 Cougar. One type of piston-engined attack bomber, the durable and beloved 'Able Dog,' the Douglas AD-1 Skyraider, lasted for years, but in the early 50s was succeeded by the tiny delta-wing and thermonuclear-armed A4D Skyhawk jet and by the large twin jet A3D Skywarrior, looking for all the world like a scaled-down B-47. Indeed, the same Navy model was procured by the Air Force as a long-range reconnaissance aircraft, the RB-66 Destroyer.

All these aircraft, although jet-powered, possessed speeds of less than 760 mph at sea level, and are therefore considered to be *subsonic*. The speed of sound varies with the density of the air, this in turn depending to a large extent on altitude, and to some degree on temperature and humidity; but it is such a vitally important parameter in the design and performance of today's jet aircraft that it has its own expression as a constant—the Mach number. Named for Ernst Mach, the Viennese physicist and philosopher who had interested himself in supersonic motion, the Mach number expresses velocity relative to the speed of sound, regardless of how the latter figure varies with conditions. Thus Mach 1 is the speed of sound, Mach 2 is twice the speed of sound, and near approaches to the speed of sound are indicated by Mach 0·8, Mach 0·85, etc.

The significance of this figure for fast jet aircraft is the sudden difference in the behaviour of air at the speed of sound—which is simply the velocity at which *any* disturbance is propagated in air. The reason for this is first, that with an aircraft travelling at the speed of sound (Mach 1), the disturbance which it produces cannot radiate and dissipate ahead of it, because the aircraft is travelling at the same speed as the disturbance it creates. This effect causes the air displaced by the aircraft to pile up, as it were, and compress, forming so-called *shock waves* which greatly increase the drag, or resistance, of the craft to passage through the air. Indeed, this sudden increase of drag with the approach of Mach 1 may prevent the aircraft from going any faster—the so-called 'sound barrier' of the newspaper writers—unless an enormous increase in power is available. Secondly, the properties of air are altered at supersonic speeds, rendering useless all aerodynamic design knowledge based on subsonic studies and tests. For instance, we were taught in school that when a stream of air is compressed, its velocity increases and it rarefies. At supersonic speeds, however, it is slowed by compression and its density increases. Where expanding air ordinarily slows and becomes more dense, at supersonic speeds the opposite is the case.[5] Complicating the problem is the great difficulty of studying air flow experimentally at supersonic speeds. Large wind tunnels, with air driven by huge fans through the constricted supersonic portion, tend to suffer from 'choking' of the piled-up flow proximal to the constriction, with subsonic velocities in the test section; or after the choking clears itself, the flow is supersonic, with no intermediate velocity in the *transonic* range, so critical for aircraft design. Small wonder that critical early studies on supersonic flight were carried out with full-sized manned aircraft.

The deadly change in aerodynamic forces and actions at the speed of sound had been known even before the jet age. With the development of fast all-metal monoplanes in the 1930s, unexpected control and vibration problems occurred at high speed, particularly in dives. These were attributed to 'compressibility,' and indeed, the compression of the air ahead of the wings and tail, and where it was constricted in its flow around the fuselage, played a part in the problem. Sometimes it was found that the aircraft became nose-heavy in a dive, and even more disturbing to the pilot, the elevator controls were ineffective. Moving the stick produced no elevator response; alternatively, the stick froze immovably, or moved by itself without action by the pilot. Severe vibrations in the tail, or even in the entire aircraft, could tear it to pieces. With further research, it was discovered that even though the entire aircraft might not be flying at supersonic speed, the air at certain points—particularly the leading edges of wings and tail—could be accelerated to supersonic speed, with the formation of shock waves. On the tail, the shock wave at the leading edge could blanket the elevators, so that they operated ineffectively in stagnant air. As the shock wave moved aft, it might 'freeze' the elevator, or even cause it to move by itself. The shock wave on the leading edge of the wing grossly altered its lift characteristics; in fact, with the customary thick wing used then, with blunt leading edge and cambered upper surface, the lift forces reversed themselves at supersonic speed, the force on the wing became downward instead of upward, with the result that the plunging aircraft finally achieved equilibrium in an inverted dive—with no hope of recovery because of the ineffectiveness of the elevators. These deadly phenomena were known collectively as the 'shock stall.' As speed built up, the aircraft, before striking the ground, might be torn to pieces by aerodynamic forces that it was not built to withstand.

Changes in design were in order if faster aircraft, particularly jet-propelled, were to fly, and fly under control, at speeds of Mach 1 and over. Part of the problem, it must be remembered, was that the supersonic aircraft spent most of its flying life operating at subsonic speeds, and had to have lift and control at these velocities also. The first advance was in aerofoil design. The reversal of lift forces on the conventional cambered wing suggested the thin, biconvex wing with sharp leading and trailing edges, piling up less air ahead of it in the leading edge shock wave, and developing lift at both subsonic and supersonic speeds. A straight wing of this section lifted the experimental Bell X-1, which, powered with rocket engines as the jet power plants of the day were too feeble, was first through the 'sound barrier' in level flight on 14 October, 1947 and reached a velocity of Mach 1·04. But the straight wing, with a shock wave along its entire width, carried an enormous mass of air along with it, and the next step, following German research, was the swept-back wing. While the centre of the swept-back wing gives off shock waves, the swept-back portion of the wing, travelling inside the Mach cone, is in effect working in subsonic air, with much less shock drag at supersonic speed than with the straight wing.

With the thin, biconvex, swept-back wing and a powerful jet engine, the Pratt & Whitney J-57 of 11,700 pounds thrust, the North American F-100 Super Sabre was the first American fighter to exceed the speed of sound in level flight—but only with the additional use of an afterburner which conferred an additional thrust of 5300 pounds. This was a simple device for spraying raw fuel into the tail pipe of the jet engine, creating an earth-shaking roar and an impressive tail of flame. The afterburner is in fact a necessary adjunct for reaching supersonic velocity, but its fuel consumption is enormous. With air-to-air refuelling from tanker aircraft, the Super Sabre ranged all over the world for Tactical Air Command, making mass flights in a period of hours to troubled areas, and the 'hardware' hung under the wings included up to 7500 pounds of nuclear weapons, bombs and rockets.

The San Diego plant of the Convair firm had developed a sleek delta-winged fighter, the F-102, which was also expected to exceed the speed of sound. The advantage of the delta design is that not only does the delta's leading edge have the shock-stall avoiding qualities of the swept-back wing, but the filling-in of the space to the rear strengthens the wing tips against torsional deformity, and permits a greater thickness of the centre section, which can be used to carry fuel. When first flight tested on 24 October, 1953, however, the sleek new F-102 failed to pass Mach 0·9.

A young member of the National Advisory Committee for Aeronautics, thirty-three-year-old Richard Whitcomb, thought he had the answer in the so-called 'area rule' he had evolved from his studies in the Committee's eight-foot diameter transonic wind tunnel. Whitcomb's research had indicated that a massive shock wave developed at the joint where the wing attached to the fuselage, due to the sudden increase in cross-sectional area of the wing/fuselage combination at this point. On the other hand, if the cross-sectional area of the entire aircraft were smoothly varied at succeeding stations from nose to tail, the massive shock waves whose drag prevented passing the 'sound barrier' did not develop. A corollary of the 'area rule' was that where the wings attached to the fuselage the cross-sectional area of the fuselage should be reduced, while the diameter of the body might actually be increased anterior and posterior to the wing. The result was the popularly-called 'coke bottle' or 'wasp-waisted' fuselage.

Thus, the biconvex wing swept back inside the Mach cone, combined with the 'area rule' fuselage and high-powered turbojet engines with afterburner, provided the successful formula for attaining continuous supersonic flight in a level attitude. One further feature was added to the formula: the all-flying tail, a single, movable horizontal surface replacing the fixed stabilizer to which a movable elevator is attached. The all-flying tail eliminates the problem of loss of elevator control due to shock waves on the leading edge of the stabilizer.

A whole generation of truly supersonic aircraft has followed the F-100 Super Sabre. The Convair F-102A Delta Dagger entered service with Air Defence Command, armed only with rockets, and equipped with automatic guidance and fire-control systems that led it to its target. In 1956 a much more powerful modification, the F-106 Delta Dart, attained a velocity of more than Mach 2. Lockheed also produced the F-104 Starfighter, another Mach 2 interceptor for Air Defence Command—a jet-powered projectile fifty-five feet long with small fins for wings giving it a span of only twenty-two feet. One of these aircraft, an F-104C, set an altitude record of 103,389 feet on 14 December, 1959. Following the F-100 Super Sabre, there came for TAC in 1955 the McDonnell F-101 Voodoo, originally conceived as a long-range escort for SAC bombers. In 1958 this was supplemented by the Republic F-105 Thunderchief, a monster grossing over twenty-four tons loaded, driven at Mach 2 by a Pratt & Whitney J-75 turbojet providing 26,500 pounds of thrust with afterburner. In the TAC fighter-bomber role, the F-105 was able to carry over 14,000 pounds of 'external stores'—the current euphemism for bombs and rockets. And SAC, too, received a supersonic aircraft, perhaps the most remarkable of the series, the Mach 2 Convair B-58 Hustler, the biggest supersonic aircraft in regular service anywhere. With its delta plan form, area rule fuselage, and four General Electric J-79 jets hung under the wing in separate pods, the Hustler looked like a scaled-up Delta Dart fighter, but carried a crew of three and a thermonuclear weapon.

The US Navy, too, is supersonic, The modern large carrier's 86-plane air group today includes the Mach 2 Chance-Vought F8 Crusader with 15,000 pound thrust Pratt & Whitney J-75 turbojet which solves the problem of lift and control at low speed by varying the angle of attack of its wing; and the McDonnell F4 Phantom II, with two J-79 engines of 16,000 pounds thrust, able to reach Mach 2·5. In an unprecedented step, the Air Force procured a quantity of these Navy-designed fighters as the F-110, complete with tail hook for operation from land bases. The Navy also developed a supersonic attack aircraft, the Mach 2 A5 Vigilante, but with strategic bombing deleted from the Navy's mission, the few aircraft procured were diverted to the reconnaissance role.

A corollary of the jet age, with higher speeds, greater altitude, longer range and more crowded air space, is the steady aggrandizement of ground controllers at the expense of the initiative and independence of the pilot. Given the limitations of the human senses, reasoning power and reaction time, this progression is inevitable, but has taken away still more of the romance and emotional satisfaction of flying as it was. The pilot's own role is increasingly usurped by the 'black boxes' which fly the aircraft automatically, and through radar control will even lead it through fog and darkness to an unseen target, as fitted in the newest interceptors. Yet as long as national defence depends on aircraft for two-way missions, instead of one-way missiles, brave men will still be needed, and will be found, to make the decisions and to take them over and back.

Still more powerful jet engines will be built. Ahead lies Mach 3, the thermal barrier, heat-resistant titanium structures, the Lockheed A-11, the Air Force F-111 and the Navy F14 with variable-sweepback wings. Technology never stands still, and medical science must keep pace with its demands.

Medically, the turbojet posed few novel problems, and even eliminated one old one—the carbon monoxide menace, associated from the earliest days with the piston-type internal combustion engine. Burning a 'rich' mixture, with an excess of fuel in relation to air, the piston engine could produce as much as 8·75 per cent by weight of carbon monoxide in the exhaust at takeoff, and 3·03 per cent when cruising. By contrast, the jet engine, burning its fuel in a huge blast of compressed air, has very low carbon monoxide levels in the exhaust. Over ninety-five per cent of this is air, and the latest Air Force Flight Surgeon's Manual holds that 'the probability of toxic levels of carbon monoxide being present is remote.'[6]

The only significant new medical problem has been that of jet engine noise. For years it has been known that prolonged exposure to loud noises could cause permanent hearing impairment ('boilermakers' disease'), and it was known that particularly in open-cockpit flying, the aviator was exposed to high noise levels from the engine exhaust, propeller and slipstream. In older aircraft the noise level could easily reach 100 decibels; in more recent propeller aircraft, such as the Navy's F4U Corsair at 2900 rpm and 35 in. manifold pressure, the noise level could reach 120 decibels.

The decibel figure is meaningless to the layman unless comparisons are made. It is a logarithmic measure of noise intensity. A whisper registers twenty decibels; ordinary conversation forty to seventy decibels; a home, forty decibels; an office, sixty decibels. It would be a mistake, however, to conclude that the office is fifty per cent noisier than the home. Actually, *a three-decibel increase at any point on the scale equals a doubling of the sound level in terms of the energy output*—and energy input at the human ear. The Corsair cockpit, by this criterion, is not twice as noisy as the office, but twenty times as noisy—a quantity of energy sufficient to cause damage to the delicate detecting mechanism of the human ear, and to the auditory nerve overloaded by the resulting stimulation. The jet engine is even noisier, and unlike the piston engine, producing a fluctuating noise of relatively low frequency, the high-pitched whine of the jet covers all frequencies. Recording instruments indicate well over 130 decibels of sound emitted by the earth-shaking roar of the F-100 Super Sabre engine operating with afterburner, even with the device located a hundred feet from the aircraft. At closer distances the intensity is of course higher, reaching at least 140 decibels. Such an intensity not only produces severe pain in unprotected ears, but even with ear defenders, may produce such generalized symptoms as disorientation, nausea and vomiting. At 150 decibels, enough energy is absorbed by the skin in the form of sound to stimulate the heat receptors in the skin, with a sensation of warmth in the affected areas.

Flight-crew members of jet aircraft are not exposed to the full noise energy output of the power plants. In fact, the major noise source affecting jet air crew is the slipstream, the noise of air flowing past at high speed, a continuous rushing sound, which increases with speed but diminishes with altitude and decreased air density. With pressurized cabins, as used at present, the noise may be greatly increased by the whistling sound of air leaking out through a faulty cockpit seal. The resulting noise in the tail gunner's position of the North American B-45 Tornado, an early jet bomber, reached 130 decibels. Noise level is lowest in the cockpit of jet aircraft, where the whine of the jet engine is masked by the slipstream noise. At supersonic velocities the jet engine in the rear is totally inaudible, its noise being unable to 'catch up' with the cockpit ahead. A single-seater, single-jet aircraft such as the Lockheed F-104A Starfighter, generates up to 110 decibels in the cockpit with afterburner at 19,000 feet. In the B-47 Stratojet, pilot and co-pilot receive 100 to 110 decibels in level flight, and 110 to 120 decibels during takeoff. On the flight deck of the B-52, readings vary from 86 decibels while taxiing to 100 during a climb. Crew men in the rear fuselage of large multi-jet aircraft experience higher noise levels, 108 decibels for instance in the B-52's tail-gunner compartment.

The real risk of serious hearing loss is run by ground-crew members working around jet aircraft on the ground. These include not only flight crews assigned to particular aircraft, but also alert crews servicing the aircraft on the line; repair and installation personnel working around aircraft, fuel-truck and tow-truck drivers, and air policemen standing guard on the flight line. As suggested above, noise levels above 130 decibels may well be experienced close to jet aircraft on the ground running at full power, particularly with afterburner, and some men actually making adjustments to engines running at full power are exposed at very close range to intensities of 140 decibels or more. A specially complex problem occurs aboard modern Navy carriers, where catapult and handling crews, on duty on the restricted and crowded area of the flight deck, must work within a few feet of big jet engines screaming at full power.

Against these extreme noise readings must be set the medical finding that with sound intensities above 95 decibels, there is a risk of permanent damage to the ear, with resulting hearing loss, in individuals exposed eight hours a day, five days a week, for a working lifetime. At higher levels protective equipment must be worn. In earlier periods, this was not regularly issued as a matter of policy; in the jet-age Air Force, this is a significant part of the flight surgeon's duty. Initially, there were the usual 'wise guys,' the old-timers who, not recognizing the degree to which they had lost hearing acuity, boasted that they had never worn protective equipment and were able to 'take' the howling jets in stride. Nowadays noise-protective equipment is generally accepted; indeed, the veriest recruit becomes aware that without it, near-by jet-engine noise is actually painful to the ears. 'Ear defenders,' or ear plugs, made of neoprene or vinylite in three sizes, are standard issue and are fitted by the medical department. These must be used with caution, however, by flight personnel, as the pressure increase during a descent may force the defender into the ear canal. Ear muffs may be worn over the external ear, with or without the inserted ear plugs. Paradoxically, in a high-intensity noise environment speech will be heard better when wearing defenders. With very loud noises, however, communication is possible only by signs.

As with any strange and frightening novelty, there have been rumours about mysterious, dangerous and even lethal effects of jet-engine noise. As early as 1945, German Me 262 pilots were worriedly telling each other that they could father only girl babies as a result of exposure to jet-engine noise.[7] Particularly feared have been the so-called ultrasonic frequencies of the jet engine—those too high to detect with the ear, above 20,000 cycles per second. These anxieties were encouraged by the known fact that small fur-covered animals could be killed by exposure to such ultrasonic frequencies at intensities of 150 decibels. This was a result of their absorbing the ultrasonic energy in the form of heat, and being unable to radiate it fast enough. Tests with appropriate instruments, however, show much less intensity of ultrasonic radiation from jet engines, and in newer and larger power plants, there is progressively less radiation energy at ultrasonic frequencies and more at low frequencies. Fear of the unknown may explain some of the more bizarre complaints of ground personnel working around jet aircraft, such as fatigue, weakness and disturbance of vision. Often a rash of such complaints appear when a new, unfamiliar and perhaps more powerful aircraft arrives at a base. They gradually disappear as the new type becomes better known.

Other problems of long standing are aggravated with the jet age, as turbine power plants drive aircraft ever higher and faster, and for longer distances. With service ceilings in even the F-80A Shooting Star equalling 45,000 feet, and going up to 60,000 feet in the B-58 Hustler, anoxia can occur despite the use of oxygen equipment and pressure breathing introduced towards the end of World War II. The pressure cabin, first used as regular service equipment in the B-29, provided an answer not only to anoxia, but also to dysbarism ('the bends'). Crew comfort was enhanced, and fatigue reduced, as oxygen equipment did not have to be worn continuously, and air temperature, humidity and ventilation could be controlled as desired. Fur-lined flight clothing and electrically-heated gloves, boots and underwear became historical curiosities. The advantages of pressurization overruled the disadvantages: increased weight and bulk of fuselage structure designed to withstand the internal pressure; the maintenance work required, particularly on seals and locks; and the medical risk of decompression.

On many high-altitude flights made today in pressurized aircraft, oxygen is not required; but pressurization does not eliminate the need for oxygen, it simply raises the ceiling at which it must be used. The decisive factor is the maximum differential pressure permissible between the inside of the cabin and the outside atmosphere. This in turn is determined by the structural design of the aircraft. Early jet fighters, such as the F-80 Shooting Star and the F-84 Thunderjet, had a differential pressure of only 2·75 pounds per square inch, permitting

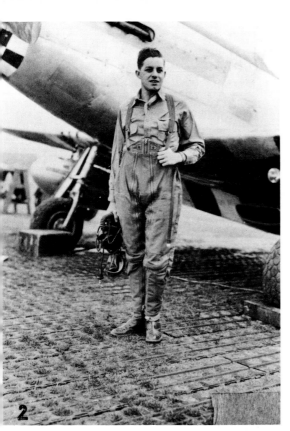

32. 'G suit' worn by P-51 Mustang pilot. Fabric outer garment covering lower half of body contains single piece bladder to compress abdomen, thighs and calves when acceleration in flight manoeuvres exceeds 2 G. Hose to air pressure source appears by pilot's left knee (1944). (Air Force Museum)

33. Testing the downward firing M-4 ejection seat, with the MA-I automatic lap safety belt and lap tiedown straps (1947). (Air Force Museum)

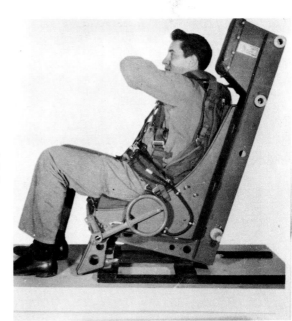

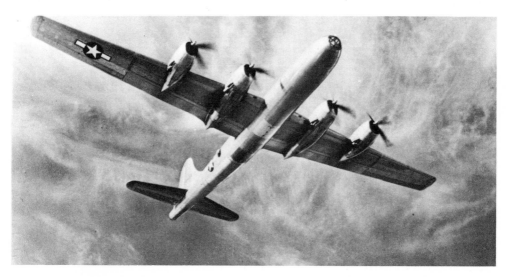

34. Boeing B-29 Superfortress, mainstay of the U.S. Army Air Forces in the bombing of Japan. First pressurized aircraft produced in quantity. Pressurized compartment in nose, and another behind the wing, were connected by a tunnel through the bomb bay, while the tail gunner had a separate pressurized compartment (1944). (Air Force Museum)

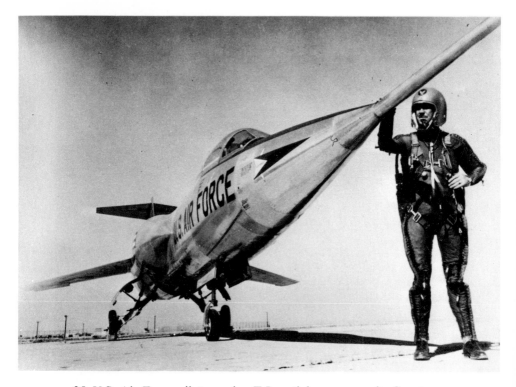

35. U.S. Air Force pilot wearing T-I partial pressure suit. Capstans to tighten the fabric of the suit are visible on outer borders of the arms and legs. The aircraft is the Lockheed F-104 Mach 2 fighter, with cabin pressurized to a differential of 5 psi (1956). (Air Force Museum)

the pilot to maintain in the cockpit a pressure of 10,000 feet—the maximum permitted without oxygen—till reaching 18,000 feet. Beyond here, the cockpit pressure fell, but was always 2·75 psi higher than that outside. By breathing oxygen (once again carried in liquid form, whereby tremendous quantities can be made available in a small, light-weight unit) through the World War II type A-13 mask and A-14 diluter-demand regulator, or the improved D-2 regulator, the pilot could progressively raise his ceiling within the limitations of his equipment. At 51,000 feet, however, the cabin pressure was equivalent to 30,000 feet, the level at which dysbarism and its symptoms ('bends,' 'chokes') might occur. Theoretically the pilot could ascend indefinitely and still not attain a cockpit altitude of 40,000 feet, the maximum height at which man can function with one hundred per cent oxygen by mask without pressure. Because of the dysbarism problem, newer fighters such as the F-86 Sabre and later, have a differential pressure of 5 psi. This permits a 10,000-foot pressure to be maintained to 26,500 feet, and in ascents beyond this altitude, the cabin pressure never falls below 27,000 feet—well below the threshold for onset of the 'bends.' Bombers, with their more massive structure, have always had a higher pressure differential. In the B-29, first pressurized aircraft in regular squadron service, the differential was 6·55 psi, and this was also the value for the B-50, the B-36, and the first mass-produced jet bomber, the B-47 Stratojet. With this differential, the B-47 at its ceiling of 40,500 feet had an equivalent cabin altitude of 12,500 feet, which of course required the wearing of oxygen masks. Later jet bombers, with higher ceilings, had stronger cabins and a higher differential pressure. The intercontinental B-52, with a differential pressure of 7·45 psi, is unpressurized up to 8000 feet. From here it maintains an 8000-foot equivalent pressure up to 35,000 feet, and at its ceiling of 55,000 feet, the cabin pressure equals 13,500 feet. The B-58 also has a differential pressure of 7·45 psi and a cabin pressure of 13,000 feet at its 60,000 foot ceiling. Thus, the crews of the bombers on which we depend for our deterrent capacity are never exposed to the 'bends,' and need oxygen only during the maximum-altitude portions of their operations.

On the other hand, the high altitudes now attainable with jet power set a limit to the use of the pressure cabin as we know it today, with a pressure differential maintained by compressing the thin outside air. Beyond 70,000 feet the pressure ratio between the atmosphere and that designed to support life within the cabin rises rapidly towards infinity, requiring an exorbitant expenditure of power in the compressors, accompanied by a degree of heating of the compressed air which would amount to 600 degrees F at 75,000 feet with a pressure ratio of 20. The solution, of course, is the completely sealed cabin with self-contained oxygen and air-purifying equipment, as first used by Professor Piccard in 1931 in his stratosphere balloon flights.

Above 50,000 feet there is also a rapid build-up of the ozone content of the air. This gas, a modified form of oxygen, most highly concentrated at 75,000 feet, is formed by the action of ultraviolet radiation on atmospheric oxygen, and by filtering out the major portion of the fierce ultraviolet rays from the sun, makes possible life on earth. Ozone is toxic in low concentrations, and in commercial jet airliners crossing the Atlantic has been found in appreciable concentrations in flights at 39,000 to 41,000 feet. Much of the ozone taken in by the compressors is broken down by heat, however, and in the latest military jets catalytic filters eliminate ozone in the air taken in at high altitude.[8]

The most serious problem in flying with pressurized equipment is the possible loss of cabin pressure through accident or by enemy action. The time required for the internal and external pressure to equalize depends on the size of the opening, the volume of the pressurized compartment, the pressure differential, and the flight altitude at which decompression takes place. The decompression is termed *explosive* if equalization takes place in less than one second, and *rapid* if the duration is between one and five seconds. Obviously the fighter-type aircraft, with its small-volume cockpit space, is at a disadvantage compared to the large bomber (though the B-47 bomber houses its two pilots in tandem under a fighter-type canopy). A further disadvantage of the fighter is that decompression frequently takes place through the canopy blowing off, providing a large opening. In early pressurized bombers such as the B-29, B-50 and B-36, lookouts and gunners were stationed in large hemispherical plastic domes which, in case of failure, provided a large opening for explosive decompression. In later aircraft such as the B-52 and B-58, the windows and other vulnerable areas are smaller.

Because loss of cabin pressure is especially likely to occur in combat, from penetration of the cabin by bullets or shell fragments, the Air Force attempts to mitigate the effects of explosive decompression by decreasing the pressure differential during combat. This requires the use of oxygen masks at lower altitude than with full pressurization, but the violence of expansion of internal gases, and of air blast within the cabin, are decreased if the pressure differential is less. The special setting with reduced differential pressure is called *combat override*. In fighters, the differential pressure is reduced from 5 to 2·75 psi; in the B-47 from 6·55 to 2·35 psi; in the B-52, from 7·45 to 4·5 psi, meaning that at a flight altitude of 50,000 feet, the internal equivalent altitude is 22,000 feet. Oxygen masks must of course be worn.

An explosive, or even a rapid decompression is a dramatic event. A loud booming noise is instantly followed by a violent 'whoosh' of outrushing air, which irresistibly drags with it papers, articles of clothing and loose objects such as pencils and flashlights, and even heavier items with such violence that a 'honey bucket' (portable toilet) with its contents was wrapped around a stanchion in an incident aboard a B-36. Some of these, such as walk-around oxygen bottles, can be dangerous missiles. The sudden drop in pressure, and expansion of the remaining air in the cabin, causes an abrupt fall in temperature, and frequently the moisture in the air condenses as fog. Formerly it was believed that serious injury could result from sudden expansion of gas in the intestines and of air in the lungs; usually, however, the former is vented harmlessly, and the expanded air in the lungs is exhaled automatically. Very rarely, severe lung damage, with rupture of the alveoli and air embolism, occurs when the breath is held during decompression. It is now recognized that at altitudes below 40,000 feet, the greatest medical hazard results from the rush of air. Men were blown incontinently overboard through ruptured plastic blisters in the B-29s and B-36s, until they learned to use restraint harnesses and to wear their parachutes at all times in such exposed positions. The narrow tube connecting the pressurized fore and aft spaces of B-29s and B-36s was a particularly bad place to be at such a time, the unfortunate occupant being shot like a projectile from a gun into the decompressing compartment, and sometimes right out the opening. Only recently a B-52 navigator, wearing neither harness nor parachute, was hurled through an opening hatch at 39,000 feet. Usually the defect in newer bombers is too small to permit the passage of a human body, but one B-52 crewman, sucked against the opening by his posterior, was unable to free himself, even with the assistance of his crew mates, until the aircraft had descended to a lower altitude. By then the pressure differential he had sustained had provoked in him the first case of aerospace haemorrhoids on record!

At flight altitudes above 40,000 feet, anoxia is a severe threat. Here the partial pressure of oxygen is so low that when breathing *air,* the 'time of useful consciousness' after decompression is only twenty seconds at 40,000 feet, and fifteen seconds at 45,000 feet. In a Royal Canadian Air Force experiment in the pressure chamber, in which thirty cadets were rapidly decompressed from 8000 to 40,000 feet in two and a half seconds, three of them were unable to apply their masks within five seconds after equalization of pressure. With *one hundred per cent oxygen* by mask (without pressure), consciousness can be retained indefinitely at 40,000 feet, for one hour at 41,000 feet, for one-half hour at 43,000, and for five to ten minutes at 45,000 feet.

Therefore, when flying between 26,000 and 35,000 feet and pressurized to 10,000 feet, the helmet should be worn and the mask be attached thereto, close to the face. Above 35,000 feet the mask should be fastened to the face.

Even when breathing one hundred per cent oxygen, the time of useful consciousness falls rapidly above 45,000 feet, and at 52,000 feet is again down to fifteen seconds—obviously not enough time for the pilot to take effective action to bring his craft to a safer and lower level. Pressure breathing is the only answer, and is responsible for the Air Force regulation that pressure suits will be worn on any flight planned to altitudes above 50,000 feet. Mention has been made of early, crude experimental pressure suits evolved in the 1930s, and of the counterpressure corsets devised for use with pressure oxygen masks late in World War II. The jet age, with the advent of regular flights above 50,000 feet, forced the development of a practical pressure suit.

The partial pressure suit (so called because it does not cover the hands and feet), developed shortly after World War II and widely used even today, is designed to furnish oxygen under pressure at any altitude, equivalent to the pressure of one hundred per cent oxygen at 43,000 feet; and the counterpressure needed to prevent serious or even fatal effects from unbalanced pressure in the lungs. These could range from overexpansion of the chest, with rupture of the alveoli in the lungs and air embolism, to the body fluids being driven into the extremities, with a resulting state of shock and collapse.

Pressurization of the lungs is assured by the pilot wearing an oxygen-tight helmet, with an easily inserted transparent face plate heated by fine electric wires to prevent fogging (with a small port in its lower portion, sealed by a hinged flap, through which tubes can be inserted for taking liquids or *puréed* foods by mouth). The helmet is sealed around the neck by a thick, tight-fitting rubber diaphragm, and pressurized by an inflatable bladder nestling inside the hard outer shell. With one hundred per cent oxygen being piped into the helmet, a pressure of 50 mm of mercury matches 43,000-foot conditions at 60,000 to 65,000 feet; 100 mm provides the same equivalent at 70,000 to 75,000 feet; and 150 mm offers adequate blood oxygenation in space. Counterpressure over the body is provided by large rubber bladders covering the entire torso front and back, and extending down over the upper thighs. The bladders are prevented from expanding outward by the snug-fitting, tightly-laced, non-stretching but porous nylon fabric of the suit. Since the helmet and the bladders are interconnected, the wearer enjoys an exact balance between the pressure in the lungs and the pressure on the chest and abdominal wall. And to prevent swelling of the arms and legs from fluid driven into the extremities by the pressure in the lungs, the suit is drawn tight by pressurized tubes, or *capstans,* running down the outside of the arms and legs. The capstans are inflated separately from helmet and bladders, with the rule of thumb being that 5 psi should be used with 50 mm of pressure in the helmet and bladders; 10 psi with 100 mm, and 15 psi with 150 mm. Tightly-laced flight boots on the feet, and gloves with bladders in the back, pressurized by an 'anti-pinch' bladder running down the arm, complete the ensemble. In flight operations, the suit inflates automatically through aneroid control if the cabin pressure falls below 40,000 feet, and maintains the proper pressure regardless of flight altitude. Thus it protects completely against anoxia, but not against dysbarism, which may show itself at equivalent altitudes of 30,000 feet or more.

Through the courtesy of Captain William J. Sears of the Physiological Training Unit, Carswell AFB, Fort Worth, Texas, I was permitted to experience pressurization in an MC-3A partial pressure suit with MA-1 helmet. The garment chosen for me had originally been tailored in March 1960 to fit a U-2 pilot, and to give me the snug fit required, AIC Michael L. Weston spent forty-five minutes lacing up my arms, legs and body. With helmet and bladders pressurized to 150 mm with one hundred per cent oxygen, and the capstans inflated to 15 psi, I experienced no difficulty in breathing. I was wearing only slippers on my feet however, and at these high pressures the feet swelled with fluid, with discomfort and itching, due to the internal pressure being unbalanced externally. Afterwards I noted that where creases had occurred in the smooth 'long john' underwear which I had worn next to my skin, there were capillary haemorrhages caused by the uncompensated internal pressure. The chief source of discomfort was immobility of the suit at high pressures. Though I was seated, the pressure inside the suit tended forcibly to extend my body. It was impossible to turn my head with the helmet, and I could only look straight ahead. I could not really bend my arms at the elbow or legs at the knees, and could not bring my hands together in the centre line. Obviously, it would be very uncomfortable to wear this suit pressurized at high altitudes for any length of time; but this discomfort would be preferable to loss of useful consciousness from anoxia above 50,000 feet, or vaporization of the body fluids beyond the 'Armstrong Line' at 63,000 feet.

The full-pressure suit, in which the entire body—arms and legs as well as the torso—would be under counterpressure from oxygen at the same pressure as the helmet and lungs—has long appeared the ideal type of protective garment. The chief difficulty has been that with a gas-tight envelope completely covering the body, heat and perspiration could not escape, and these could rise to intolerable levels even when the suit was uninflated. Recent progress in full-pressure suit design—as attested to in the Introduction, describing the flight of Ross and Prather to 113,000 feet in such garments—has depended largely on efficient ventilation and air conditioning of the suit. The resulting benefits include protection against the 'bends,' for the suit can be set to inflate automatically above 27,000 feet, well below the threshold for dysbarism and its effects.

To the jet pilot, fully enclosed in a pressurized, air-conditioned cockpit and protected against wind blast, speed constitutes no serious medical problem. It is true that at supersonic velocities, there may be some distortion of forward vision through the shock wave given off by the nose of the aircraft, as the compressed air in the shock wave is denser than that before or behind it. Indirectly, however, the jet age has aggravated a secondary effect of the speed of flight, by shortening the time available to the pilot in which to perceive an object ahead and to take appropriate action. This can create dangerous possibilities for the air crew of a jet travelling at supersonic speed—say 1800 mph, or half a mile per second. While the speed of the aircraft has increased, the reaction time of the human operator remains a constant, as a function of his biological mechanisms. Air Force studies show that it will take about 0·4 seconds merely to see an object ahead, and about one second to recognize it, during which time the supersonic aircraft will have travelled nearly 3700 feet. This means that if two aircraft flying at 1800 mph on a collision course both emerged from clouds 3000 feet apart, they would collide before their pilots could take any action, and if they were initially 500 feet apart, they would crash before their pilots could see each other. Even the simple operation of shifting focus from distant to close vision to read an instrument in the cockpit, and accommodating again to distant vision, takes 3·39 seconds, during which time the 1800 mph aircraft will have travelled 6336 feet. Inevitably this will require the development of an automatic avoidance mechanism activated by ahead-warning radar—one more black box encroaching on the absolute independence that once was the pilot's.

Acceleration—radial, angular and linear—poses medical problems that are exaggerated in jet aircraft. In fact, the inability of the human pilot to tolerate radial forces in excess of six G (positive) limits the manœuvrability of high-performance jet aircraft. It will be remembered that the G forces developed with any change of direction increase as the square of the speed, or inversely as the radius of the turn. Thus, the pilot of an aircraft making a turn of one mile radius at 600 mph experiences a force of four G, but if the radius is halved to one-half mile, or the speed doubled to 1200 mph, the acceleration rises to sixteen G—far beyond the tolerance of the human pilot, not to mention that of the aircraft structure. Higher speeds require even larger turning radii. A pilot will experience six G—sufficient to produce blacking out even with an ordinary G suit—with turns of the following radii at the following speed:

250 mph	686 feet
500 mph	2,740 feet
750 mph	6,170 feet
1000 mph	11,132 feet (2·1 miles)
1500 mph	25,074 feet (4·75 miles)
2000 mph	44,530 feet (8·45 miles)

For today's fighter pilots, handling the supersonic F-104 Starfighter, the F-106 Delta Dart, or the F-110 Phantom II, the dogfighting style of World War I and II is physically impossible.

The crouching position and the G suit are still in use to increase pilot tolerance to G forces. The latest model G suit has an abdominal bladder and capstans running down the legs, both automatically inflated whenever the acceleration exceeds two G. For pilots wearing partial-pressure suits, the abdominal bladder and leg capstans are part of the suit. Otherwise no practical progress had been made in dealing medically with the problem of radial acceleration in flight. Theoretical solutions still seem attractive in the laboratory, such as the prone or supine positions, but have not been accepted for service aircraft. Considering that flying on one's back or stomach involves many disadvantages in exchange for an advantage useful only during brief seconds of high-speed manœuvres, these positons probably never will be accepted. Another attractive theoretical solution—to enclose the upright pilot in a water-filled vessel wherein the G forces on the column of water will exert counterpressure against the lower part of his body—will certainly encounter even more user resistance. Pilots as a group are conservative, and the seventy years since Kitty Hawk have been long enough for the growth of a considerable tradition.

Much research has been done on the effects of radial G force on the human body, notably in the human centrifuge at the Naval Air Development Center, Johnsville, Pennsylvania. With an arm fifty feet long, carrying a closed gondola for the test subject which can be evacuated to simulate an altitude of 60,000 feet, the centrifuge develops up to forty G with a rate of change of ten G per second. The beneficiaries, however, have been the astronauts of the space programme. Having no control functions to perform during the lift-off for orbital flight, or during the re-entry into the atmosphere, they can tolerate the ten to twelve G involved by lying supine on moulded body-contour couches.

Medical problems of linear acceleration have been aggravated by the increasing performance of jet aircraft. In normal flight there are no unusual linear loads on the pilot—acceleration during jet takeoff being notoriously less than with a propeller, due to the very low efficiency of jet propulsion at speeds below 400 mph. Even present-day catapult launchings and arrested carrier-deck landings impose on the human body not more than five G of linear force in either direction.

An aircraft crash, particularly at the flight speeds now attainable, produces accelerations (or more properly, decelerations) of quite another order. It must always be remembered that the kinetic energy absorbed by the decelerating object—either the aircraft itself, or the pilot enclosed in its cockpit—varies as the square of the velocity. In the stick-and-wire days, a pilot might expect to walk away from a crash at 80 mph. At 640 mph the kinetic energy of his moving body is sixty-four times greater, providing that much more potential for injury when his motion is abruptly halted. This can lead to disintegration of the human frame as well as that of the aircraft. 'In a recent accident a jet bomber (evidently a B-47) nosed in from low altitude at more than 500 mph. Only 19,000 pounds of fragments, none bigger than one man could carry, were all that could be found of the 193,000 pound aircraft. The unidentifiable remains of the three crew members totalled $9\frac{1}{2}$ pounds.'[9]

One man who believed that something might be done about deaths and injuries in aircraft crashes was Colonel John P. Stapp USAF (MC), who eventually became Director of the Aero Medical Laboratory at Wright-Patterson AFB, Ohio. While a subordinate member of that facility, be initiated a study in August 1945 designed to determine by experiment the tolerance and survival limits of flight personnel in emergencies to 'decelerative forces of abrupt onset, high magnitude and short duration.'[10] A machine was developed to produce on the ground 'linear deceleration similar to that encountered in crashes, ditchings, rocket-powered capsule ejections and parachute-opening shocks.'[11] This was a 1500-pound slipper mounted sled running on 2000 feet of track and propelled by one to four solid fuel rockets, each having 1000 pounds thrust for a duration of five seconds. A series of friction brakes were located along fifty feet of track at a point 1250 feet from the starting point. The rockets gave the sled a maximum velocity of 214 mph, and with a speed of 164 mph, the brakes were able to stop the sled within a distance of eighteen feet, producing a sustained force of 66·2 G. As will be seen later, the apparatus could readily be adapted to the study of wind blast on human subjects at high velocities.

Between April 1947 and June 1951 254 runs were made with the sled at Edwards AFB, some with parachute dummies. The most strenuous studies were done on chimpanzees, but human volunteers, including Colonel Stapp, made runs subjecting themselves to as much as 46·6 G in seats facing both forward and backward. More important than the sustained G level was the rate of change of deceleration. When the brakes produced decelerations with a rate of change of less than 500 G per second, the subjects generally tolerated this well, though Colonel Stapp, after a run in which forty-five G was experienced in the forward-facing position, with a rate of onset of 500 G per second, developed a retinal haemorrhage which partly obscured lateral vision in the right eye, and only after ten weeks did normal sight begin to return. In a forward-facing experiment where thirty G was experienced with a rate of onset of 1000 G per second, Colonel Stapp reported:

Subject felt a very hard, well-distributed impact on hitting the brakes. The winter coveralls worn for this run seemed to gather under the leg straps and pinch very painfully at the inner aspects of the thighs under impact. This pain overshadowed other sensations, and was confined to the skin. Immediately following the second, rather pronounced impact in the emergency arresting cable, scintillating spots in the peripheral field of vision, lasting about 30 seconds, were noted. Subjective sensations, usually associated with dropping blood pressure and fast pulse, were also noted. There was darkening and narrowing of the field of vision. This vasomotor reflex could have been due to the considerable pain of the pinching of the inner aspect of the thighs, or possibly a generalized effect of the severe impact. In two minutes the reaction was over and the subject was able to return to his duties. The inner aspect of the thighs had solid purple bruises 3 by 6 inches in extent the following day.[12]

The sled run described above had been made with the subject fastened to the seat with 3-inch nylon webbing harness consisting of shoulder straps, chest belt, lap belt, two leg straps and emergency chest straps. In order to evaluate further the efficiency of the harness in preventing injury with high rate of change of deceleration, Stapp made some further tests with anaesthetized hogs, seated facing forward or backward in a carriage suspended from a 30-foot monorail. An ejection cartridge with variable charge gave the carriage a velocity of 9·5 to 33·4 mph, but it was then abruptly decelerated against a lead cone three to seven and a half inches long. The resulting violent jolt produced forces up to 300 G within 0·01 to 0·08 seconds, with onset as high as 48,000 G per second. With suitable positioning and restraint. the hogs survived ninety-seven G with onset at 21,000 G per second facing rearward, and in the forward-facing position, 125 G with onset at 10,500 G per second when wearing a three-way harness consisting of lap belt, shoulder harness and leg straps. With the leg straps omitted, there was a higher rate of fatality, and no survivors of two experiments with lap belt alone. Paradoxically, though Colonel Stapp has elsewhere written in favour of the rear-facing seat giving a higher crash survival rate than the forward-facing seat with lap belt alone, he demonstrated in these experiments that the forward-facing position with extensive restraints was even safer, due to the elasticity of the nylon webbing. By contrast, the colonel readily demonstrated that with forces which the properly restrained hog could easily survive, death resulted when the animal was allowed to smash forward against a simulated instrument panel, control wheel or stick, or an automobile steering wheel.

Summing up, Colonel Stapp asserted that values of fifty G for tolerance of deceleration, and 100 G for survival, were 'conservative estimates,' and threw down a challenge to the aircraft industry:

> For uninjured survival of forces considerably in excess of those usually encountered in crash conditions, short of immediate total destruction of the airframe, the properly supported body requires no more attenuation than from a $\frac{1}{2}$ inch thickness of felt as a back cushion in a steel aft-facing seat, or from 8300 pounds test nylon webbing of thirty-five per cent total elasticity in the restraints for the forward-facing seating position. It thus becomes evident that structural limitations of aircraft rather than human tolerance and survival limits will determine the maximum anti-crush force protection which can be incorporated into aircraft design. Until effective protection against dynamic loads imposed on seats, crash restraints and cabin inclosures reaches the equivalent of fifty G at 500 G per second for 0·25 second duration, human tolerance is not the criterion. The most enlightened approach should be to provide the maximum protection against crash forces which can be obtained in any particular aircraft without compromising its performance.[13]

With the more classic physiological problems of aviation medicine such as anoxia, dysbarism, wind blast and low temperatures being eliminated by such technical developments as the fully enclosed, pressurized and soundproofed cabin, the elusive problem of fatigue is coming more to the fore. The question for this chapter is whether the advent of the jet aircraft has caused increased fatigue for its pilots, and the answer would seem to be a guarded 'yes.' Certainly a consensus is developing among commercial jet aircraft pilots that they experience more fatigue than when operating piston equipment—a consensus reinforced by a number of professional articles by airline flight surgeons and other medical men. Relatively little has been published about fatigue in military jet operations compared to piston-engined aircraft. An RAF study showed that 'measurable performance deterioration occurred after ten hours in a multi-engine piston aircraft;

after six hours in jet bombers; was greater during night-flying operations; progressed in severity during four consecutive fifteen-hour night missions; was present though not subjectively noted after three (jet) fighter sorties; and was noted to vary widely among individual pilots flying under the same circumstances.'[14] In 1958, the Air Force conducted a study, 'Operation Head-Start,' to evaluate the responses of B-52 crews flying repeated twenty-hour missions over a three-month period. Some objective measurements of stress were derived from in-flight assay of urinary hydroxycorticosteroid levels, reflecting the adrenal hormone output of the individual. Flights which upset the biological rhythm, particularly those starting at 8 pm and 4 am, were most disliked. At the end of the three months, seventy-five per cent of the crews stated that the missions should be reduced to fifteen hours. As for rest periods after the three-month tour of duty, thirty-four per cent stated they would be ready to resume such missions after thirty days, twenty-nine per cent after three months and fourteen per cent desired a year's rest.

Why should flying a jet aircraft be more fatiguing than operating a piston-engined one? At first glance, this would seem paradoxical when so many causes of acute fatigue have been eliminated by advances in design and technology. Thus, vibration—always perceptible in piston-engined aircraft, and often severe—has been greatly reduced with the turboprop power plant, and practically eliminated with the turbojet. Noise levels have gone down with better soundproofing and elimination of the propeller with its noisy tip vortices. Cockpits have been designed for safety and comfort, instruments better grouped and made more readable.

Certain constant problems contributing to fatigue—both acute and chronic—have continued from previous eras, but are beginning to get more attention. These include time on duty before and after flight; living conditions away from the home base; the burden of responsibility on all members of the flight crew, particularly the captain; and non-flying situations productive of tension, such as domestic and financial problems. Lastly, it must be remembered that the new jets, both Air Force and commercial, are being flown by an ageing pilot population, many in their fifties. They 'can fly better than ever although there is no denying they can take less of it.'[15] One very possible cause of fatigue, more chronic than acute, is the relative anoxia experienced by operators of pressurized equipment. Is the partial pressure of oxygen in pressurized cabins at equivalent altitudes of 8000 or 10,000 feet adequate to maintain all physiological and psychological functions at normal level? We know already that night vision is seriously impaired through relative anoxia at these altitudes, and there may be more to the story. More attention is being given to smoking and anoxia in air crew. For cigarette smokers who inhale, blood carboxyhaemoglobin levels may reach eight per cent, and the reduction in oxygen-carrying capacity of the blood can equal an increase in altitude of 5000 feet or more. Thus, a heavy-smoking pilot in a pressurized cockpit at 8000 feet equivalent altitude will experience a blood oxygen level equivalent to that at 13,000 feet—well within the zone of clinical anoxia.

On the other hand, certain factors having a bearing on the fatigue problem have undoubtedly been aggravated by the increased performance of jet aircraft. Writings on the subject make much of the disturbance of the body's biological rhythm in operations across the world's twenty-four time zones, and anyone with jet travel experience will agree that it takes between one and two days to adjust to the local day and night cycle after being hurried across five or more time zones in only a few hours. It would seem self-evident that an American pilot making an 8 am landing at Frankfurt will not be at his best when every cell in his body is protesting that it is really 2 am at home in New York, and he belongs in bed. Fatigue will be further aggravated when flight personnel are unable to get adequate rest away from home because their own biological rhythm has not adjusted to the day and night pattern of their destination. The 'physiological clock' is in phase with local time during north and south flights, and it has been noted that more experienced jet aircraft crews prefer such runs. 'Flying to Buenos Aires,' says one veteran pilot, 'my bowels stay on Eastern Standard Time.'

For the jet aircraft flight crew, it would seem that the chief aggravating cause for fatigue is the increased tempo of decision-making, the more rapid presentation of cues and stimuli, and the more rapid responses required, with the increasing speed of aircraft. In 1947, DC-6 flight crews were crossing the North American continent in ten hours; today they travel the same distance in five. In half the time they fly the same number of miles, make the same (or possibly more) number of decisions concerning power settings, course and altitude changes, and send and receive the same number of radio messages. In other words, the tempo of activity for these busy specialists, bearing a crushing weight of responsibility, has speeded up, has doubled. This is true of military jet pilots equally with civilian airline personnel. As the Flight Surgeon's Manual observes under the heading 'Speed and Load':

Speed is so great that flight controls must give advance information. The load is so high that computer systems have become standard equipment, relieving the pilot of many steps in controlling the aircraft. The increase in speed, with resultant narrower margin of control lead and the increasing mass of simultaneous stimuli all produce tension, a higher pitch of work, a push for greater alertness, and a naturally stepped-up tempo for fatigue.[16]

Despite intensive effort by many dedicated men acting alone and in concert, escape equipment has often failed to keep pace with the incredible performance of jet aircraft as they exceed supersonic speed and reach out towards the 'thermal barrier' at Mach 3. This is perhaps inevitable, considering that the primary mission of air forces is protecting the security of the state, and saving the lives of air crew in emergencies must be a secondary consideration. Yet the sheer dollars-and-cents value of a trained pilot, radar bombardier or defence-systems operator would seem to justify greater attention to survival equipment in a period when new advances in aircraft performance have created new and serious problems in this area, not to mention the effect on morale of attention to survival.

The parachute continues to be the flyer's ultimate means of salvation, and certain advances have been made since World War II. Parachute canopies are now larger than the standard twenty-four foot 'chute of World War II; the recent C-8 and C-9 'chutes, made of 1·1 oz nylon, are twenty-eight feet in diameter, and the newest C-10 and C-11 canopies are thirty feet in diameter. This is because during parachute deployment at high altitude, the larger diameter canopy sets in motion a larger mass of air, whose inertia reduces the velocity of the falling man–parachute combination before the 'chute fully deploys and develops its highest opening shock forces. Packing the new parachutes in 'quarter bags' housing the bottom quarter of the canopy permits a smooth rather than sudden deployment of the 'chute. Pockets or guide extensions at the edges of the canopy opposite every other gore reduce the speed of opening at high altitude, and hence the opening shock, while they also stabilize the parachute and minimize oscillations during descent which otherwise can severely injure the parachutist by swinging him violently against the ground.

Despite these measures, designed to reduce the violent opening shock of the twenty-four foot parachute at high altitude, free fall is still the procedure taught for escape from aircraft above 20,000 feet. This is because free fall rapidly takes the escaping airman through the least dense portion of the atmosphere, where anoxia and low temperatures may well prove lethal to a man slowly drifting down beneath an open canopy. The time of free fall from 40,000 feet is approximately two and a half minutes, while with open parachute the time reaches twenty-five minutes—long enough to exhaust the ten-minute supply of the bail-out oxygen bottle.

Because of the possibility of the jumper losing consciousness at high altitude, free fall was hazardous until the development of the automatic

230 THE DANGEROUS SKY

parachute rip-cord release. This mechanism can be pre-set to a lower altitude to open the parachute automatically, eliminating the hazard of the jumper misjudging his altitude, and also permits an unconscious man to be thrown overboard by his mates in an emergency, with assurance that his parachute will open at lower altitude. The earliest automatic releases, introduced in 1946, were fired by a small explosive squib. The current F-1B release is spring-actuated, the spring being wound by pulling an arming handle just before bail-out. Two dials appear on the face of the release mechanism, one a timer reading from nought to thirteen seconds, the other an aneroid reading from 5000 to 20,000 feet. The usual setting is five seconds and 14,000 feet. When jumping below 14,000 feet, the release opens the parachute five seconds after arming. In high-altitude bail-out, the 'chutist will fall free to 14,000 feet, where the barometric feature actuates the release. Five seconds later—at about 10,000 feet—the 'chute will open.

Jet aircraft, carrying men to extreme heights, have added another hazard to high-altitude bail-out—spinning of the body in free fall. Rates for tumbling (head over heels) and spinning (with arms and legs extended in the horizontal plane) at 40,000 feet are double those at sea level for the same air speed. Early experiments with dummies indicated that at 83,000 feet, the body might spin at 465 rpm. Such high rates could produce not only unconsciousness, but also death, by draining the blood and body fluids away from the heart and into the extremities, with severe blood-vessel injuries. In human subjects, spinning at 160 rpm produced unconsciousness in three to ten seconds. At 125 rpm, haemorrhages in the eyelids, swelling of the orbital tissues and pain and diffuse headache resulted. It was in testing the Beaupré multistage parachute—designed to stabilize the free-falling parachutist in high-altitude bail-out—that Captain Joseph W. Kittinger made the balloon flights to 102,000 feet (described in Chapter 1) that won him the Harmon Trophy in 1960. The Beaupré 'chute had two timers, the first releasing the pilot 'chute, eighteen inches in diameter, sixteen to eighteen seconds after arming. This pulled out the stabilizing 'chute, six feet in diameter, which pulled the twenty-eight foot diameter main parachute three-quarters of the way out of its bag. The resulting ensemble holds the parachutist upright as he free falls to a lower altitude. Here the second timer releases the last portion of the main 'chute from the 'quarter bag,' and the flyer floats down to land.

The landing is still a risky procedure even though the larger twenty-eight foot canopy has a descent rate at sea level of nineteen feet per second compared to the twenty-four feet per second of the old twenty-four foot diameter 'chute. Ninety per cent of non-fatal injuries in recent emergency bail-outs were caused in landing, and sixty per cent of the non-fatal major injuries were the result of faulty landing technique. The current Class V nylon webbing harness has quick releases on both shoulders so that the canopy can be jettisoned immediately on landing, preventing the jumper from being dragged along the ground in a wind. The canopy releases have safety covers, lest the parachute be detached in the air with disastrous results.

Leaving the plane in an emergency is made more difficult by the greater air speed, and the greater accelerations, developed by jet aircraft. One is no longer able, as in the open-cockpit days, to climb out on the wing and dive off. At present-day speeds, one would be smashed against the tail surfaces or some other part of the aircraft. And G forces developed in a spin can pin a man helplessly in his seat. Though one may maintain consciousness with radial accelerations up to five G, one may still have great difficulty moving about at two G, and at three and a half G will be unable to stand or move. Where men have to walk from their stations and escape unaided from a hatch designed for the purpose, the blast of the slipstream may be broken by spoiler doors on the leading edge of the hatch, as in the early B-47 bombers, or they may swing from a bar and fall out feet first through an escape tunnel, as in the KC-135 jet tanker. Such devices do not eliminate the great risk to life and limb involved in going out into an airstream velocity of 300 to 600 mph. The slipstream may catch the feet of the air-crew member and slam his head into the spoiler door designed to protect him. When exiting from a belly hatch, it is safest to squat at the rear edge of the hatch, knees under the chin and arms clasped around the legs, and roll forward and out head first in the 'cannon-ball' attitude. This posture, by increasing the ratio of mass to area, causes the jumper to decelerate less rapidly, with less likelihood of injury from wind-drag deceleration. Not only may a man find it physically difficult to reach the escape hatch and fling himself out, but fear, panic and confusion may cause the air-crew member to hesitate until it is too late. Early in the jet age, between 1946 and 1949, there were 1054 attempts to escape from USAF aircraft in an emergency without assistance, with only 52·2 per cent getting down uninjured, while 10·2 per cent ended fatally. Fifty-three and three-tenths per cent of the deaths were caused by jumping too low, or by being struck by the aircraft.

Assisted escape was the answer, particularly for aircraft with a cockpit covered by a transparent canopy—as in all fighters and such bombers as the B-47 Stratojet. In 1945, shortly after V-E Day, a team headed by Colonel R. W. Lovelace brought back from Germany a Heinkel He 162 ejection seat, as used late in the war in German fighter aircraft, and a Swedish J-21 ejection seat. The German model was copied for the Air Force, and on 17 August 1946 the ejection seat was first used in a test flight at Wright Field. For some time F-80 Shooting Star and F2H Banshee pilots had to continue to fight their way over the sides of their aircraft in an emergency—often with fatal results—but on 8 August 1949 a Navy pilot saved his life by using the ejection seat for the first time in an emergency.

Strapped to his seat, the ejecting pilot is literally 'shot from a gun,' as the impelling force, whereby he overcomes G accelerations and is lofted over the tail surfaces of his aircraft, comes from a smokeless powder cartridge. This, fired inside an inner tube, blows upward the outer tube, fitted snugly over it, to which the seat is attached. A large enough propellant charge can easily lift the loaded seat with occupant (estimated weight 350 pounds) to a sufficient height, but the designer has to take into account the fragility of the human load, and its tolerance for G forces in the upward direction. The limits for upward ejection have been calculated at thirty-three G with onset at the rate of 500 G per second. The M-1 upward ejection seat, originally developed, gives an acceleration of fifteen G for about 0.2 second, and achieves a terminal velocity of fifty-seven feet per second. For upward ejection in large bombers with tall tails, such as the B-47 and B-52, the M-3 catapult, with longer tubes providing a longer stroke, accelerates to eighteen G for 0.3 seconds, with a terminal velocity of eighty feet per second. The M-5, the successor to the M-1 in fighter aircraft, gives an upward acceleration of sixteen G for 0.2 seconds, and a terminal velocity of sixty feet per second. Although *prolonged* forces of five G may cause blacking out, the higher forces imposed by the catapults do not have this effect, as they are applied so briefly that the blood does not have time to drain from the head.

In some large aircraft, such as the B-47 and the B-52, the navigator and other crew members are on the lower deck and cannot eject upwards, so for them the downward-ejecting M-4 catapult was provided.[17] Tolerance for negative G forces is of course less than for positive, the limit being considered to be sixteen G with a rate of onset of 200 G per second. Working with gravity, the M-4 can meet operational requirements with an acceleration of eight G for 0.1 second, and a terminal velocity of forty feet per second, well within these limits.

Severe injury has resulted, however, from the pilot ejecting when not properly restrained in the seat, or when he has not taken the optimum position. This is particularly important when ejecting downwards. Obviously, very severe injuries will occur if the air crew member's feet catch on the sides of the cockpit as he is fired downwards. In preparing to eject downwards, the crew member positions his feet on foot rests,

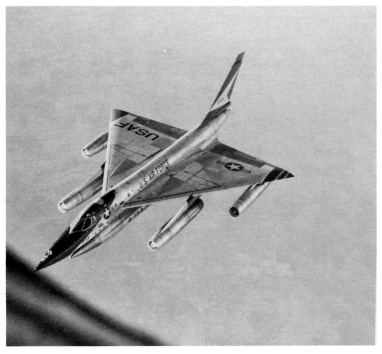

36. The General Dynamics B-58 Hustler, first large aircraft with supersonic capability, able to achieve Mach 2.5 above 35,000 feet, and with a ceiling of 60,000 feet. Weapon and fuel carried in streamlined pod underneath the fuselage (1959). (General Dynamics)

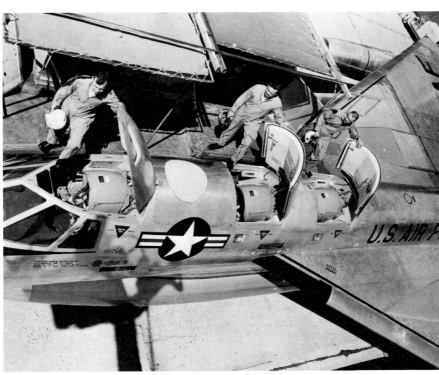

37. The supersonic environment: crew members of the B-58 Hustler stand beside their cockpits, to which they are confined for eight hours of flight (up to twelve hours with air refuelling). Each cockpit contains an escape capsule, rocket powered, the first fitted in an operational aircraft. Left to right: pilot, bombardier/navigator, defense systems operator. (General Dynamics)

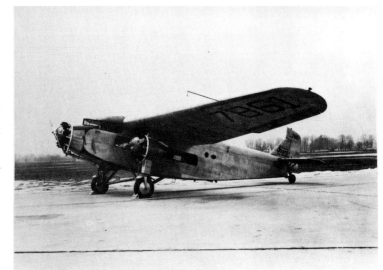

38. Ford trimotor, 4-AT-B type, carrying ten passengers, with three 220 hp Wright Whirlwind engines. This aircraft was completed in December 1928. (Air Force Museum)

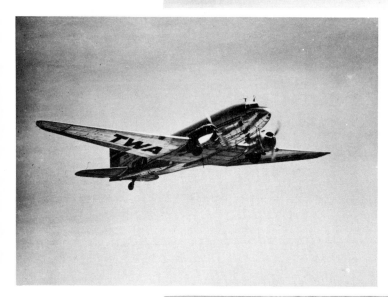

39. The Douglas DC-3, first appearing in 1935 with two Pratt & Whitney 1200 hp engines and carrying 21 passengers. Known around the world in World War II as the C-47 and the Dakota. (Air Force Museum)

40. The world's first jet transport aircraft, the De Havilland Comet I. Photo shows the two prototypes, and in foreground, the first production aircraft, G-ALYP, which on 10 January 1954, was lost off Elba in the first pressure cabin explosion. (De Havilland photo)

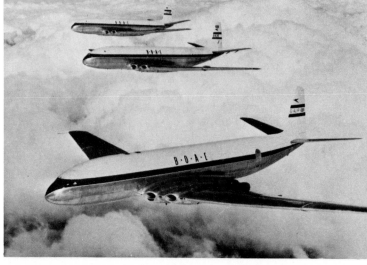

then moves retaining devices which clamp the feet just above the ankles, while also tightening a V-belt running from between the legs up to the lap belt. With feet and pelvis thus restrained, the flyer is prevented from rising off the seat as it accelerates downward.

In the upward-firing seat, position of the body is almost equally important. The spine should be as straight as possible, the buttocks pressed firmly against the seat back, the head pressed back against the head-rest and the chin tucked in. If bent forward, the flyer risks having his vertebrae fractured by the upward thrust on the buttocks being applied unequally to the forward edge of the vertebral bodies. A 1957 study of 633 non-fatal ejections showed that fourteen (2·2 per cent) had such fractures. In some cases, faulty position was the cause, in others, separation from the seat. Paradoxically, a too-thick cushion under the buttocks can cause such fractures. Instead of smoothly accelerating upwards, the cushion-user receives a severe jolt on his posterior as the seat, getting a head start, strikes him after compressing the cushion. In upward ejection, it is not so necessary for the feet to be positioned on the foot-rests. They may be left on the rudder pedals during firing, and will then merely swing back against the foot rests, causing nothing worse than bruising of the calf. Elbows should be on the arm rests, lest they strike the sides of the cockpit. Usually they are properly positioned, as the left arm rest moves to fire the canopy and lock the shoulder harness, while the right arm rest fires the catapult.

Initially, it was expected that once thrown clear of the aircraft, the flyer would free fall, still strapped to his seat, to an altitude where aneroid controls would release the man from the seat and open his parachute. In test drops from above 25,000 feet it was found, however, that tumbling was severe about the head-to-foot axis, even with a small stabilizing parachute. Present doctrine is to separate from the seat as promptly as possible. Formerly the flyer had to unfasten his lap belt and kick the seat away; at present an explosive charge severs the lap belt automatically within one or two seconds of leaving the aircraft. The F-1B automatic parachute release is armed as the seat falls away. At higher altitudes, the flyer then free falls to 14,000 feet, where the parachute opens automatically; below that level, the timer opens the 'chute within one or two seconds.

Ejection at low altitude is always a critical problem, yet frequently must be resorted to with engine failure or other emergencies at takeoff. Despite technical advances, the results too often are fatal. Between 1 August 1949 and 30 June 1958 there were 1462 ejections from USAF aircraft, of which 294, or twenty per cent, resulted fatally. Two hundred and thirty-six of these deaths, or eighty-four per cent, were caused by 'violent contact with ground or water.' In 128 cases, the dead flyer was still strapped in his ejection seat, and in ninety-nine cases, separated from the seat but with the 'chute not deployed. The greatest cause of this death toll is bail-out at low altitude, 126 of the 294 deaths resulting from ejection below 1000 feet. With the 'one and zero' system the D-ring of the parachute is now connected by a lanyard to the automatic lap-belt release when flying below three hundred feet; on ejection, the seat separates one second later, and the 'chute opens instantly. With the M-3 catapult and a quick-opening flat circular canopy, a man may eject and survive when his aircraft is on the runway and doing 120 knots.

Low-altitude ejection has been made safer by newly-developed rocket escape catapults. First fitted in the F-102 in 1958, the 'B' type rocket ejection seat has also been used in the F-106 and in later models of the F-104. The rocket has the advantage over the powder-cartridge catapult that the thrust can be continued much longer at tolerable G forces, thus carrying the escaping flyer much higher and faster (to a height of 300 feet above the level of ejection when flying at 200 knots), without exceeding twenty-two G.

The latest ESCAPAC 1C-3 rocket-propelled ejection seat has zero-zero capability, in other words, it will fire the pilot high enough to save his life even when the aircraft is stationary on the ground. The seat is fired either by an overhead handle or by an 'alternate' handle between tne legs. As the seat ascends to a height of 200 feet, it is held vertical by a DART lanyard attached to the cockpit floor, with a snubber reel under the seat which slightly retards the rapid feed-out of the lanyard. A self-contained oxygen supply, good for ten minutes, is actuated as the seat ejects. One second after ejection, a nitrogen-inflated bladder separates the crew member from the seat. Three-quarters of a second later the parachute opens automatically if the altitude is below 14,000 feet; otherwise the pilot free falls to that altitude where the 'chute is opened by a barometric release.

In supersonic aircraft, the ejection seat is semi-streamlined and its design affords considerable protection against wind blast and wind-drag deceleration. These are by far the most deadly medical phenomena to accompany the jet age. To eject at 600 knots indicated air speed has been compared to 'hitting a brick wall.' Possibly falling from a height into water would be a better simile; in either case, fluids ordinarily considered yielding can inflict severe injuries in violently decelerating a moving body. Here, at least, there is an advantage in ejecting at high altitude, for the 'q force,' or pounds per square foot of ram air pressure against the surface of the body, is a function of speed and density. At Mach 0.9 the total force on a human body (assuming its area to be four square feet) is 4960 pounds at 5000 feet, but only

632 pounds at 50,000 feet. (At supersonic speeds, the q force is not only higher, but is increased by the pressure of compressed stagnant air over the anterior surface of the body.) Without special protection to the face, from hard helmets with visors, eyelids may be torn, the mouth cannot be held closed, and lungs and stomach may be overdistended by ram air forced into the mouth. Wind-blast erosion, so called, produces flailing motion of unrestrained arms and legs, far beyond the ability of the flyer to resist with his muscles, leading to severe fractures and dislocations. Even restraints may be torn free at supersonic speed. Lastly, there is wind-drag deceleration, with a prolonged duration of G loads reaching as high as thirty-five G, the maximum that can be tolerated, and which is already being reached at indicated air speeds of 575 to 725 knots.

Colonel Stapp, whose rocket-sled investigations of linear deceleration have already been referred to, made a number of experiments on chimpanzees, and on 10 December 1954 on himself, designed to simulate wind blast and wind-drag deceleration encountered in an ejection at 1600 knots at 40,000 feet. This could be reproduced with a speed of 562 knots at sea level. This was achieved with a two-unit sled, the rear propulsion unit of which was driven by nine solid-fuel rockets providing a 40,000 pound thrust for five seconds. Colonel Stapp took his place in a seat on the forward sled, with no windshield. He was wearing a wind-proof fibre-glass helmet with plexiglas visor, secured to the head rest; teeth protected by a bite block; standard wool flying coveralls; flying gloves and shoes; and 6000-pound test three-inch-wide nylon webbing was used for shoulder straps, chest belt, lap belt and inverted-V tie-down. To prevent flailing of arms and legs, 1000-pound one-inch webbing was used to tie the feet to the footrest, hands to the colonel's knees, and elbows to the back of the seat. Eighty minutes were spent in making all the straps fast.

With burnout of the rockets after five seconds, the maximum speed was 562 knots (Mach 0·85). After 0·1 second the two sleds were separated by the rear one entering water brakes; after 0·3 second the test sled, having been decelerated by wind drag to 508 knots in a distance of 310 feet, entered water brakes and was stopped in a further 380 feet within 1·1 second. G forces incurred reached peak levels of thirty-five to forty G.

Colonel Stapp wrote of his own subjective sensations:

At the instant of burnout the pressure of acceleration against the back instantly disappeared as forces were reversed, and the wind-drag and rail-friction effects decelerated the sled in the power off phase at about 5·5 to 16·8 G. The instant that forces reversed and harness pressure could be felt on strap impingement areas, there was a very rapid transition from black to yellow in visual perception, followed by a brief view of the track and water brakes, somewhat like a stroboscopic flash, before entry into the water brakes threw the subject's body violently forward against the harness. Up to this point there is a vague recollection of wind pressure being felt as a fluttering of the shoulders of the coveralls but without buffeting or unpleasant sensation.

On entry into the water brakes, the face immediately felt congested with severe pain around the eyes, as though they were being pulled from the sockets. Vision became a shimmering salmon-coloured field with no images—evidently the pupils were impinged against the stretched upper eyelids and the visual sensation was caused by light coming through the lids. The congestion and pain increased noticeably during the exposure to more than twenty-five G for more than one second. Sensation in the eyes was somewhat like the extraction of a molar without an anaesthetic. This pain was sufficient to over-ride sensations caused by impingement on harness straps even though later abrasions and contusions were visible at all strap pressure areas.

When the sled stopped the visual impression of shimmering salmon colour not only persisted but was present when the eyes were forced open. There was a marked exophthalamos which made it difficult to open the eyes without using the fingers. The chest strap was so tight that it was extremely difficult to breathe. Mental confusion like that of struggling against the onset of anaesthesia was present. As soon as the chest strap was loosened, and the bite block removed, normal respirations were possible and the confusion diminished. There was no loss of consciousness at any time.[18]

Colonel Strapp's courageous experiment had reproduced accurately the prolonged, intense G forces that would result from wind-drag deceleration in high-speed bail-out. Six months later came a demonstration of how punishing they could be in actual supersonic bail-out, and of how much a determined man could take, and live. On the morning of 26 February 1955 George Smith, a civilian test pilot from North American Aviation, was forced to abandon his F-100A Super Sabre over the Pacific Ocean when the controls locked. With the aircraft in a near-vertical dive, the altitude approximately 6000 feet and the Mach meter reaching 1·05 (giving a true air speed of 675 knots), Smith blew off the canopy and fired his ejection seat. Unfortunately he did not have time to tighten his shoulder straps, with the result that he not only was injured during ejection, but also tumbled with his body bent double. Instantly he lost consciousness as q forces of 1280 pounds per square foot smashed at his body, while he experienced a peak wind-drag deceleration force of sixty-four G with a rate of onset of 700 G per second, with a duration of 0·12 second above thirty-five G and 0·29 second above twenty G. This ripped off his helmet and oxygen mask. Very fortunately, Smith had one of the early ejection seats with automatic lap belt, which fired two seconds after ejection. Two seconds thereafter his automatic parachute release pulled the D-ring, a four-second delay which should have permitted Smith's battered body to decelerate to 140 mph, a safe velocity for parachute opening. But the fact that a third of the panels were torn suggested that the 'chute had deployed at higher speeds—possibly ripped from its pack by wind blast. In any event Smith was still alive, though unconscious, when he parachuted into the water, providentially close to a fishing boat which picked him up in less than a minute. Within ninety minutes he was getting expert attention in hospital.

The badly injured pilot arrived in deep shock, with a variety of grave injuries, mostly caused by wind-drag deceleration. His head and face were severely swollen, there were haemorrhages in the eyelids and in the retinas, blood in both middle ears, and his stomach had been inflated and distended by air rammed into his mouth and down his throat. The small intestine had been ruptured, probably by his being doubled over the lap belt during ejection. Flailing of the legs had caused dislocation and sprain of the hip joints. Miraculously, no bones were broken. Abdominal surgery, jaundice due to liver damage, and weight loss of sixty-five pounds complicated a recovery which lasted for months. Eventually this indestructible man was able to return to testing high-performance aircraft.

Experiences such as George Smith's, many of which did not end so happily, demonstrated that the ejection seat did not provide adequate protection at air speeds in excess of 600 mph. In particular, recent animal experiments with rocket sleds reaching Mach $1 \cdot 7$ demonstrate that with one-second exposure at this speed, the q forces acting on the skin can raise its temperature to 300 to 320 degrees F, sufficient to cause severe third-degree burns.

Thus, some type of closed system will be needed for successful escape at supersonic speeds. It has been argued that such a complicated procedure is hardly justified when aircraft with supersonic capability fly by far the greater part of the time at subsonic velocities. The Flight Surgeon's Manual is undoubtedly correct, however, in its rebuttal:

On the contrary, operating stresses on the aircraft (at supersonic speeds) and the time available to take corrective action places unusual demands on the human operator. This increases the chances for mechanical failure or human error during maximum performance flight, and the probable development of an emergency escape situation.[19]

At the present time, the Air Force's Handbook of Information for Aircraft Designers specifies that 'any aircraft flying above 50,000 feet or above 600 knots indicated air speed must provide an enclosed escape system, or capsule.'[20] The wind-drag deceleration forces will remain a problem—though a more favourable mass/drag ratio with suitable capsule design may mitigate the problem—but the occupant will be well protected against blast and wind erosion, as well as anoxia. The first supersonic aircraft to be fitted with the capsule was the three-place B-58 Hustler.

The 'ultimate' aircraft—the one whose performance made the greatest demand on its flight crew, and engendered the most complex medical problems—is, in the author's opinion, the Convair (General Dynamics) B-58 Hustler, now being phased out of the Strategic Air Command inventory as it cannot be modified to carry terrain-following radar. A few aircraft go faster, some go higher, but the Hustler is one of the very few large supersonic aircraft in regular service in the world today. With the Mach 3 B-70 relegated to experimental testing, it is possible that the B-58 will be the last of the manned bombers.

With its sharp pointed nose, slender, 'area-rule' fuselage, tall, swept-back fin and rudder, and thin delta wing, the Hustler looks like an overgrown fighter. It is in fact an enlargement, scaled up 1·4 times, of Convair's F-102A Delta Dagger, and flew for the first time less than two years after the fighter, on 11 November 1956. Yet, even though the B-58 is considered small compared to the B-52 Stratofortress, it is still a large aircraft—96 feet 9 inches long, 56 feet 10 inches across the delta wing, and measures 29 feet 11 inches from the ground to the tip of its fin. At takeoff it grosses 163,000 pounds, of which about 100,000 pounds is jet fuel, much of it carried in the delta wing. In flight the B-58 can be further fuelled to a gross weight of 176,890 pounds. Power to drive the B-58 comes from four General Electric J-79 turbojets, producing 15,600 pounds thrust each with afterburner, which are carried in separate pods under the wing. Beneath the fuselage is a long, slender, streamlined pod designed to carry fuel and a thermonuclear weapon to the target, and then to be released for a clean getaway for home. In newer versions the pod is in two parts—a larger, lower fuel compartment which is detached before the run up to the target, and a smaller, upper component containing the weapon.

Three men handle this monster. In the nose sits the pilot, who is aided in flying the plane by autopilot equipment providing constant Mach control, altitude control for penetration missions 'on the deck' at speeds of 700 mph, and automatic heading controls, as well as automatic ILS coupling. Foot pedals control the rubber, and the stick operates a pair of horizontal surfaces—'elevons'—at the trailing edge of the delta wing—these acting together as elevators, and differentially as ailerons. The surfaces are hydraulically actuated, with a back-up hydraulic system; if both fail, the crew must eject as it is impossible to control the aircraft by muscle power. On the pilot's instrument panel the engine instruments are grouped to the right, the flight instruments to the left. These include Mach meter, indicated airspeed meter, rate of climb altimeter, two attitude gyros, angle of attack indicator, accelerometer and an elevator position indicator. This latter instrument—showing the elevator angle being set by the autopilot to hold the aircraft in straight and level flight—is made necessary by the fact that the centre of pressure of the delta wing may shift aft several feet at supersonic speed. This is compensated for by pumping fuel aft, and the necessary amount is automatically programmed in a panel on the right side of the cockpit. Should the centre of gravity coincide with the centre of pressure, the aircraft loses stability and may spin with disastrous results. The position of the centre of pressure and its distance from the centre of gravity, as well as the air speed, determine the elevator setting needed to compensate for these factors.

There is little time to investigate in case of trouble, so two warning lights are located in plain sight of the pilot at the upper left-hand side of the instrument panel. The upper one directs his attention to a panel to his right, were one of about thirty signs will light up to indicate the cause of trouble. In addition, a woman's voice—pre-recorded, of course—breaks into the masculine chatter in the pilot's earphones to tell him what is wrong. This gets instant attention. Imagine yourself at Mach 2 and 60,000 feet and hearing a soft female voice warning, 'Check for engine fire'!!

Behind the pilot, and separated from him by a star-tracker and computer, is the cockpit of the bombardier/navigator. His equipment, comprising a doppler-inertial-stellar system, is designed to provide a continuous record of the aircraft's position at supersonic or subsonic speeds, at 60,000 feet or on the deck. The position is computed by dead reckoning from data provided by the star tracker, which indicates heading; from a high-resolution Ku-band doppler radar which senses speed and drift; and from the inertial system which senses attitude and acceleration. An integrating computer-display-and-control unit ties together all sensing units to feed information to the bombardier/navigator. He controls the aircraft's heading during the bomb run, and can arrange for automatic bomb release by target-sighting, offset or check-point methods. The bombardier/navigator has little outward visibility from the two tiny windows on each side of his cockpit, but obviously he is too busy watching his radar equipment to look out in any case.

Behind the bombardier/navigator is the cockpit of the defence systems operator. He remotely controls the 20-mm 'Gatling gun' cannon mounted in the extreme tail, plays the role of co-pilot in broadcasting information and position reports, and operates deceptive electronic devices to confuse enemy radar. These involve noise jamming and 'track breaking,' the B-58 countermeasures system being the first where 'the range gate of the tracking radar is captured and led away from the attacker.'[21]

After extensive testing by the manufacturer, and then by the Air Force, the B-58 entered regular service with the 43rd Bomb Wing at Carswell AFB, Texas, on 15 March 1960. A second wing, the 305th at Bunker Hill, Indiana, also operates the Hustler. Partly because of teething troubles with the aircraft, particularly in the hydraulic and electrical systems, and partly because Air Force bomber commanders expected it to be succeeded shortly by the Mach 3 North American B-70 Valkyrie, only one hundred and sixteen B-58s have been built. Each wing operates about forty of the bombers and three TB-58A trainers, in which an instructor's cockpit replaces that of the bombardier/navigator.

By the end of 1963, Air Force crews had made over 10,500 flights in the B-58, for a total of 53,000 hours of flying time. 1150 of these hours were supersonic, and 375 hours at Mach 2. At present, each B-58 is capable of flying SAC missions every other day, and the whole wing can, if necessary, take off within the 15-minute warning time given by the Ballistic Early Warning System. Typical training missions last six or seven hours, but can be extended by air refuelling to ten to twelve hours. Refuelling from KC-135 tankers takes place at moderate altitudes below 40,000 feet; usually there is also a low-level penetration run on the deck just below Mach 1, and a high-altitude bomb run at Mach 2 above 35,000 feet.

The B-58 originally came out with the ejection seat and the M-3 catapult, and admittedly, successful ejections have taken place, without injury, at air speeds below 300 mph. On occasion crew members have ejected successfully also in takeoff emergencies on the runway. Several unfortunate incidents served notice early in the development programme that the ejection seat would not enable personnel to survive at air speeds above 600 mph. On 16 December 1958 a B-58 being flown by an Air Force evaluation crew went down in Deaf Smith[22] County, Texas. All three crewmen ejected; the pilot's parachute 'streamed' (i.e. tore in so many places, due to high air speed at deployment, that it failed to fill) and he did not survive. The other crew members suffered severe flailing injuries of arms and legs, with fractures and dislocations, and spent months in hospital. The investigators concluded that the defence systems operator ejected at Mach 1·3, and the navigator and pilot at Mach 1·6. The protective measures recommended were to improve restraint mechanisms for the arms and legs, but safety personnel still worried that the head might be battered by the wind blast—and effective head restraints would unacceptably restrict the pilot's vision.

On the night of 4 June 1960 a shocking catastrophe overtook a crack Convair test crew, convincing the company's design-safety specialists that a closed escape system must be provided for the B-58 as urgently as possible. For reasons never ascertained, the aircraft, leaving light cloud formations at 42,000 feet, found itself confronted by a huge thunderhead towering to 50,000 feet instead of the forecasted 40,000 to 45,000 feet. Due to the B-58's very high speed, the pilot was unable to turn or climb to avoid the cloud, and though the aircraft did not break up, it was undoubtedly damaged in some way by turbulence or hailstones, possibly losing cabin pressure. The three crew members ejected, with fatal results, between 26,000 and 16,000 feet while the bomber was rolling to the left in a steep dive at supersonic speed, and the aircraft struck the ground in an inverted attitude, at a 70-degree angle, making a crater thirty feet deep and sixty feet wide.

The three bodies showed an extraordinary degree of violent injury, caused by wind-blast erosion and wind-drag deceleration, and by bombardment with hailstones at supersonic velocity. Leg and arm restraint straps failed, permitting severe flailing injuries of the extremities, and in two cases the heads were violently battered by side-to-side oscillations, with severe brain damage. Helmets with visors and oxygen masks, designed for protection in subsonic escape, failed completely at supersonic speed. In the case of the occupant of the No. 2 position, the left leg straps of the ejection seat failed, permitting the left leg to flail upwards and over the left shoulder. Smears of shoe polish were found on the head rest of the ejection seat, there were fractures of the left leg and separation of the symphisis pubis. The flying clothes were almost entirely torn off by wind blast, and the remaining clothing was tattered and punctured by hailstones which produced macerated pits through the skin of the face, upper arms and thighs. The occupant of the No. 3 position had ejected upward with signs that the aircraft had been rolling violently to the left, as he had been thrown against the right side of the cockpit with severe injuries on that side. His 'chute had opened at supersonic velocity—possibly deploying prematurely in the cockpit—though the shock had not ruptured the 9000-pound test webbing harness. The canopy had streamed, with severe hailstone damage, and a mass of hailstones was found in the crown. The man's head and neck had been bent up over the back of the headrest, with fractures and dislocation of the cervical vertebrae; the leg-restraint straps had failed and the legs flailed upward under the thigh restraints sufficiently to break them. There was massive congestion of the head and face, with the outline of the oxygen mask imprinted thereon. The pilot in the No. 1 positon had ejected last, apparently in an inverted position, for a compression fracture of the eighth thoracic vertebra suggested that the seat had slammed down on his buttocks. Wind blast during deceleration had battered his head with such force that dents matching the rivets holding the sun visor to his helmet were stamped in the duralumin head rest, the right arm had torn loose from its restraints and flailed, and there were macerated pits in the face caused by hailstones. His parachute had eventually deployed at a speed of less than 333 knots.[23]

The escape capsule, of which three have been fitted in each B-58 Hustler since early 1964, provides complete protection against loss of cabin pressure at high altitude, wind blast and wind-blast erosion, and thermal injury. Though flight-crew members still wear helmets and oxygen masks, they can enjoy a 'shirt-sleeve environment,' dispensing with uncomfortable pressure suits, flotation vests, exposure suits, personal parachutes and survival gear. The rear of the capsule is packed with rations, water, radio, fishing gear, foul-weather clothing, an M-4 rifle, water desalting kit, etc., and the capsule itself provides shelter on land, and will float in water. In case of loss of cabin pressure, a pull on one of two pre-ejection handles convenient to the right and left hands, initiates closing of the capsule. The door, in four overlapping segments like those of a lobster's tail, starts downward from behind the man's head. Automatic leg retractors draw his knees up and tuck his feet under, clear of the descending lower edge of the door. The restraint harness pulls back on his shoulders. In one second the door has fully closed and pressure starts building up from the capsule's own high-pressure oxygen supply. Within seven seconds—well within the limit of useful consciousness—the capsule is fully pressurized. In this situation, the bombardier/navigator and defence-systems operator are cut off from the outside world, and informed of events only by an amber alert light and a red bail-out light actuated by the pilot. The latter, though physically cut off from his cockpit, can see essential instruments through a transparent panel in the door, and can control the aircraft through the massive, pistol-grip stick inside the capsule. Buttons on the stick permit him to disconnect the autopilot, shift the centre of gravity and retard the throttles, enabling him to fly the bomber down below 40,000 feet and decapsulate. If the worst should develop, he can signal the crew to bail out through another button on the stick, and after red lights show that they have done so, the pilot can eject himself.

Triggers under the pre-ejection handle cause the canopy over the cockpit to blow off and fire a catapult which shoots the closed capsule up a track and out of the cockpit. A stabilization 'chute deploys and rockets fire as the capsule leaves the catapult, lofting over the tall, swept-back tail in a great arc. G force builds up as wind-drag deceleration batters at the capsule, retarding its forward flight, and flinging the man brutally against his retaining straps. During the 0·4 second that the rocket fires, a pair of stabilization frames, with small fins, thrust out from the rear of the capsule, to hold it straight in flight and to prevent it from tumbling. At 2·6 seconds after the trigger is pulled, the capsule has slowed to near terminal velocity and the recovery 'chute—a 41-foot-diameter Pioneer Wind Sail—deploys. At 5·4 seconds the 'chute 'disreefs,' changing the lead of its shroud lines, so that the capsule descends with the occupant facing upwards and prepared to take the landing impact on his back. This is reduced—if it descends on land—by knives slicing for six inches through aluminium cylinders and shear plates.[24]

Fantastic? Incredible? Yes—but also urgently necessary for survival in the jet age. And early in 1964 the capsule proved itself in a manned test ejection from a B-58 flying over Fort Worth.

In July 1964 I was privileged to spend an afternoon with Captain John W. Joyce (MC) USAF, flight surgeon of the 43rd Bomb Wing at Carswell AFB, Texas, to discuss with him medical problems of the B-58 crews, to meet crew members of the Wing's 63rd Squadron, and to examine a Hustler in the shops. The *élan* of the members of this outstanding unit, their enthusiasm for their work and their pride and confidence in their aircraft made an indelible impression. The 80-ton supersonic bomber is very much a 'pilot's aeroplane' and greatly liked by its crew. (They laughed indulgently when I related a rumour I had heard, that the B-58 is too fast and complex for human control, and is automatically operated in flight by a tape-fed programmer!) I was assured that the aircraft handled well in the air, and in 'going supersonic' there was little or no buffeting compared to lighter fighters. There was no perceptible sensory awareness of flying at supersonic speed, except that on looking out along the delta wing, a shock wave was visible by virtue of the greater density of the compressed air—the shock wave initially standing ahead of the wing, and at speeds approaching Mach 2, moving back to the leading edge and bending more sharply to the rear. All sound, including that of the four J-79 turbojets, is left behind at supersonic speed. The approach and landing are unusual, but I was told that it was perfectly safe with the delta wing, which cannot stall even in extreme nose-high attitudes, though the aircraft then sinks rapidly. The approach is made at an angle of

12·5 degrees on the angle-of-attack indicator. There are no flaps, the entire delta aerofoil serving as a giant flap as the nose is raised higher, slowing the aircraft to a landing speed of 155 knots. During the roll-out a high-drag parachute deploys from the tail and the nose is pulled up to fifteen degrees, gradually dropping again as speed decreases. Admittedly the view ahead is poor at the fifteen-degree nose-up angle.

Dr Joyce, who had flown as a passenger in the TB-58A trainer, obviously enjoyed the full confidence of his flight crews. He was particularly concerned about fatigue, to which the narrow fighter-type cockpits of the Hustler contribute. Space is even further limited by the capsule in each cockpit. Pilots agreed that the cramped quarters, sitting in the same position with no opportunity to move around during missions which might last for twelve hours with air to air refuelling, was the chief cause of acute fatigue. Dr Joyce commented on the tired state of crews which had been flying all-night missions when they came in to land at sunrise. Pilots themselves did not admit lasting fatigue, and claimed that they felt fresh after twenty-four hours' rest. But a defence-systems officer, pointing out that he was 'busy every moment from takeoff to landing' with calculations, admitted fatigue lasting for several days afterwards. Fortunately, chronic fatigue is unlikely in these crews as they fly only two to three missions per month—not enough to keep them in practice, so that they resort to simulator training.

Because they were sometimes used in World War II under close supervision of flight surgeons, I asked about amphetamines ('pep pills') to ward off fatigue on long missions. Flight personnel have never used the stimulant, however, and Dr Joyce was emphatically opposed to their use.

He expressed much concern that there was literally no room in the pilot's cockpit for nourishment. Water carried in a plastic bottle strapped beneath the canopy flowed down through a tube, but frequently the water tasted vile. Dr Joyce hoped to find space for a thermos of coffee, but the only storage spot available was in the pilot's map case, measuring about $16 \times 12 \times 5$ inches, and there would then be no room for the flight maps. With sandwiches tending to fall onto the floor of the cockpit when personnel were busy with their duties, meals were being issued in individual bite-sized morsels. With pressurization, the relief tube is a thing of the past, and a plastic 'duck' with stopper takes its place.

Busy indeed is Dr Joyce, watching over the health, well-being and morale of the flight crews of one of the elite groups of the Strategic Air Command—today America's first line of defence. Concerned as he is with supersonic flight, pressurization, capsule escape and crew fatigue, he sometimes may look back to the beginning of the story at whose end he stands today. In the year 1783 Professor Charles suffered the first attack of aero-otitis media during the first flight of a hydrogen balloon. The intervening hundred and ninety years have seen a myriad of fascinating developments, as aviation medicine has kept pace with the progress of flight.

[1] An alloy of cobalt 55 per cent, tungsten 15 to 25 per cent, chromium 15 to 25 per cent and molybdenum 5 per cent. Too hard to machine, turbine blades made of this material have to be cast by the lost-wax process.

[2] See Grover Heiman, *Jet Pioneers* (New York: Duell, Sloan & Pearce, 1963).

[3] Kenn C. Rust and William N. Hess, 'The German Jets and the U.S. Army Air Force,' *Journal of the American Aviation Historical Society,* vol. 8, no. 3, Autumn 1963, p. 155.

[4] Ernest R. McDowell, 'Ryan's Fireball,' *Journal of the American Aviation Historical Society,* vol. 8, no. 4, Winter 1963, p. 231. Also Ernest McDowell, personal communication.

[5] W. F. Hilton, *High Speed Aerodynamics* (London: Longmans, Green & Co., 1951), p. 180.

[6] Flight Surgeon's Manual, AF Manual 161–1, Department of the Air Force, 17 January 1962, p. 12–1.

[7] Hubertus Strughold, 'Development of Aviation Medicine in Germany,' *German Aviation Medicine in World War II,* Prepared under the auspices of the Surgeon General, USAF (Washington: Government Printing Office, 1950), vol. I, p. 24.

[8] *Journal of the American Medical Association,* 20 July 1964, editorial, 'Ozone in Aircraft,' p. 232.

[9] John P. Stapp MD, 'Effects of Linear Acceleration,' *Aerospace Medicine,* ed. Major General Harry G. Armstrong USAF (Baltimore: Williams & Wilkins Co., 1961), p. 265.

[10] John B. Stapp MD, 'Tolerance to Abrupt Deceleration,' *Collected Papers on Aviation Medicine* (London: Butterworth Scientific Publications, 1955), p. 122.

[11] *ibid.,* p. 122.

[12] *ibid.,* p. 158.

[13] *ibid.,* p. 138.

[14] Flight Surgeon's Manual, 1962, pp. 10–13.

[15] Marius Lodeesen and James E. Crane, 'Tired Jet Pilots' *(Airline Pilot,* reprinted from *Flying),* March 1963, p. 16.

[16] Flight Surgeon's Manual, 1962, pp. 10–13.

[17] Most unfortunately, the downward-ejecting seat had to be fitted to earlier models of the supersonic F-104 Starfighter, as even the M-5 would not throw the pilot clear of the high *T*-shaped tail with the high speeds attainable by this aircraft. The downward-ejecting seat practically eliminated the pilot's chances of escape in case of trouble at low altitude. Later models of the F-104 have been fitted with the more powerful upward-firing rocket ejection catapult.

[18] Stapp in Armstrong, p. 279.

[19] Flight Surgeon's Manual, 1962, pp. 7–10.

[20] *ibid.,* pp. 5–29.

[21] Lieutenant Colonel Henry R. Hirsch, 'The B-58,' *Air University Review,* September–October 1964, p. 57.

²² Pronounced DEEF Smith.

²³ Niess, Lentz, Townsend, Davidson and Chubb, 'The Role of the Physician in the Investigation of Aircraft Accidents,' *Journal of the American Medical Association,* vol. 184, no. 9, 1 June 1963, p. 701.

²⁴ USAF Hospital, Carswell AFB, Texas, 'B-58 Escape Capsule,' 8 October 1963.

7

Mass Movement around the Earth: Commercial Air Transport, 1910–

In the two decades since World War II ended, the aeroplane has wrought a revolution in commercial transportation. Usurping the traditional roles of the steamship and the railroad train, today's jet and turboprop transport fleet carry more travellers across the ocean than go by sea, and have driven the railroads out of the long-haul passenger business. Aviation medicine and safety engineering have played a significant part in the creation of today's high-speed, high-altitude airliners, particularly through the development of the pressure cabin, without which our modern globe-girdling network of airlines would not exist today.

The first aerial mass transport medium was the Zeppelin airship. More as a propaganda stunt than as a serious means of aerial commerce, Count Zeppelin founded the *Deutsche Luftfahrt Aktien-Gesellschaft* (DELAG) in November, 1909. Seven passenger airships operated between then and 1 August 1914 from hangars near large German cities. Yet this was not a scheduled service, but involved mere joyrides of two hours' duration in good weather in the neighbourhood of the hangars, for which patriotic Germans were more than willing to pay fifty dollars per person. The Zeppelins were primitive and crude, with a speed of no more than 47 mph, but they carried up to twenty-four passengers in large enclosed cabins amidships, with wickerwork chairs and tables, and fine wines and cold platters were served by a steward from a buffet in the rear.[1]

Immediately after the Armistice the Zeppelin Company operated a small, efficient passenger airship, the *Bodensee,* on a regular schedule seven days a week between Friedrichshafen and Berlin, until the Interallied Commission of Control forced suspension of the flights in December 1919. Meanwhile, the weight-lifting bombing aircraft of World War I were available for conversion to passenger carrying, and European airlines were off to an early start, remaining ahead of American competition until the early 1930s. The British and French had produced large twin-engined bomber designs, several of which, such as the Handley-Page 0/400 and the Farman Goliath, were carrying ten to fourteen passengers between London and Paris in enclosed cabins only a few months after the Armistice.

Within a few years economics, geography and national policy had forced the amalgamation of the early, struggling individual airlines. Errors of policy denied to the British air transport industry the predominance which the nation enjoyed at sea. Initially, the pioneers, forced to 'fly by themselves' in the words of Winston Churchill, then Secretary of State for Air, failed in competition with the heavily subsidized French. Later, Imperial Airways, established in 1924, found it impossible to connect the Empire, or even the nations of Europe, by air because of nationalistic rivalries. As late as 1937, air travellers from England to India had to cross Europe by train from Paris to Brindisi, and the journey from London to Karachi took five and a half days. After 1932, there was an airline from Alexandria through Africa to Cape Town, and after 1935, to Australia. During their first decade Imperial Airways, following a policy of 'safety first,' relied on huge, boxy, angular biplanes, innocent of nearly all pretence of streamlining, which by virtue of their maze of struts and wires, uncowled engines hung between the wings, and elephantine fixed landing gears, cruised at no more than 100 mph. An ambitious replacement programme featuring the sleek Empire flying boat, civil forerunner of the Short Sunderland, was overtaken by World War II before it could be fully realized.

The leader in European commercial flying was Germany. Aggressively air-minded, both her people and her financiers—the latter secretly encouraged by the German War Ministry—established a network of inter-city routes out of Berlin within a year of the Armistice. By 1924 their operations extended to London, Zürich, Budapest, Stockholm, Helsinki and (via the German-backed Russian airline DERULUFT) to Moscow. In the year 1926 the State-owned 'chosen instrument,' *Deutsche Lufthansa,* was formed by amalgamation of the pioneer firms, and particularly after the rise of the Hitler regime, proceeded to expand into foreign lands. After 1931 the South American branches were connected to the Fatherland by the passenger airship *Graf Zeppelin,* and after 1934 by flying boats. On the North Atlantic run, the giant airship *Hindenburg* in 1936 carried fifty passengers at a time in incomparable luxury from Frankfurt to Lakehurst—antedating aeroplane passenger service across the North Atlantic by three years—only to burn on her first landing in America in 1937, bringing an end to the passenger airship era.

German predominance in European air transport resulted not only from government encouragement of a potential military asset, but also from superiority in aircraft design. As previously noted, World War I had fostered an ambitious programme of 'Giant' aircraft production which eventually bore fruit technologically if not militarily. Contracts signed in 1917 for high-performance day bombers had inspired several firms, notably Junkers, Dornier and Zeppelin-Staaken, to do considerable work on clean, all-metal, unbraced cantilever-wing monoplanes.[2] The latter firm in 1919 had constructed an all-metal monoplane, the Staaken E 4/20, with four Maybach engines mounted in the leading edge of the thick cantilever wing, twelve passengers in a comfortable cabin, and two pilots in a fully-enclosed cockpit forward. This airliner, years ahead of its time, was scrapped by order of the Interallied Commission of Control, but similar all-metal Junkers, Rohrbach and Dornier monoplanes, as well as rugged Dornier flying boats, not only carried the German flag around Europe, but also overseas—many serving foreign airlines.

The other major countries of Europe were also-rans in the period before 1939. Air France, the national line organized in 1933, inherited '259 aircraft of thirty-five different types, of which no less than 172 were single-engined machines, which alone would seem to be ample excuse for amalgamation.'[3] In the six years before World War II, Air France made a start at introducing high-speed metal monoplanes, including the 212 mph Bloch 220 in 1938. Air France had also inherited an overseas empire—Aeropostale, crossing the South Atlantic to Buenos Aires, Air Orient, terminating in Saigon, the capital of French Indo-China, and Air Afrique, crossing French Equatorial Africa to Madagascar. These colonial systems existed for prestige and national purpose, rather than commercial profit, and the same was true of the Italian lines extending into Ethiopia, operated by Ala Littoria, the Italian national airline which Mussolini organized in 1935.

Far more passengers were carried by the airline of one of the 'small' nations of Europe—Holland's *Koninklijke Luchtvaart Maatschappij*. Founded in 1919, it preceded the State-owned networks of the subsequent subsidized period, and as a monument to free enterprise survives to this day, calling itself 'the world's oldest airline.' By 1923, KLM covered northern Europe from Copenhagen to London and Paris. In 1931 it opened an all-air route to Batavia, the capital of the Netherlands East Indies, and in 1933, beat the British into their own colony of Singapore by seven months. Much of KLM's commercial success and appeal to international passengers resulted from their virtual partnership over twenty years with a Dutch aircraft factory which acquired a world-wide reputation—the NV Nederlandsche Vliegtuigenfabriek, which was a 'front' for none other than that flamboyant genius, Anthony H. G. Fokker.[4] During the years in which Fokker had equipped the German Air Force he had learned to build his fighter aircraft fuselages of welded-steel tubing and the thick, unbraced cantilever wings of Lithuanian birch plywood covered with veneer. This simple, sturdy and economical formula he followed for twenty years in producing a famous line of high-wing cabin monoplanes. With one of the first of these, an eight-passenger F VII, a KLM crew flew to Batavia as early as November 1924. Hanging three 200 hp American Wright radial engines on this aircraft, Fokker created the F VIIA-3M a year later and invaded the American market. American-built Fokker F 10 and F 10A trimotors equipped many of the early American airlines, and the automotive giant, Henry Ford, paid Fokker the ultimate compliment by bringing out a similar all-metal trimotor. Fokker's star began to set in 1931 when the legendary Notre Dame football coach, Knute Rockne, was killed in the crash of a TWA Fokker trimotor which was blamed on a wing failure.[5] But the Fokker formula had been rendered obsolete by developments abroad, whence now came the new, fast, all-metal transports which henceforth equipped not only KLM, but many other European airlines.

The American air transport industry was much later starting than those of Europe. In general, US Government policy in the early 1920s did not encourage passenger airline development, and neither the public nor the financiers were impressed by the aeroplane, which was regarded as a dangerous toy in the hands of irresponsible adventurers. Yet the United States Post Office laid the foundations for passenger flying by developing and operating a trans-continental airway for carrying airmail from New York to San Francisco. As early as July 1919 Chicago and New York were linked, and by September 1920 the system was extended to the west coast. Short-range, open-cockpit, war-surplus De Haviland DH 4s with Liberty engines made sixteen stops along the route, which gradually was marked by beacons every fifteen miles. After July 1924 flights were made by night as well as by day, and the schedule eastbound became 29 hours 15 minutes, and 34 hours 20 minutes westbound. When the post office routes were turned over to private operators in 1927 under the terms of the Kelly Air Mail Act, the airfields and hangars built by the government served the new operators. These were further encouraged by the Air Commerce Act of 1926, assigning to the Department of Commerce regulatory powers over civil aviation (including for the first time examination and licensing of both aircraft and pilots), and by Post Office mail payments which encouraged the development of large passenger carrying aircraft.

A tremendous stimulus to aviation in America was the solo flight of the 'Lone Eagle,' Charles A. Lindbergh, from New York to Paris on 20–21 May 1927 and the wave of public enthusiasm which followed. Even more important, Wall Street bankers were persuaded—perhaps prematurely—that air transportation might be a new and profitable industry. By mid-1929 the first adequately financed and equipped transcontinental passenger airline—Transcontinental Air Transport—was in operation. True, the journey began with the Pennsylvania Railroad from New York to Columbus, Ohio; from Columbus to Waynoka, Oklahoma, by Ford 5-AT aircraft; from Waynoka to Clovis, New Mexico, via the Santa Fe railroad; and from Clovis to Los Angeles by aeroplane. Though TAT called itself 'The Lindbergh Line,' and the Lone Eagle handled the controls in the first eastbound flight from Los Angeles, wags averred that the initials meant 'Take A Train' and the total travel time was 48 hours. Within a year, with night flying introduced, TAT was purchased by United Air Lines, and passengers were flying from coast to coast in 36 hours. In the same year two more lines—Transcontinental and Western Air, and American Airways—were flying competing transcontinental routes. With Eastern Air Transport, flying from New York to Miami, these were the original 'Big Four' of American domestic commercial aviation which, with variations of name, have survived to the present day. And a fifth—a true giant—represented the commercial power of the United States abroad, and was the 'chosen instrument' of American policy in South America, Asia and Europe. Pan American Airways originated in 1927 with a route from Key West to Havana, opened up South America during the 1930s, instituted a scheduled service across the Pacific in 1935 from San Francisco to Hong Kong via Hawaii, Midway, Wake, Guam and Manila, and in 1939 opened a route across the Atlantic. Initially this proceeded via Bermuda and the Azores to Lisbon, and a few months later via Shediac in Nova Scotia, Botwood in Newfoundland, Foynes in Ireland, to Southampton in England.

The first generation of American passenger transport aircraft followed the trimotor motif introduced by Tony Fokker, and touted by Henry Ford in the name of safety. It is difficult to grasp today how small were the total number of aircraft which established the American air transport industry. Only thirty-five fourteen-passenger Fokker F 10 and F 10A trimotors were serving Pan American, TWA and American Airways at the time of the Rockne crash.[6] The Ford Motor Company produced 199 of its similar fourteen-passenger 'tin geese,' ugly but beloved, and resembling the German Junkers in the use of metal spars and structure, and corrugated metal covering.[7] These craft had cruising speeds between 110 and 140 mph, depending on model and year; the range was 500 to 600 miles, and service ceiling not much over 15,000 feet, though the aircraft were never flown this high on scheduled passenger runs. Pan American Airways, operating over water around the Caribbean and between the continents, flew from marine bases and relied on flying boats. For their first passenger route across the Pacific from San Francisco to Hong Kong they procured the Martin M 130 Clipper.[8] For the North Atlantic route, Pan American went to Boeing for twelve B 314s, true flying ships which carried seventy-four passengers and a crew of six to ten on two decks. The Boeings marked the peak of American passenger flying-boat construction, for with the development of faster four-engined land planes, PAA felt obliged to substitute these for the 165 mph flying boats.

The revolution in air transportation in the thirties was wrought by the Douglas Aircraft Company of Santa Monica, California, but Boeing was the trail blazer. In 1930 the Seattle firm had broken with the biplane tradition to produce the Monomail to a new high-speed formula—unbraced cantilever wing of metal with smooth metal skin; streamlined circular monocoque fuselage; landing gear retracting into the wing; and 575 hp Pratt & Whitney 'Hornet' engine in a low-drag Townend ring. Top speed was 158 mph. The 186 mph Boeing B-9 bomber of 1931 was in effect a twin-engined Monomail. Finally, in 1933, a ten-passenger civil version of the B-9 appeared—the Boeing 247. Only seventy-five were built altogether, but with a 200 mph top speed, they gave an inestimable competitive advantage to United Air Lines, which purchased the first sixty of them.[9] Suddenly the safe, slow, 140 mph Fords and Fokkers were obsolete.

Douglas, heretofore a builder of military aircraft, rolled out their DC-1 on 1 July 1933. Designed under a contract with TWA, the one and only '1' was a twelve-passenger low-wing all-metal monoplane which cruised at 170 mph, and which a few months later set a transcontinental speed record from Los Angeles to Newark of thirteen hours and four minutes. Numerous modifications caused the twenty-five production aircraft for TWA to be labelled the DC-2. Unlike the Boeing, the Douglas craft featured trailing edge flaps, which enabled it to combine a high top speed with a reasonable landing speed. Other lines, hastening to replace their Fords and Fokkers with the 200 mph fourteen-passenger speedster which climbed on one engine, flooded the Santa Monica plant with orders. Then, in redesigning the '2' to serve American Airways as a fourteen-passenger sleeper, the DST (Douglas Sleeper Transport), Douglas created a yet more famous plane, the DC-3. Larger, carrying twenty-one passengers in the day version, with a maximum speed of 230 mph and a service ceiling of 24,000 feet, it permitted the airlines at last to develop into a major industry. So complete was Douglas predominance that in 1942, out of 322 commercial airliners in service in the United States, 260 were DC-3s and eight were DC-2s. In addition, many foreign lines purchased them, notably KLM and also Swissair and the Polish LOT.

Many other changes took place in commercial flying in the years between 1933 and 1939, marking aviation's transition from the era of the open cockpit and the daredevil pilot flying by the seat of his pants, to the modern swift, comfortable public transportation medium handled by grey-haired veterans with literally years in the air. Taking a leaf from the book of their European competitors, who had had cabin attendants since the early nineteen-twenties, United Air Lines, in June 1930, hired eight graduate nurses to be the first stewardesses. Load limitations required that they weigh no more than 130 pounds, and the successful candidates averaged five feet three inches in height and were between twenty-one and twenty-seven years old. The stewardesses took tickets, showed passengers to their seats, checked their destinations, provided reading and writing material, served luncheons and answered questions about the terrain and the aircraft. Even more important than their assigned duties was their morale-building function. If frail young girls thought nothing of flying every day, why should the public be afraid to follow suit? And what passenger could feel panicky when being ministered to by a registered nurse? ('Men are embarrassed to be airsick in front of a stewardess.'[10]) Competing airlines perforce followed suit, though Eastern for some years preferred male stewards.

Other technological advances were introduced during these years—the autopilot, de-icing equipment, instrument flying techniques, and radio aids to navigation. 'Flying the beam' entered the popular vernacular. The first flight engineer, aiding the pilot and co-pilot by monitoring engine instruments and fuel supply, was introduced in the Martin M 130 transpacific Clipper of 1935. In the big Boeing 314 flying boat of 1938, the 'flight deck' accommodated two pilots, a flight engineer, a navigator and a radio operator.

Another advance with direct medical implications was the introduction of 'over-the-weather' flying. In contrast to their slow, short-range predecessors, the Boeing 247s and Douglas DC-2s and 3s had the performance to ascend to altitudes of 16,000 to 20,000 feet. Here, with supercharged engines, they could fly even faster than in the denser air below. And here they would find themselves in clear, smooth air, well above the clouds and turbulence that blinded pilots and made passengers miserable.[11] Transcontinental and Western Air was particularly interested in developing 'over-the-weather' flying as a regular commercial proposition, and in 1935 and 1936 the company spent more than a hundred thousand dollars in experimental flying at high altitude. Much of this was done personally by Jack Frye, the president of the company, and by Captain D. W. Tomlinson, the Chief Engineer. With two-stage superchargers the 975 hp engines of the DC-

1 'flying laboratory' still delivered 975 hp at 20,000 feet, and with fifteen litres of liquid oxygen aboard for a crew of four, the two company officials spent twenty hours flying the speedy Douglas above 20,000 feet. Here they found most of the weather below them, but wishing to rise above all clouds, Tomlinson determined to go behond 30,000 feet. This of course was close to the ceiling for efficient human performance on one hundred per cent oxygen. With an Air Corps two-stage supercharger feeding a 900 hp Wright Cyclone in the nose of a clean all-metal Northrop 'Gamma' monoplane, and with liquid oxygen equipment, Tomlinson flew for fifteen hours above 30,000 feet around a triangular course. Here the speed at constant horsepower was thirty-four per cent greater than at low altitude. Because an effective oxygen mask had not yet been devised, Tomlinson and his observer breathed oxygen through a rubber tube and mouthpiece, biting down on the latter to conserve the gas and exhaling through the nose. One of the observers pulled the oxygen tube off the nipple at 32,000 feet and lost consciousness before he could replace it; his companion revived him by placing the tube from a second oxygen bottle in his nostril. Tomlinson himself recorded symptoms of dysbarism—pain under the knee caps and little fingers doubled at the joints—above 30,000 feet. His most remarkable feat was a flight on instruments from Kansas City to Newark, at altitudes of 30,000 to 36,000 feet, through clouds that rose still higher, on a night when all flights east of the Mississippi had been cancelled. Due to the oxygen tube and mouthpiece arrangement Tomlinson found it very difficult to use the voice radio; he had to take deep breaths of pure oxygen and then talk into the microphone. Once he inhaled air by mistake, nearly lost consciousness, and did not fully recover his faculties until five minutes later. With radio aids failing him, Tomlinson made a dead-stick landing at Princeton, New Jersey beneath a two-hundred foot ceiling, in freezing rain and quarter-mile visibility.[12]

Already considerable thought had been given to the problems of high altitude passenger flying. While a theoretical debate continued as to whether each passenger should have his own individual oxygen supply, whether the cabin pressure should be allowed to fall with altitude while the atmosphere was enriched with pure oxygen, or whether the cabin should be pressurized, some airlines were trying the former solution with the DC-3 and discovering that passengers disliked wearing masks on their faces and found the implications alarming. Frye and Tomlinson knew about the Army Air Corps pressure cabin experiment,[13] and with correct judgment, chose this solution for their own 'over-the-weather' aircraft. Pan American Airways, which had become interested in high altitude flying across the Andes in South America, joined with TWA in ordering the first commercial pressure-cabin aircraft—the Boeing S-307. Five Stratoliners were delivered to TWA in 1940, and three Stratoclippers to PAA.[14] More would have followed had not the US entry into World War II been imminent.

A civilian counterpart to the four-engined Boeing B-17 bomber, the 307 carried a crew of five or six, and thirty-three passengers by day and twenty-five as a night sleeper. The circular cross-section cabin had a pressure differential of only 2·5 psi. Ventilation rates were found rather inadequate, and temperature control not all that it should have been in the tropics or at low altitude in summer; but the 307 was a great technological advance and the envy of other airlines. Up to 8000 feet, the pressure was equal within and without the cabin, which was ventilated through a scoop in the roof of the fuselage. From eight to 15,000 feet the internal cabin pressure was held at 8000 feet, but above 15,000 feet there was a gradual drop, with 12,000 feet equivalent pressure at 20,000 feet.

World War II assured the subsequent dominance of today's global air transport industry. The United States Government in particular, spending millions as no airline could afford to do even with subsidies, created a network of routes to Europe, Asia and Africa, developed and paved dozens of airfields, erected hangars and control towers, and procured thousands of commercial-type aircraft for the military transport systems so vital to the global war effort.[15] Over 9000 of the Douglas DC-3 model were ordered, serving the USAAF as the C-47 and their allies as the Dakota. Another twin-engined aircraft, the larger Curtiss C-46, did not enter scheduled airline service after the war but made most of the 'Hump' flights from India to China at altitudes of 16,000 feet or more. Both of these aircraft could be ferried across the oceans, but lacked the fuel capacity to carry cargo over long distances. The first truly intercontinental land plane, however, became the mainstay of the Air Transport Command—the Douglas DC-4,[16] labelled C-54 or Skymaster in Army Air Force service. Originating in a contract between Douglas and five US airlines, this four-engined transport was procured to a total of 952 before V-J Day. Many of these aircraft served on a regular North Atlantic run via Goose Bay in Labrador, Gander in Newfoundland, or Lagens in the Azores to the United Kingdom; across the South Pacific via Hawaii through the Fiji Islands, Espiritu Santo and New Caledonia to Australia, and via Kwajalein and Tarawa to New Guinea, the Marianas and the Philippines. Here was the global passenger network of the future.

Though the DC-4 had been designed as a pressure-cabin aircraft, this feature was not included in the examples ordered by the Army Air Forces. At war's end, however, further commercial-type aircraft with pressure cabins were in the experimental stage. One was the Boeing C-97 Stratofreighter, a two-decked cargo version of the B-29 Stratofortress. Known commercially as the B-377 Stratocruiser, it carried sixty passengers at 300 mph. Pan American, American Overseas Airlines, and BOAC favoured it for transoceanic runs. Another was the Lockheed C-69, a commercial model on order at the time of Pearl Harbor which was not proceeded with due to the competing demand for P-38 fighters. As the L 049 'Constellation,' the Lockheed product, with cabin-pressure differential of 4·18 psi, carried fifty-four passengers at a cruising speed of 310 mph. Trans World Airlines first put this into service on its overseas and domestic services, and was followed by Eastern and KLM. Lastly came the Douglas entry, the DC-6, an enlarged and pressurized version of the reliable DC-4, with cabin-pressure differential of 4·16 psi, fifty-six passengers, and a cruising speed of 310 mph. United Air Lines took first delivery, almost every domestic airline following suit, with SABENA being a major overseas user. Safe, reliable, efficient, these magnificent aircraft dominated domestic air travel within the United States and around the world, operating routinely above the weather at 18,000 to 21,000 feet. Their successors—'stretched' modifications with more powerful engines and larger passenger capacity, the sixty-six place DC-6B, the seventy-six passenger DC-7C, the eighty passenger Lockheed L 1049G Super Constellation, and the eighty-one place L1649A Starliner, continued the American lead on the world's airways for years.

In 1952 came a dramatic challenge. Hopelessly outdistanced in the piston-engine transport race, Great Britain saw its chance to be first with pure jet passenger aircraft. While American designers were busy with military jet orders, the De Havilland company produced an aircraft of breath-taking beauty and elegance, the DH 106 Comet. With a circular cabin pressurized to 8·2 psi, and a swept-back low wing concealing four De Havilland Ghost 50 engines with a total thrust of 17,800 pounds, the prototype carried thirty-six passengers and cruised at 490 mph at altitudes up to 40,000 feet. In 1952, despite the fact that it lacked the range to fly the Atlantic, BOAC put a fleet of ten forty-four passenger Comet 1s in service on routes to Johannesburg, South Africa, and to Japan. Two years later came the end of the dream of British supremacy when two Comets broke up in the air and fell in flaming wreckage into the Mediterranean shortly after taking off from Rome. The first incident, in which thirty-five persons died on 10 January 1954 was most thoroughly investigated. Autopsies by Italian pathologists on the fifteen bodies recovered off Elba immediately pointed to the cause of the disaster—all had suffered explosive decompression and violent deceleration, and had been killed by being hurled upward and forward against the cabin roof. The Royal Navy salvage craft recovered most of the wreckage from about sixty fathoms of water, and this confirmed that there had been a massive pressure-cabin failure, which had started as a fatigue crack near a direction-finding aerial window in the cabin roof. The Comet 1 was immediately withdrawn from service, and it was not until 1958 that the larger sixty-passenger Comet 4, with heavier pressure cabin, was delivered and established the first jet service across the Atlantic. Though two British turboprop aircraft, the Bristol Britannia and the Vickers Viscount, enjoyed considerable sales, even in foreign countries, pure jet supremacy reverted to the United States.

The Boeing Company of Seattle, Washington, had an inestimable advantage over its American competitors by reason of its having produced the first successful jet bombers in the B-47 of 1947 and the monstrous B-52 of 1952. These high-speed aircraft made acute the need for a jet tanker, and in 1954 Boeing rolled out a four-jet tanker prototype, intermediate in size between the B-47 and the B-52. The design first went into production in 1956 as the KC-135, and with internal modifications, was shortly offered as a passenger transport, the Boeing 707.

The airlines hesitated to gamble on the big jets on grounds of expense but in self-defence, most had to follow suit when the giants of the industry took the plunge. In October 1958 Pan American put the Boeing 707-120 into transatlantic service, and American Airlines started competition in the transcontinental service in January 1959. This was a 132-passenger airliner cruising at approximately Mach 0·82 at 35,000 to 41,000 feet and powered by four Pratt & Whitney JT3C turbojets with 13,500 pounds thrust each. With a pressure differential of 8·6 psi, the cabin maintains sea-level pressure up to 22,500 feet, and an equivalent altitude of 7000 feet at 40,000 feet. 'Rip-stop' design and structure ensure against any major failure of the pressure cabin, and it is a fact that no pressure-cabin catastrophes have occurred in the Boeing jets, except through sabotage. Within a year Boeing introduced the long-range 707-320, able to carry up to 189 passengers in direct transoceanic flights non-stop from New York to London, Paris and Frankfurt at Mach 0·85 in eight hours or less. Simultaneously Douglas brought out a successful competing product, the DC-8, in September 1959. The rush was on, every major American airline buying one or the other, while the flag and prestige of many foreign arlines are carried by the Boeing and Douglas twins—BOAC,

Air France, Lufthansa, Alitalia, KLM, Sabena, Qantas, even Ireland's Aer Lingus. Such is the fantastic cost of developing huge jet liners, and so overwhelming the success of Boeing and Douglas, that little competition persists in the long-range field—in the Unites States, only Convair with the four-jet 880 and 990, and in Britain, BAC's rear-engined VC-10.

Yet one foreign manufacturer has shown the way in the short-haul jet field (proving, incidentally, that there was no reason for hanging jet engines under the wing except the tradition that piston engines belonged there), and American manufacturers are following suit: in 1961 France's Sud Aviation introduced their seventy-passenger Caravelle, with its twin Rolls-Royce Avon turbojets attached to the rear of the fuselage. The French transport filled a definite need, and was ordered by many foreign airlines, including United in America. Boeing, in fact, has seen fit to imitate the concept with the 727 with three jet engines in the rear, and the twin-engined Douglas DC-9 has a similar installation.

The jets have established a remarkable safety record, attributable in no small degree to the simplicity and reliability of the turbine power plant compared to the reciprocating piston engine. Yet they present several safety problems unknown in the just-ended reign of the Lockheed Super-G Constellation and the Douglas 'Seven Seas.' One is the decrease in true air speed and increase in stalling speed with increased altitude, and around 40,000 feet the two curves sometimes meet. For all their blinding speed, which has brought the continents only hours apart, the big commercial jets, because of their design and power limitations, cannot surpass the velocity of sound—making no better than Mach 0·9 at best. Decreasing air density with altitude means that the speed of sound, and the maximum speed of the aircraft, diminishes, while the stalling speed increases. And with their aerodynamically clean design and great mass of 150 tons or more, a jet liner in a stall rapidly attains supersonic velocity in the recovery dive, with loss of control and ultimately, structural failure. Experienced captains therefore keep an eye on the stalling speed and gross weight charts, and do not fly at 40,000 feet as often as they did a few years ago.

Another problem is CAT—Clear Air Turbulence. Flying above the weather at last, it was a shock to encounter turbulence at 30,000 feet or higher, striking from a clear sky without the cloud warning customary at lower altitudes. The jet streams are alleged to be responsible—the torrents of hundred-mile-an-hour winds flinging themselves around the earth in the upper troposphere—and the vortices at their boundaries constitute the turbulence. CAT has been responsible for several recent jet crashes, and still cannot be predicted with accuracy. Again, turbulence may cause an aircraft to stall, dive at a sharp angle, lose control at supersonic speed, and ultimately break up in the air. Some have had narrow escapes: in an incident involving a DC-8 in November, 1963, the big jet recovered from a supersonic dive only when the pilot put all four engines into reverse thrust, having one jet engine pod torn off in the process. This manœuvre is permitted in flight in the DC-8; in the Boeing 707, 'spoilers' on the wings would be raised to increase the drag.

For the modern airline passenger, reclining in a body-contoured seat with a cocktail in his hand as he soars miles above the weather in a sound-proofed, pressurized cabin, it is difficult to imagine the misery and discomfort visited on his predecessors of forty years ago. The early airliners, with their large wing areas, low wing loading, low speeds and flight altitudes taking them through turbulent strata near the earth, had such a reputation for airsickness that even today, many of those who refuse to fly offer this outmoded argument to justify their stand. Other predisposing factors were apprehension—first-flight passengers usually had no knowledge of aviation[17]—and frequently only dire emergencies, themselves productive of anxiety, such as a serious illness or a death in the family, were the reason for their taking such a drastic step. Noise and vibration were aggravating factors, the average airliner being quite innocent of sound-proofing, with engines located in the worst possible position from the passenger's point of view, while large resonant surfaces, such as unsupported bulkheads and fabric cabin walls, made their contributions. It was taken for granted that conversation between passengers would be out of the question. Here is a passenger's impression of a London to Amsterdam flight aboard a Handley-Page Hampstead 14-passenger airliner of Imperial Airways in the year 1926:

The rigger, who nobly fulfills his duties as master of ceremonies, makes deaf and dumb signs and motions above my head to a little receptacle containing cotton. Pulling out a bit, I obey his signs and stuff it into my ears to help deaden the maddening roar of those three powerful Jaguars, which, with their eleven hundred and fifty-eight horsepower, make more noise than ten boiler factories. The cotton to some extent reduces the terrific din, which affects the ear-drum and is thought to be partly responsible for airsickness. . . .

We swoop up and down, and lurch from side to side. Every time we plunge into a cloud or emerge from the other side of one, we get a bump. The sky bristles with invisible bumps. . . . I no longer have any interest in the scenery. I feel my first suggestion of airsickness. When I have the ambition to look around me, I discover there is a special basin under each chair. Most of the passengers are holding them in their laps now. They are ghastly green and apparently feel far worse than I do. If this merciless dipping doesn't let up, I don't care whether I land in Holland or drop into the Channel.[18]

The early American transports were no more comfortable. The Ford trimotor, pride of the 'Lindbergh Line,' 'affords an excellent example of complete acoustical neglect. . . . The noise level was estimated at about 124 db at a cruising speed of 112 mph. No sound insulation was used, nor was there any attempt to control reverberation within the cabin. Conversation was impossible even by shouting, and vibration was excessive and very unpleasant for the air traveller.'[19] To add to the passenger's miseries, three 136-gallon fuel tanks in the wing centre section leaked sickening gasoline fumes into the cabin and were the reason for a large 'No Smoking' sign on the front bulkhead. A few years later, however, in the Curtiss Condor of 1932, sound-proofing had reduced the noise level to ninety db at 150 mph, and 'it was possible to converse in normal tones.'[20] And in a 1933 lecture, Miss Rosalie Gimple RN, one of United Air Lines' first stewardesses, modestly advised her audience of flight surgeons, 'if you have not made a trip on the new Boeing 247, you don't realize the improvement we have over the Ford. It is no effort to carry on conversation across the aisle.'[21]

Miss Gimple and her early associates were directly involved in the problem of the airsick passenger. Children, she observed, were very seldom ill, probably because they did not know enough about flying to be frightened. The traveller with a hangover was highly susceptible, as was the upset individual travelling in an emergency: these benefited from sedation with sodium amytal by mouth. Miss Gimple asked her distinguished medical audience whether she should advise her airsick passengers to fix their gaze inside or outside the aircraft, and must have been annoyed when the president replied, 'I suggest that Miss Gimple suggest to airsick passengers, that instead of looking out of the window or at some point in the cabin they fix their attention on the stewardess.'[22]

In the early days of 150 mph aircraft and transcontinental journeys lasting more than a day, the 'sleeper' plane offered the acme of luxury aloft. American Airways commenced sleeper plane service with the XT-32 Condor biplane in 1934; but a year later came the first of the Douglas Sleeper Transports which enabled travellers to cross the continent in style in fifteen hours fifty minutes eastbound, and seventeen hours forty-one minutes westbound. Thus the immortal DC-3 commenced its long career as an enlarged sleeper version of the fourteen-passenger DC-2. In upper and lower berths six feet five inches long, which could be converted into seats by day, the Flagship sleeper accommodated twelve passengers. But they also underlined an annoying aeromedical problem: because sleeping passengers were unable to vent their ears during descent, the stewardesses had to awaken each of them at every landing, lest they develop a painful case of aero-otitis media.

The whole problem of the airline passenger and pressure changes in the middle ear was more acute in the days before the development of the pressure cabin. Experience indicated that passengers could not tolerate altitude changes more rapid than three hundred feet per minute, particularly in descent, and this figure in fact was embodied in a Federal Aviation Agency regulation. The resulting requirement to plan the flight for maximum passenger comfort, rather than maximum aircraft performance, led to delays and excessive fuel consumption, as airliners ascended or descended from altitude at rates lower than their performance permitted. Sometimes the results could be dangerous: no airline captain would willingly linger in an ice-forming cloud, but might hesitate to make a rapid descent that would lead to complaints from passengers. With the pressure cabin, the apparent rate of descent within the cabin was less than that of the aircraft itself.

Over-the-weather flying with high-speed, high-performance monoplanes confronted the airlines with the problem of anoxia at high altitudes in both aircrew and passengers. United Air Lines was the first to carry oxygen equipment in its Boeing 247s and DC-3s, thanks to the energy and professional outlook of its medical director, Colonel A. D. Tuttle, former Chief of the Army Air Corps School of Aviation Medicine at Randolph Field. Though his was not the first airline medical department (Eastern Air Lines had inaugurated one at Coral Gables, Florida, on 1 June 1936), Tuttle had insisted from the date of his appointment in October 1937 that United pilots use oxygen whenever they ascended above 10,000 feet.[23] The equipment was developed by W. M. Boothby and W. R. Lovelace of the Mayo Clinic, in co-operation with Northwest Airlines, which made available a Lockheed 10 on flights between Minneapolis and Los Angeles. The heart of the new equipment, in the opinion of the authors, was the B-L-B mask, which was seen as a great advance on previous masks ('a placebo for distressed passengers'), and saving one-half to two-thirds of the oxygen formerly wasted by use of the pipe-stem. To supply oxygen to passengers and air crew, a twenty-seven pound tank was provided with the gas under a pressure of 1300 psi. Flights were made with the Lockheed 10 as high as 31,000 feet, where the straight-flow equipment delivered 1·8 litres per minute of oxygen. History repeated itself in that pilots wanted to 'lay off until they felt the need,' and complained that the oxygen loosened the fillings in their teeth.

Thus, for a brief period, passengers as well as aircrew wore the B-L-B masks whenever the airliners of the day ascended above 10,000 feet. Vital as the gas was to normal function at higher altitudes, there was a great resistance to using the equipment, particularly the masks. Smoking was impossible, conversation and eating difficult. The wearer was confined to his seat, and though there were proposals that long tubing be provided to enable the passenger to move about and go to the toilet, Armstrong 'could not but agree with a certain wit who "didn't believe that anyone would want to wander around in an aeroplane with his umbilical cord dragging along behind him".'[24] Passenger acceptance alone dictated the development of pressure-cabin equipment, which at one stroke solved the problem of anoxia. With the expansion of world-wide commercial flying in the post-World War II period, the pressure cabin was universally accepted as the ideal answer to these problems.

The pressure cabin, however, brought its own medical complications. Until military experience dispelled some of the mystery, the danger of explosive decompression was overrated during the post-war years. Only eighteen such incidents occurred in United States scheduled transport aircraft up until late 1952,[25] and these showed that below 25,000 feet at least, loss of consciousness and significant anoxic symptoms did not occur. Above 25,000 feet, the short time of useful consciousness required that the air crew have military-type oxygen masks immediately at hand, and simple masks were available in emergency for the passengers also (though few airline travellers realized that the cup-like receptacles might not maintain consciousness above 33,000 feet). Among the emergency procedures that each captain and co-pilot are taught is the descent from high altitude in the event of explosive decompression—not an abrupt nose-over, which would throw the passengers to the ceiling, but a steeply-banked descending turn which presses them into their seats.

It cannot be overemphasized that with present-day oxygen equipment at high altitude, particularly that available to passengers, preservation of useful consciousness depends more on a rapid descent than on the administration of oxygen. (At an altitude of 40,000 feet, the time of useful consciousness without oxygen is approximately twenty seconds). Yet the prescribed rapid descent may be a source of danger by increasing the aerodynamic loads on the airframe. On the night of 22 May 1962, Captain Fred Gray of Continental Airlines faced a fatal option of difficulties when a dynamite bomb exploded in a washroom of his Boeing 707 jet aircraft at 39,000 feet over Missouri, causing an explosive decompression. The evidence indicates that Gray, realizing the structural integrity of his aircraft had been seriously impaired, initiated a gentle descent with minimum G loads, compared to the steep spiral descent prescribed by regulations. Actually he and his crew found time to locate an emergency check list, to lower and lock the landing gear, and to don smoke masks, which supplied one hundred per cent oxygen. After about two minutes of descent, however, the tail broke off abaft the damaged section, and the remains of the big Boeing spun down from 36,800 feet, killing the thirty-seven passengers and crew of eight. A point not discussed in the CAB accident report is the possibility that Gray lost consciousness due to anoxia, in spite of the smoke mask, and thereby lost control of the badly damaged aircraft, causing it to break up.[26]

Weaknesses of windows, navigational astrodomes, doors and door latches caused many less catastrophic accidents, and in too many instances, passengers and personnel were sucked out the aperture unless securely strapped in. Concerned with repeated door latch failures, Lockheed Aircraft Company developed for its Constellations and Electras the so-called 'plug door.' Fitted inside the skin of the aircraft, the 'plug door' cannot blow outwards as it is larger than the aperture, and is sealed all the tighter by the internal pressure. It is in fact retracted inward for opening, and then rolled upward out of the way.

The first airline medical department, as noted above, was that of Eastern Air Lines, established on 1 June 1936 the physician in charge being Ralph Greene MD who twenty years earlier had been the first Army Surgeon ordered to fly. Initially the medical department was concerned only with the air crew, Dr Greene having 129 pilots under his supervision as well as stewards and radio operators. In dealing with the flight crews, Dr Greene and his associates had to overcome the suspicion, not to say hostility, of the service flyer towards the flight surgeon: 'Pilots who are professionally advised to initiate corrective measures are not inclined to yield to methods of compulsion as quickly as they are inclined to accept fatherly medical advice.'[27] Rather, the mission of the flight surgeon working for the airline was considered preventative, and Greene was proud that two flight-crew members, found to have active pulmonary tuberculosis, were treated and found fit to fly after six months. Aside from periodic physicals, Eastern's medical department examined personnel flying the Caribbean, South American and Orient runs for tropical diseases, finding that sixteen per cent of these men suffered from amoebic dysentery, while the incidence on domestic airlines was only two per cent.

Colonel A. D. Tuttle of the United Air Lines medical department turned his attention to passengers as well as to air crew. Capitalizing on the fact that United's stewardesses were all graduate nurses, he placed in their hands on 1 January 1938 a 'Discomfort and Medication Report' to be filled out in each instance of airsickness, aero-otitis media, or other medical event.[28] These reports indicated whether at the time of the incident the air was 'smooth,' 'moderately rough,' or 'rough,' the altitude, and whether the condition existed before emplaning. The reports showed medical incidents occurring in 6·0 passengers per thousand in the year 1938, divided into 852 airsick, 247 nervous, 198 oxygen want (heart), 141 ear trouble and 122 all others.

By World War II, Eastern, United, Pan American and American Airlines had medical departments, and these sent representatives to a forum on airline medical problems held by the Aero Medical Association in Miami in 1939. The lectures emphasized maintaining the function and capability of trained pilots, and to a lesser extent, the safety and comfort of passengers. Reassuring to the medical men was the assertion by David Behncke of the Air Line Pilots' Association that 'I think pilots are definitely losing their fear of the flight surgeon. . . . In the aeronautical field, I note with satisfaction the trend is towards having flying skills compensate for a limited degree of physical deficiency. Experience is something you can't buy.'[29] W. R. Lovelace of the Mayo Clinic directed attention to the decreased altitude tolerance of flight personnel taking the miraculous new bacteriostatic drug, sulfanilamide, because it converted a significant portion of the oxygen-carrying haemoglobin to useless methaemoglobin. Ralph Greene of Eastern Air Lines told of transporting ill persons by air including a child with tetanus flown from Miami to New York, and asserted that the heart patient, ambulatory and able to manage his affairs, could travel more safely by air than by any other form of transportation. Ross MacFarland sketched the Pan American Airways medical organization, with flight surgeons' offices at the operating base at Miami, San Francisco, Brownsville and Baltimore. Pilots received semi-annual physical examinations, including electrocardiograms, chest X-ray, basal metabolic rate, blood counts, stool examination for amoebae and parasites, and blood Wassermann. Flight engineers, radio operators and stewards were examined annually. Six per cent of the pilots were found to have faulty night vision, largely due to inadequate diet. Being especially interested in fatigue, MacFarland had made appropriate physiological tests in flight on trans-Pacific crews in 1937, and on trans-Atlantic crews in June 1939. In those leisurely, gracious days, when the roomy flying boats took thirty hours to cross the Atlantic and six days to island-hop across the Pacific, MacFarland could advise that 'experience in transoceanic operations seems to justify the belief that fatigue can be reduced to a minimum by increasing the size of the crews.' Indeed, the huge Boeing B-314 flying boats carried two men for each flight crew position—pilot, co-pilot, navigator, radio operator and flight engineer—with bunks for the watch off duty. MacFarland also emphasized job security, and claimed that Pan American was able to place every grounded pilot in a position with the company where his ability, training and experience could be used to the best advantage.

Pan American Airways, 'chosen instrument' of the United States Government for aerial expansion overseas, had a unique medical problem in the protection of its passengers against infectious disease at stop-overs abroad. Starting in 1927 as a link between Miami and Havana, PAA ten years later was carrying 70,000 passengers annually to the Caribbean countries and South America. For their protection, it was necessary for the chief steward to maintain a constant check on the food and drinking water supplied in foreign countries. Airport managers were ordered to obtain water from the safest sources, and food prepared in a sanitary manner, but 'at best it was on a hit-or-miss basis.'[30] Because local agents did not do it properly, stewards aboard company aircraft were trained to collect water samples at airport stops and deliver them to Miami for testing. With in-flight meals being prepared by local hotels and restaurants (except in Rio and Miami, where they were packed in company kitchens), there was sometimes trouble with establishments which did not maintain acceptable standards of cleanliness. If complaints to the local authorities did not bring results, the airline sometimes had to exert economic pressure.

With the passage of the years, and the virtual elimination from the modern transport aircraft of such purely physiological stresses as wind blast, noise, anoxia and low temperatures, airline medical departments have been increasingly concerned with the problems of ageing in pilots, and fatigue.

The situation of the older flyer was highlighted in this country by a Federal Aviation Agency order of 1960 forbidding pilots older than sixty years of age to fly passengers in aircraft exceeding 12,500 pounds gross weight; but even before World War II the airlines were concerned to maintain the physical and physiological efficiency of their senior captains—some of them pioneers from the early days of aviation—with the goal of keeping them productive as long as possible, both for their own sake and that of their employers. Where the World War I ideal was the perfect young physical specimen, it was recognized in the mid-thirties that these same flawless youths, now twenty years older, could no longer focus their eyes on close objects. It was a relief to airline pilots and executives when corrective lenses were permitted for this group. Ralph Greene of Eastern Airlines' medical department fitted his farsighted pilots with lower lenses only to minimize the reflection from standard eyeglasses in night flying, but 'recommended that they do not wear the moon-shaped lower segments in the presence of passengers, for in the case of middle-aged pilots there is a patriarchal suggestibility created by the grandfatherly type of eyeglass that might not be particularly comforting or reassuring to the nervous type of passenger.'[31] Nowadays, of course, many airline passengers realize that the captain may literally be a grandfather, and think nothing of it.

As early as 1940—thirty-seven years after the Wright Brothers' first ascent at Kitty Hawk—Ross MacFarland of Pan American Airways, after noting that 'many of the ablest pilots are between forty and fifty years of age,'[32] dared to suggest that they might continue to fly until age fifty-five or even longer with moderate living and regular exercise. This prediction has been borne out, and as MacFarland himself relates, 'in aviation it would be appropriate to say that an airman is as old as his vision, his motor skill, or his mental adaptability as they relate to the performance of his duty in flight.'[33] Chronological age, as is well known, is no indication of an individual's physical or mental powers, and the author knows of airline pilots over sixty who continue to fly large transport aircraft, either with freight or carrying passengers under foreign flags. And in the year 1965, incredulous Federal Aviation Agency physicians spent three days examining Dr A. McGarvey Wallace of Gate City, Virginia, who has been flying since 1935 and at ninety years of age is still able to pass the Class III physical examination.[34]

Fatigue among airline pilots is a many-sided subject these days, with a multiplicity of views relating to its cause reflecting the subjective experience of the writers, and even their prejudices (one airline chief pilot advised the author, 'this has been the subject of years of research and study by all of the airlines and regulating agencies in the world and to my knowledge nothing of any value has been produced to this time.') Though possibly present during the early open-cockpit days of commercial aviation, fatigue did not receive scientific attention until long-range aircraft were developed with continuous flight endurance of up to twenty-four hours—such as the Martin M 130 'China Clipper' flying boat of 1935, used on Pan American's transpacific route. Initially it was assumed that time on duty was the sole causative factor in fatigue, and in 1938 the Civil Aeronautics Board limited pilots on international flights to eight hours' flying in one day, thirty-two hours in a week, and one hundred hours in one month. In 1944 similar restrictions were applied to pilots on domestic

United States airlines. In actual practice, during the propeller-driven era, commercial United States airlines flew their pilots for roughly eighty hours per month, a figure now tending to decline to nearer sixty hours with the advent of faster jet aircraft.

An early and ambitious attempt to study fatigue in flight was made by MacFarland and a colleague who, in August 1937, performed a large number of physiological and psychological tests on the eight-man crew (and eleven passengers) of a Pan American Martin 130 flying boat during actual flight from California to Manila and back, and at the stop-overs en route.[35] The mean altitude was 9500 feet, the total flying time $122\frac{1}{2}$ hours, and the total distance over 14,000 nautical miles. The flight crew had alternate shifts of two to four hours on duty, and one to two hours off duty. Aboard the roomy Clipper the investigators tested visual function and verbal facility at altitudes up to 12,000 feet, while arterial and venous blood samples were taken immediately after a twelve-hour flight at 11,000 feet from Honolulu to Alameda, and after a seven-hour flight at 8000 feet between Midway and Honolulu. Most of the findings simply duplicated those in pressure-chamber volunteers at the same simulated altitude, and did not show any fatigue effects. Urine output of flight-crew members increased during the early stages of a flight, reflecting the initial tension of men in a position of responsibility (the observers had no such response). This was held to be the result of increased secretion of adrenal cortical hormone under stress—the measure of which is still the best objective indication of the emotional strain a man may have experienced.

Further appraisal of the fatigue problem in commercial air crew indicates that other experiences besides the start of a flight are stressful. Thus, there is a considerable area of agreement that landings, particularly under adverse circumstances, such as darkness or poor visibility, are even more stressful than takeoffs and departures, and more fatiguing to flight-crews than time spent in flight at altitude. Inadequate rest facilities at stop-overs or layovers away from home are stressful, as is the experience of delay on the ground due to scheduling, weather or mechanical difficulties. Relative anoxia at flight altitude may be physiologically stressful and contribute to fatigue. Conversely, boredom may be a cause of fatigue. MacFarland reports that 'airmen flying on the west coast of South America where the weather is often faultless day in and day out have, on occasion, threatened to resign simply because of sheer monotony. As experienced by one pilot, "not even a fish jumped" during the entire flight.'[36] On the other hand, fatigue is blamed in commercial air crashes only when the flight crew has flown for an obviously excessive length of time, usually with inadequate rest beforehand. Thus, the crash of a DC-4 at Gander in 1946 which MacFarland attributes to fatigue occurred after the pilot had been on duty for twenty-three hours and had logged sixteen hours of flight time, the last portion at 11,000 feet without oxygen.[37]

Fatigue is being actively discussed among commercial airline pilots at present, the most urgent question being whether flying turbojet aircraft is more fatiguing than handling piston and propeller aircraft. The consensus seems to be that the jet is harder on its crews, some of the data being positively alarming. Thus, one survey of pilots' *wives* indicated that after their husbands transitioned to jets, fifty-seven per cent were irritable, seventy-five per cent complained of being tired, thirty-two per cent had a changed attitude towards sex, and thirty-nine per cent did not enjoy the children so much.[38] Emphasis has been placed on the effect of dislocating the air crew's biological rhythm with the zone changes in east to west flight, which are undoubtedly more rapid in turbojet aircraft. On the other hand, at least one physician intimately involved in the problems of many airline pilots feels that the above complaints simply reflect the anxieties, tensions and conflicts of men in their forties and fifties adapting to equipment that is twice as heavy and twice as fast as anything they have ever handled previously. The process of adaptation, in his opinion, takes six to twelve months for a captain and three to six months for a co-pilot, but 'after they get used to it they do very well.'[39]

Airline medical departments were initially concerned with the care and efficiency of the flight crew, but very soon became involved with the passengers. A perennial question for the medical department was whether persons with certain chronic diseases should fly. As early as 1938, Dr Tuttle of United Air Lines maintained 'if it is safe for a heart case to walk, it is equally safe for him to fly,'[40] which corresponds to one of the latest pronouncements, 'does he look normal? Does he act normal? Can he walk up the steps of a plane?'[41] Whereas my own professor of obstetrics advised in 1936 that 'in pregnancy, generally speaking, carriage transportation is safer than motoring,'[42] his successors prefer their patients to travel by air up to the eighth month because it is less time-consuming and fatiguing than going by road. One particular problem, however, is well known to be aggravated by flying, namely, any condition where air is trapped in some body cavity and expands with increased altitude. One such case, which ended in death, was reported in 1945: a passenger on a trans-Canadian flight who, after an ascent to 16,000 feet, lost consciousness and died in convulsions twenty-eight minutes later despite a prompt descent with full oxygen to 4000 feet. An investigation showed that the dead man suffered from tuberculosis and had had a pneumothorax—air injected into the chest cavity to collapse the diseased lung. During the climb to altitude the air trapped in his chest had expanded to nearly twice its sea-level volume.[43]

And now, with the jet age well established in commercial air transportation, there looms the glamorous and incredibly expensive supersonic transport, flying at twice or thrice the speed of sound at 75,000 feet. Aside from the problem of the supersonic boom and its effects on those on the ground, the supersonic transport will introduce some new aeromedical problems for its occupants. Flying well above the 'Armstrong Line,' oxygen masks will be useless in the event of loss of cabin pressure; but it is probable that an air scoop, automatically extending into the air stream, will maintain an equivalent cabin altitude below 30,000 feet with ram air. Cosmic and solar ionizing radiation will obviously have a greater effect on an aircraft flying in air one-seventh as dense as that supporting present-day jet aircraft.[44] And indubitably, the 'physiological time clock' will be even further dislocated by an aircraft capable of flying from Los Angeles to Rome in four and a half hours. 'Are we really going to save time . . . or just lose sleep?'[45]

General aviation, which includes both private flying and the operation of small business aircraft, forms a considerable segment of civil aviation activity, particularly in the United States. Yet until recently, it has had less than its share of medical problems, inasmuch as most general aviation flying has been below 10,000 feet. Within the past five years, however, powerful, fast, twin-engined business aircraft such as the Aero Commander, Beechcraft Baron, Cessna Skyknight and Piper Aztec—some with supercharged engines—have been attaining altitudes where oxygen is indispensable. An educational campaign is in progress to acquaint the private flyer with the dangers of flying above 10,000 feet without oxygen, and numerous kits are on the market, featuring compressed oxygen tanks, regulators (usually of the straight-flow type) and simple masks. The truly sophisticated business jets, such as the Lear Jet, North American Sabreline, and Lockheed Jet Star, are pressurized to fly above 40,000 feet, and with accommodation for eight to twelve, are jet airliners in miniature.

One department of general aviation is of special medical interest—crop dusting. A rapidly expanding but highly risky activity, crop dusting requires the aviator to fly at the lowest possible altitude above the field to be treated, zoom and turn at the end without stalling, and demands the utmost in skill, precision and knowledge of the aircraft. Traditionally the last stronghold of the open-cockpit biplane, especially suited to this dangerous game because of its all-round visibility and low wing loading, the usual aircraft for crop dusting was the Stearman PT-17 trainer of the World War II period. Another favourite, a 'souped-up' version of the moth-like Cub, the Piper Super-Cub with a husky 150 hp Lycoming in the nose, is still in production. More recently, special aircraft have been built for crop dusting, single-seaters with big hoppers ahead of the cockpit, such as the Call Air A-9 which can lift 1350 pounds of dust off a 1000 foot runway. Agricultural planes must be built to crash, with a welded tubing 'bird-cage' above the pilot shielding him in the event of a turnover, and reinforced cockpit structure. For Grumman Aircraft to be able to claim that its 'Ag-Cat' cockpit can withstand loads of forty-five G in a crash is a valuable selling point.

The medical problem in crop dusting lies in the toxic effect of the insecticides used. If they can poison bugs, they may also poison people. That these substances—the chlorinated hydrocarbons such as DDT, lindane and chlordane, and the organophosphates such as parathion and TEPP (tetraethyl pyrophosphate)—have toxic effects on persons handling them has been well known for years in the industry, but it took a recent investigation by the Federal Aviation Agency to prove that pilots could be intoxicated by these chemicals to the point of being unable to control their aircraft. Beyond doubt, a certain proportion of fatal crop-dusting crashes have been caused by the insecticide used.

Formerly it was considered that persons on the ground would not be affected by the chemical-laden cloud (over ninety-five per cent of which is inert talc dust), but a recent report cites brief illness in persons, and fatalities in cattle, caused by two aircraft spraying TEPP on hop fields in the State of Washington. Forty-one persons exposed to the dust clouds complained of tightness in the chest and shortness of breath and were examined at a local hospital, and three of them were admitted overnight for observation. Cattle were made much more ill, fifteen showing symptoms and two of these dying in convulsions. These alarming results must, however, be attributed to unusual meteorological conditions, for on the day of the incident there was no wind, an inversion, and a temperature of ninety-six degrees F, causing the dense clouds of TEPP dust to persist for up to two hours in the same location. The authors of the monograph on the State of Washington incident recommend that people and cattle be evacuated when clouds of insecticide dust persist as on this occasion.[46]

The medical problems of one group in aviation deserve more attention even though they are not flight-crew members—the control personnel in the FAA-manned towers at large airports, and in the air route traffic control centres responsible for the spacing on the airways of aircraft flying under instrument conditions. Conscientious and dedicated men, they feel intensely the strain of responsibility and decision-making involved in tracking, separating and safely bringing to the ground traffic which may include large airliners moving at nearly the speed of sound with over 150 passengers aboard. Ulcers, hypertension and occasionally severe emotional reactions are the penalties for a certain number, and must be considered incurred in line of duty.

Lastly, a salute to our sisters, the ladies who fly. Their numbers are small (probably due to the difference between the sexes in psychosexual drives, goals and attitudes), but they never fly while intoxicated, never perform aerobatics recklessly at low altitude, and competently handle everything from two-seater Cubs on Sunday afternoons up to (in Russia, at least) the monstrous Tupolev TU 114 four-engined turboprop transport in international service.

Women do have their special medical problems, and those who fly may be amused, and certainly will be annoyed, to learn how long Victorian attitudes towards menstruation prevailed among aeromedical authorities. As recently as 1935 the Medical Division of the Department of Commerce solemnly warned, 'all women should be cautioned that it is dangerous for them to fly within a period extending from three days prior to three days after the menstrual period. Many women pilots have fainted when flying during this period with fatal results.'[47] Another release by R. E. Whitehead, Medical Director of the Department of Commerce, blamed three accidents on the menstrual period. In the first, the twenty-eight-year-old student, who 'fainted' at 1000 feet and spun in with minor injuries, confessed 'I was feeling unwell that day and should not have gone up, but wanted to practise a little as I was supposed to complete the test for private pilot's licence the following day.'[48] Two deaths—one occurring when the girl stunt pilot abandoned her plane at 600 feet but failed to open her parachute, and the other involving the crash of an experienced girl pilot during a closed-circuit air race—were blamed on the fact that both were menstruating at the time. 'Although many women hesitate to speak freely about the effect menstruation has on their emotional and mental make-up, still the importance of this subject should be brought to their attention,' wrote Dr Whitehead. 'The emotions and the mind are more or less correlated in flying and anything, therefore, that interferes with the normal emotional and mental reactions of an individual are bound to disturb that individual in skilfully controlling and manœuvring an aeroplane.'

Higher marks for open-mindedness and scientific objectivity must go to Dr Raymond S. Holtz, Assistant Chief Flight Surgeon of the Connecticut Department of Aeronautics: instead of pontificating, he asked the ladies about their problem. From the answers of many women pilots to a questionnaire, he concluded:

In the vast majority of instances women who were practically free from symptoms during the menstrual period experienced no ill effects while flying during this time. Furthermore, many of the outstanding races and endurance flights were flown during some phase of the menstrual cycle with very little if any effect on the pilots. The minority of those heard from readily admitted that they refrained from flying during their hours of distress and voluntarily grounded themselves until 'the storm was over.'[49]

No medical authority has seen fit to dispute this eminently sensible evaluation of the problem.

Today, seventy years after the Kitty Hawk, air transportation has not only come of age—it is an integral part of the lives of every one of us, and the means whereby the world is shrinking almost daily, until a journey round its circumference is measured in hours instead of miles. Advances in aviation medicine, pioneered by military researchers and adapted by civilian engineers and medical men, have made it safe for women, children and babes in arms to hurtle through the hostile stratosphere at altitudes where brave men a few short years ago perished of anoxia and cold. Supersonic passenger flight, and possibly even the commercial utilization of space, may come in our own lifetime. When they do, aviation medicine will be found ready.

[1] Douglas H. Robinson, 'Barnstorming With Champagne,' *Journal of the American Aviation Historical Society,* vol. 7, no. 2, Summer 1962, p. 100.

[2] See G. W. Haddow and Peter M. Grosz, *The German Giants* (London: Putnam, 1962).

[3] R. E. G. Davies, *A History of the World's Airlines* (London: Oxford University Press, 1964), p. 93.

[4] Since Fokker's death in 1939, increasing evidence has come to light that the design genius of the Fokker works was not Fokker himself—who was contemptuous of engineers and theoreticians—but one Reinhold Platz, a welder lacking any formal engineering training, who none the less designed all Fokker aircraft after 1916. For a well-documented account favourable to Platz, see A. R. Weyl, *Fokker: the Creative Years* (London: Putnam, 1965).

[5] Another Fokker aircraft figured in the first prominently-reported aerial suicide when the Belgian financier, Alfred Loewenstein, disappeared on 4 July 1928 while flying the Channel from London to Brussels in his personal F VIIB-3M.

[6] Henri Hegener, ed. Bruce Robertson, *Fokker—the Man and the Aircraft* (Letchworth, Herts., England: Harleyford Publications Ltd, 1961).

[7] William T. Larkins, *The Ford Story* (Wichita: The Robert R. Longo Co., 1957), Introduction.

[8] Robert H. Scheppler and Charles E. Anderson, 'The Martin Clippers,' *Journal of the American Aviation Historical Society,* vol. 10, no. 3, Autumn 1965, p. 172.

[9] Victor D. Seeley, 'Boeing's Pacesetting 247,' *Journal of the American Aviation Historical Society,* vol. 9, no. 4, Winter 1964, p. 239.

[10] Rosalie Gimple, 'Air Passenger Travel from the Standpoint of the Nurse,' *Journal of Aviation Medicine*, vol. 4, no. 4, December 1933.

[11] This has proven generally true, though with the recent operation of jet aircraft at altitudes of 35,000 to 40,000 feet, it has been found that thunderstorms may extend even higher, up to 75,000 feet.

[12] D. W. Tomlinson, 'Development of Stratosphere Flying,' *Journal of Aviation Medicine*, vol. 12, March–December 1941, p. 136.

[13] See p. 133.

[14] Robert H. Scheppler, 'The Boeing Stratoliner,' *Journal of the American Aviation Historical Society*, vol. 8, no. 1, Spring 1963, p. 23.

[15] American dominance of the post-war commercial aircraft market was assured by the fact that nearly all transport-type aircraft used by the United Nations were American-built, though this was not, as is widely believed, the result of a prior agreement with Great Britain (Davies, p. 239).

[16] Not to be confused with the earlier—and larger—triple tailed DC-4E of 1938, a failure which, sold to the Japanese, served its native country by transmitting its faulty lubrication system and other defects to its Japanese progeny, the four-engine bomber code-named 'Liz.'

[17] Even in the year 1965 an acquaintance taking a jet flight reported the little old lady in the next seat complaining to the stewardess, 'where are the propellers? I paid for propellers!'

[18] Lowell Thomas, *European Skyways* (Boston and New York: Houghton, Mifflin & Co., 1927), pp. 49, 57.

[19] Ross A. MacFarland, *Human Factors in Air Transport Design* (New York and London: McGraw-Hill Book Co., Inc., 1946), p. 269.

[20] MacFarland, p. 269. The real aviation history buff will remember that there were two distinct types of Curtiss Condors—the CO, the eighteen-passenger bomber conversion of 1929 with two Curtiss Conqueror liquid-cooled engines, and the entirely different XT-32 of 1932, a biplane with two Wright Cyclones and retractable landing gear. One night at East Boston Airport (now Logan Airport) I was privileged to sit in the right-hand seat of an XT-32 of American Airways while the pilot warmed up the engines, but how or why the invitation was extended I cannot remember.

[21] Rosalie Gimple, *op. cit.*

[22] *ibid.* He might have quoted Armstrong: 'Having the passenger fix his eyes on definite objects on the terrain is of great benefit in most cases' (Harry G. Armstrong, *Principles and Practice of Aviation Medicine* (Baltimore: Williams & Wilkins Co., 1939), p. 241).

[23] Colonel A. D. Tuttle, 'Safety and Comfort Aloft,' *Journal of Aviation Medicine*, vol. 10, March–December 1939, p. 27.

[24] Armstrong, p. 315.

[25] Ross MacFarland, *Human Factors in Air Transportation* (New York: McGraw-Hill & Co., 1953), p. 688.

[26] Civil Aeronautics Board, Aircraft Accident Report, File no. 1-0003, 1 August 1962. During the uniform descent to 36,800 feet the G loads did not exceed 1·23 G, according to the flight recorder.

[27] Ralph Greene, 'Air Transport Flying from the Medical Standpoint,' *Journal of Aviation Medicine*, vol. 10, March–December 1939, p. 12.

[28] A. D. Tuttle, 'Safety and Comfort Aloft,' *Journal of Aviation Medicine*, vol. 10, March–December 1939, p. 72.

[29] 'Forum on Air Line Medical Problems,' *Journal of Aviation Medicine*, vol. 11, March–December 1940, p. 2.

[30] William K. McKittrick, Chief Steward, Pan American Airways, 'Sanitary Precautions on International Airways,' *Journal of Aviation Medicine,* vol. 10, March–December 1939, p. 87.

[31] Ralph Greene, 'Air Transport Flying from the Medical Standpoint,' *op. cit.*

[32] 'Forum on Airline Medical Problems,' *op. cit.*

[33] MacFarland, *Human Factors in Air Transportation,* p. 391.

[34] AOPA Pilot, vol. 8, no. 2, February, 1965, p. 68.

[35] MacFarland and Edwards, 'The Effects of Prolonged Exposure to Altitudes of 8000 to 12,000 feet During Trans-Pacific Flights,' *Journal of Aviation Medicine,* vol. 8, March–December 1937, p. 3.

[36] MacFarland, *Human Factors in Air Transportation,* p. 328.

[37] *ibid.,* pp. 357–8.

[38] Marius Lodeesen and James E. Crane MD, 'Tired Jet Pilots,' *Airline Pilot,* March 1963, p. 14.

[39] John Minnett MD, Dallas, Texas. Dr Minnett also emphasized the unnecessary strain on pilots of being harassed by government regulatory personnel—'I'm bothered most by trying to stay legal,' was the commonest answer to a questionnaire.

[40] A. D. Tuttle, 'Safety and Comfort Aloft,' *Journal of Aviation Medicine,* vol. 10, March–December 1939, p. 72.

[41] James J. Hutson MD, *Medical World News,* 29 January 1965, p. 93.

[42] Frederick C. Irving, *A Textbook of Obstetrics* (New York: Macmillan Co., 1936), p. 86.

[43] K. E. Dowd, 'Report of Death of Passenger under Treatment by Pneumothorax,' *Journal of Aviation Medicine,* vol. 16, February–December 1945, p. 346. (The direct cause of death in this case undoubtedly was an air embolism from the thorax to the brain.)

[44] Donald H. Stuhring MD, 'The Medical Aspects of Supersonic Flight,' *Journal of the American Medical Association,* vol. 185, no. 1, 6 July 1963, p. 14.

[45] Marius Lodeesen and James E. Crane MD, 'Racing the Sun,' *Airline Pilot,* January 1964, p. 23.

[46] Griffith E. Quinby and Glenn M. Doornik, 'Tetraethyl Pyrophosphate Poisoning Following Airplane Dusting,' *Journal of the American Medical Association,* vol. 191, no. 1, 4 January 1965, p. 1.

[47] *Journal of Aviation Medicine,* vol. 6, no. 3, March 1935, p. 71.

[48] R. E. Whitehead MD, 'Women Pilots,' *Journal of Aviation Medicine,* vol. 5, no. 2, June 1934.

[49] Raymond S. Holtz MD, 'Should Women Fly During the Menstrual Period?' *Journal of Aviation Medicine,* vol. 12, March–December 1941, p. 300.

Bibliography

(A) AVIATION

CHAPTER 1

Dr Bröckelmann, *Wir Luftschiffer.* Berlin and Vienna: Ullstein & Co., 1909.

Henry Coxwell, *My Life and Balloon Experiences.* 2 vols. London: W. H. Allen & Co., 1889.

James Glaisher, Camille Flammarion, W. de Fonvielle, and Gaston Tissandier, *Travels in the Air.* Philadelphia: J. P. Lippincott & Co., 1871.

John Jeffries, *A Narration of the Two Aerial Voyages of Doctor Jeffries with Mons. Blanchard.* London: J. Robson, 1786.

Captain Joseph W. Kittinger Jr USAF with Martin Caidin, *The Long, Lonely Leap.* New York: E. P. Dutton & Co., 1961.

Kriegswissenschaftliche Abteilung der Luftwaffe, *Die deutschen Luftstreitkräfte von ihrer Entstehung bis zum Ende des Weltkrieges 1918. Die Militärluftfahrt bis zum Beginn des Weltkrieges 1914.* Berlin: E. S. Mittler & Sohn, 1941.

F. Marion, *Wonderful Balloon Ascents.* New York: Charles Scribner & Co., 1870.

National Geographic Society–U.S. Army Air Corps Stratosphere Flight of 1935 in the Balloon 'Explorer II.' National Geographic Society, Washington, DC, 1936.

Auguste Piccard, *Earth, Sky and Sea.* New York: Oxford University Press, 1956.

Lieutenant Colonel David G. Simons (MC) USAF with Don A. Schanche, *Man High.* New York: E. P. Dutton & Co., 1961.

Kurt Stehling and William Beller, *Skyhooks.* New York: Doubleday & Co., Inc., 1962.

John Wise, *A System of Aeronautics.* Philadelphia: Joseph A. Speel, 1850.

CHAPTER 2

General H. H. Arnold, *Global Mission.* New York: Harper & Brothers, 1949.

R. Dallas Brett, *History of British Aviation.* 2 vols. London: The Aviation Book Club, n.d. (1933).

John R. Cuneo, *Winged Mars: The Growth of the German Air Weapon, 1870–1914.* 2 vols. Harrisburg: Military Publishing Co., 1942–47.

C. H. Gibbs-Smith, *Sir George Cayley's Aeronautics*. London: HM Stationery Office, 1962.

C. H. Gibbs-Smith, *The Aeroplane: an Historical Survev*. London: HM Stationery Office, 1960.

Claude Grahame-White, *The Story of the Aeroplane*. Boston: Small, Maywood & Co., 1911.

Historical Division of the Italian Air Force, *The First War Flights in the World, Libia, MCMXI*. Rome: 1953.

Allen H. Wheeler, *Building Aeroplanes for 'Those Magnificent Men.'* London: Foulis, 1965.

Arch Whitehouse, *The Early Birds*. New York: Doubleday & Co., 1965.

CHAPTER 3

Karl Bodenschatz, *Jagd in Flanderns Himmel*. Munich: Verlag Knorr & Hirth, 1935.

Benedict Crowell, *America's Munitions 1917–18*. Washington: Government Printing Office, 1919.

Sholto Douglas, *Years of Combat*. London: Collins, 1963.

G. W. Haddow and Peter M. Grosz, *The German Giants*. London: Putnam & Co., Ltd, 1962.

Ira Jones, *King of Air Fighters*. London: Ivor Nicholson & Watson Ltd, 1935.

W. Geoffrey Moore, *Early Bird*. London: Putnam & Co., 1963.

Sir Walter Raleigh and H. A. Jones, *The War In The Air*. 6 vols. Oxford: at the Clarendon Press, 1922–35.

Douglas H. Robinson, *The Zeppelin in Combat*. Henley-on-Thames: Foulis, 1962, revised edition 1972.

Elliott White Springs, *War Birds: Diary of an Unknown Aviator*. New York: George H. Doran Co., 1926.

Rudolf Stark, *Jagdstaffel Unsere Heimat*. Leipzig: Verlag von K. F. Koehler, 1932.

Fritz Strahlmann ed., *Zwei deutsche Luftschiffhäfen des Weltkrieges, Ahlhorn u. Wildeshausen*. Oldenburg: Oldenburger Verlagshaus Lindenallee, 1926.

US Navy, *Rigid Airship Manual*. Washington: Government Printing Office, 1927.

CHAPTER 4

'Aireview', *The Fifty Years of Japanese Aviation, 1910–1960*. Tokyo: The Kantosha Co., Ltd, 1961.

Richard Sanders Allen, *Revolution in the Sky*. Brattleboro, Vermont: The Stephen Greene Press, 1964.

Edward Arpee, *From Frigates to Flat-Tops*. Published by the author, 1953.

Andrew Boyle, *Trenchard*. New York: W. W. Norton & Co., 1962.

Harry Bruno, *Wings Over America*. New York: Halcyon House, 1944.

A. J. Jackson, *De Haviland Aircraft*. London: Putnam & Co., Ltd, 1962.

Isaac Don Levine, *Mitchell: Pioneer of Air Power*. New York: Duell, Sloan & Pierce, 1943.

Charles A. Lindbergh, *The Spirit of St Louis*. New York: Charles Scribners Sons, 1954.

Henry R. Palmer Jr, *The Story of the Schneider Trophy Race*. Seattle: Superior Publishing Co., 1962.

Jean du Plessis de Grenedan, *Les Grands Dirigeables*. 2 vols. Paris: Plon–Nourrit & Cie, 1925.

CHAPTER 5

The Staff of 'Aireview,' *General View of Japanese Military Aircraft in the Pacific War*. Tokyo: Kanto-Sha Co., Ltd, 1956.

Martin Caidin, *Black Thursday*. New York: E. P. Dutton & Co., Inc., 1960.

Wesley Frank Craven and James Lea Cate, *The Army Air Forces in World War II*. 7 vols. Chicago: The University of Chicago Press, 1948.

Lovat Dickson, *Richard Hillary*. London: Macmillan & Co., 1951.

Sholto Douglas, *Years of Command*. London: Collins, 1966.

James Dugan and Carroll Stewart, *Ploesti*. New York: Random House, 1962.

Robin D. S. Higham, *The Armed Forces in Peacetime*. Hamden, Connecticut: Archon Books, 1962.

Sir Charles Webster and Noble Frankland, *The Strategic Air Offensive Against Germany*. 4 vols. London: HM Stationery Office, 1961.

CHAPTER 6

Grover Heiman, *Jet Pioneers*. New York: Duell, Sloan & Pierce, 1963.

W. F. Hilton, *High Speed Aerodynamics*. London: Longmans, Green & Co., 1951.

CHAPTER 7

R. E. G. Davies, *A History of the World's Airlines*. London: Oxford University Press, 1964.

Henri Hegener and Bruce Robertson, *Fokker—the Man and the Aircraft*. Letchworth, Herts: Harleyford Publications Ltd, 1961.

William L. Larkins, *The Ford Story*. Wichita: The Robert R. Longo Co., 1957.

Lowell Thomas, *European Skyways*. Boston and New York: Houghton, Mifflin & Co., 1927.

(B) MEDICINE

H. Graeme Anderson, *The Medical and Surgical Aspects of Aviation*. London: Henry Froude and Hodder & Stoughton, 1919.

Captain Harry G. Armstrong, *Principles and Practice of Aviation Medicine.* Baltimore: Williams & Wilkins Co., 1939.

Major General Harry G. Armstrong (ed.), *Aerospace Medicine.* Baltimore: Williams & Wilkins Co., 1961.

Louis Bauer MD, *Aviation Medicine.* Baltimore: Williams & Wilkins Co., 1926.

Robert J. Benford MD, *Doctors in the Sky: the Story of the Aero Medical Association.* Springfield, Illinois: Charles C. Thomas, 1955.

Kenneth G. Bergin, MD, *Aviation Medicine.* Bristol: John Wright & Sons Ltd, 1949.

Paul Bert, *Barometric Pressure. Researches in Experimental Physiology.* Trans. Mary Alice Hitchcock and Fred A. Hitchcock. Columbus, Ohio: College Book Co., 1943.

Edward Bishop, *The Guinea Pig Club.* London: Transworld Publishers, 1963.

Douglas D. Bond, *The Love and Fear of Flying.* New York: International Universities Press, Inc., 1952.

Bureau of Naval Personnel, *Aviation Medicine Practice. Navpers 10839-A.* Washington: Government Printing Office, 1955.

Collected Papers on Aviation Medicine. London: Butterworth Scientific Publications, 1955.

Flight Surgeon's Manual, AF Manual 160–5, Department of the Air Force, July 1954.

Flight Surgeon's Manual, AF Manual 161–1, Department of the Air Force, 17 January 1962.

German Aviation Medicine in World War II, prepared under the auspices of the Surgeon General, USAF. 2 vols. Washington: Government Printing Office, 1950.

Lieutenant Colonel Roy R. Grinker MC and Major John P. Spiegel MC, AAF, *Men Under Stress.* Philadelphia: Blakiston, 1945.

Major Donald W. Hastings MC, Captain David G. Wright MC and Captain Bernard C. Glueck MC, AAF. *Psychiatric Experiences of the 8th Air Force, First Year of Combat (July 4, 1942–July 4, 1943).* New York: Josiah Macy Jr Foundation, August 1944.

Isaac Jones, *Flying Vistas.* Philadelphia: J. P. Lippincott Co., 1937.

Der Kommandierende General der Luftstreitkräfte, Sanitäts-Abteilung, *Einflüsse des Fliegens auf dem menschlichen Körper und ärztliche Ratschläge für Flieger.* Januar 1918.

Mae Mills Link and Hubert A. Coleman, *Medical Support of the Army Air Forces in World War II.* Washington: Government Printing Office, 1955.

Ross A. MacFarland, *Human Factors in Air Transport Design.* New York and London: McGraw-Hill Book Co., Inc., 1946.

Ross A. MacFarland, *Human Factors in Air Transportation.* New York: McGraw-Hill Book Co., Inc., 1963.

Robert Maycock, *Doctors in the Air.* London: George Allen & Unwin Ltd, 1957.

Squadron Leader S. C. Rexford-Welsh, *The Royal Air Force Medical Services*. 3 vols. London: HM Stationery Office, 1955.

War Department, Air Service, Division of Military Aeronautics, *Air Service Medical*. Washington: Government Printing Office, 1920.

William J. White, *A History of the Centrifuge in Aerospace Medicine*. Santa Monica: Douglas Aircraft Co., Inc., 1964.

William H. Wilmer, *Aviation Medicine in the AEF*. Washington: Government Printing Office, 1920.

PERIODICALS

(A) AVIATION

AOPA Pilot.
Air Power Historian.
Airline Pilot.
Air University Review.
Cross & Cockade.
Journal of the American Aviation Historical Society.
National Geographic Magazine.
Wingfoot LTA Society Bulletin.

(B) MEDICINE

Journal of the American Medical Association.
Journal of Aviation Medicine (now *Journal of Aerospace Medicine*).
Air Surgeon's Bulletin.

INDEX

281